Key Clinical To

Plastic and
Reconstructive Surgery

Key Clinical Topics in

Plastic and Reconstructive Surgery

Tor Wo Chiu BMBCh (Oxon) **FRCS** (Glasg) **FHKAM** (Surg)
Consultant in Plastic Surgery
Director of Burns Service
Prince of Wales Hospital
Chinese University of Hong Kong
Hong Kong SAR
PR China

Tze Yean Kong BA MB BCh BAO (Hons) MA MRCS FRCS (Plast)
Associate Consultant
Department of Plastic Surgery
KK Women's and Children's Hospital
Singapore

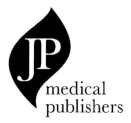

JP
medical
publishers

London • Philadelphia • Panama City • New Delhi

© 2015 JP Medical Ltd.
Published by JP Medical Ltd,
83 Victoria Street, London, SW1H 0HW, UK
Tel: +44 (0)20 3170 8910   Fax: +44 (0)20 3008 6180
Email: info@jpmedpub.com   Web: www.jpmedpub.com

The rights of Tor Wo Chiu and Tze Yean Kong to be identified as authors of this work have been asserted by them in accordance with the Copyright, Designs and Patents Act 1988.

All brand names and product names used in this book are trade names, service marks, trademarks or registered trademarks of their respective owners. The publisher is not associated with any product or vendor mentioned in this book.

Medical knowledge and practice change constantly. This book is designed to provide accurate, authoritative information about the subject matter in question. However readers are advised to check the most current information available on procedures included and check information from the manufacturer of each product to be administered, to verify the recommended dose, formula, method and duration of administration, adverse effects and contraindications. It is the responsibility of the practitioner to take all appropriate safety precautions. Neither the publisher nor the authors assume any liability for any injury and/or damage to persons or property arising from or related to use of material in this book.

This book is sold on the understanding that the publisher is not engaged in providing professional medical services. If such advice or services are required, the services of a competent medical professional should be sought.

Every effort has been made where necessary to contact holders of copyright to obtain permission to reproduce copyright material. If any have been inadvertently overlooked, the publisher will be pleased to make the necessary arrangements at the first opportunity.

ISBN: 978-1-907816-24-6

British Library Cataloguing in Publication Data
A catalogue record for this book is available from the British Library

Library of Congress Cataloging in Publication Data
A catalog record for this book is available from the Library of Congress

Commissioning Editor:	Steffan Clements
Editorial Assistant:	Sophie Woolven
Design:	Designers Collective Ltd

Foreword by Fu-Chan Wei

Key Clinical Topics in Plastic and Reconstructive Surgery provides plastic surgery trainees, medical students, nurses and general practitioners with a concise yet essential framework for learning. The relevant content, clear descriptions and lists of important points make this book unique and valuable. Drs Tor Chiu and Tze Kong, recognised specialists in plastic and reconstructive surgery, are to be congratulated for their great contribution to the education of our field and beyond.

I believe that *Key Clinical Topics in Plastic and Reconstructive Surgery* will serve as a vital tool for all plastic and reconstructive surgery students and trainees around the world.

Fu-Chan Wei MD, FACS
Professor, Plastic and Reconstructive Surgery
Taipei, Taiwan

Foreword by Taimur Shoaib

The FRCS(Plast) exam is arguably the toughest exam any plastic surgeon in training is likely to sit. Authoring a book on such a huge subject matter is, therefore, a major undertaking.

The authors, Drs Kong and Chiu, both specialist plastic surgeons, have worked hard to condense plastic surgery into key topics. I have had the pleasure of working with both of them during my career, both as a plastic surgeon in training and subsequently as a consultant plastic surgeon. It comes as no surprise to me that they have been able to convey the clarity of thought which is so important when it comes to successfully passing any plastic surgery exam, but more so the FRCS(Plast) exam.

The book summarises the vast subject of plastic surgery in alphabetically arranged topics. Each topic is presented from a starting point of knowledge that would be held by a senior plastic surgeon in training. It also aids the more junior plastic surgeon who is studying clinical cases prior to seeing procedures in the operating theatre and patients in out-patient clinics.

It is, of course, difficult to know where to stop writing such a potentially large book. In one volume it would be impossible to discuss the technical aspects of operative procedures, the scientific knowledge that plastic surgeons require in relation to research and ethical aspects of plastic surgery, and other subjects that constitute a plastic surgeon's lifelong education. However, the authors have achieved a good balance between discussing aspects of plastic surgery that could be considered minutiae, and topics that are either too large to condense into a book of this size or are better taught in clinical environments.

In summary, the book delivers core knowledge that all plastic surgeons need, without inappropriately burdening them with detail they are likely to obtain in clinical and surgical settings. The level of information delivered is high, but it is delivered with just the right amount of detail.

Taimur Shoaib MD, FRCSEd(Plast)
Consultant Plastic Surgeon
Glasgow, United Kingdom

Preface

This book came about from regularly teaching plastic and reconstructive surgery to medical students and surgical trainees in the United Kingdom and Hong Kong. This makes it fundamentally different from many of the other short books that tend to be a set of revision notes, usually more useful to writer than reader.

The main text is a focused and concise distillation of current knowledge, while lists are also used for clarity. Numerous figures have been included to clarify key points. Relevant and key articles are discussed and further reading suggestions are included at the end of each topic. Discussion is to be encouraged; the systematic critical evaluation of the literature is an important skill to acquire.

Tor Chiu
Tze Kong
August 2014

Acknowledgements

To my mentors: Arup, who enabled me to process my thoughts more efficiently; Ben, whose invaluable insights dissect difficult problems down to their finest detail; Eva, who showed me what precision and consistency can achieve; Miki and Alain, whose support and nurturing took me to where I am today. Last, but not least, to Cristina for putting up with me when I was doing all of this, and even more when I was not.

Tze Kong

The publishers wish to thank Series Advisors Dr Tim M. Craft and Dr Paul M. Upton for their assistance during the planning of the *Key Clinical Topics* series.

Dedications

In memory of my father
謹以此書獻給先父
Tor Wo Chiu

For my parents who nourished me in unison
Tze Kong

Contents

Abbreviations

5FU	5-fluorouracil
ABI	ankle brachial index
AFB	acid fast bacilli
ALT	anterolateral thigh
AP	anteroposterior
ARDS	acute respiratory distress syndrome
ASIS	anterior superior iliac spine
ATLS	Advanced Trauma Life Support
BAPN	beta-aminopropionitrile
BCC	basal cell carcinoma
BCG	Bacillus Calmette–Guérin vaccination for tuberculosis
BCS	breast conservation surgery
BSA	burn surface area
CFNG	cross-facial nerve grafting
CL	cleft lip
CL/P	cleft lip with or without associated cleft palate
CNS	central nervous system
CO	carbon monoxide
CP	cleft palate
CPO	cleft palate alone
CSF	cerebrospinal fluid
CT	computed tomography
CXR	chest X-ray
DD	Dupuytren's disease
DIEP	deep inferior epigastric perforator
DIPJ	distal interphalangeal joint
DNA	deoxyribose nucleic acid
DVT	deep vein thrombosis
ECG	electrocardiogram
EM	erythema multiforme
EMG	electromyogram
EMLA	eutectic mixture of local anaesthetics
ENT	ear, nose and throat

ER	extensor retinaculum
FDA	Food and Drug Administration
FDP	flexor digitorum profundus
FDS	flexor digitorum superficialis
FFP	fresh frozen plasma
FNA/C	fine needle aspiration/ cytology
FTSG	full-thickness skin graft
HBO	hyperbaric oxygen
HIV	human immunodeficiency virus
HLA	human leukocyte antigens
HPV	human papilloma virus
ICP	intracranial pressure
ICU	intensive care unit
IGF	insulin-like growth factor
IgG	immunoglobin G
IJV	internal jugular vein
IMA	internal mammary artery
IMF	intermaxillary fixation
INR	international normalised ratio
KA	keratoacanthoma
LD	latissimus dorsi
LDI	laser doppler imaging
LMWH	low molecular weight heparin
MALT	mucosa-associated lymphoid tissue
MCPJ	metacarpophalangeal joint
MGH	Massachusetts General Hospital
MM	malignant melanoma
MRI	magnetic resonance imaging
MRM	modified radical mastectomy
MRND	modified radical neck dissection
MRSA	methicillin resistant *Staphylococcus aureus*
MWL	massive weight loss
NA	needle aponeurectomy
ND	neck dissection
NF	necrotising fasciitis

NF1	neurofibromatosis type 1
NICE	National Institute for Health and Care Excellence
NPWT	negative pressure wound therapy
OPG	orthopantomogram
ORIF	open reduction and internal fixation
PCR	polymerase chain reaction
PCWP	pulmonary capillary wedge pressure
PDE	phosphodiesterase
PDGF	platelet-derived growth factor
PDS	polydioxanone suture
PE	pulmonary embolism
PEEP	positive end expiratory pressure
PIPJ	proximal interphalangeal joint
PSA	pleomorphic salivary adenoma
PUVA	psoralen ultraviolet A
PVD	peripheral vascular disease
QS	Q-switched
QSRL	Q-switched ruby laser
RCT	randomised controlled trial
RFFF	radial forearm free flap
RND	radical neck dissection
RSTL	relaxed skin tension line
RTA	road traffic accidents
SCC	squamous cell carcinoma
SIGN	Scottish Intercollegiate Guidelines Network
SJS	Stevens–Johnson syndrome
SNB	sentinel node biopsy
SPE	streptococcal pyrogenic exotoxins
SPF	sun protection factor
SSD	silver sulphadiazine
SSG	split skin graft
TCA	transverse cervical artery
TCS	Treacher–Collins syndrome
TEN	toxic epidermal necrolysis
TFL	tensor fascia lata
TGF	transforming growth factor

Introduction

Examination structure

The FRCS (Plast) Intercollegiate examination is divided into sections 1 and 2. A pass is required in Section 1 prior to being allowed to attempt Section 2. A maximum of four attempts are permitted in each section, with no subsequent possibility for entry. Fees are repayable for each attempt.

Both sections are held bi-annually and alternate sequentially. The Joint Committee on Intercollegiate Examinations (JCIE) will permit the candidate to sit Section 2 at the next sitting after Section 1 is passed. The shortest possible interval to pass both sections is 3 months, and this can be achieved by taking and passing Section 1 and 2 in the summer and autumn of the same year. The pass rates of both sections are independent of season (summer/autumn vs. winter/spring sittings) and therefore should not govern your choice of sitting.

Section 1

The Section 1 examination is entirely computer based and comprises two papers; Single Best Answer (SBA) and Extended Matching Items (EMI), which are separate mini-examination sessions on the same day, with a break in-between. The SBA will seem difficult, the EMI seemingly the easier of the two. However, most candidates score worse in the EMI.

The SBA has 110 multiple-choice questions (MCQ) with five choices (A to E) each, and is completed in 2 hours. This allows 65 seconds per question and usually means that there is little opportunity to review questions that you are unsure about. As the examination is not negatively marked, all questions should be attempted. There is a facility to flag questions for review, but a provisional answer should be entered in case of inadequate time for review. As the examination is computer-based, the time limit is precise to the second. The time pressure is greater for the SBA section than the EMI. Ensure that you are able to complete questions within the 65-second limit, otherwise guess and move on.

The EMI section comprises 45 main question headings from which an average of three questions will stem. Each of these is equally weighted, giving a total possible score of 135. These must be completed within a timeframe of 2.5 hours, averaging 66 seconds each. Again, there is little opportunity for review due to time constraints and a provisional answer should be entered before moving on to the next question.

For the Section 1 examination it should be noted that the only timer available is the countdown timer in the top right-hand corner of your screen (watches are disallowed and clocks are frequently absent). All questions must be done in sequential order, starting from 1. Pacing strategies, such as answering MCQs in reverse order (to ease computation of the number of questions remaining) are not permitted.

If you are unsure of the answer your choice should be governed by a process of elimination, based on your knowledge of the options that are definitely incorrect: choose any one of the remaining answers (remembering you will not lose marks if it is wrong).

Section 2

The Section 2 examination is split into the clinical and oral sections that are examined on two consecutive days. The clinical section is held on the first day and accounts for 64% of the total mark. Candidates often score worse in this section, implying that a good score in the oral examination on the second day is essential.

Understanding the scoring system

The examination is unconventionally marked in a custom-based system that has a minimum mark of 4 and a maximum of 8, which must be allocated as a whole number. It is vital you understand the marking descriptors for each score, as the average score of 6 required to pass requires not only the demonstration of competence but higher order thinking (see below).

The examination has a maximum score of 400 and a minimum of 200, with a rigid pass mark of 300, with no cumulative adjustment. There are thus 50 scoring opportunities. All candidates are marked in duplicate by a pair of examiners who will each give an independent score. Of the 25 events that can be scored, 16 occur in the clinical section, with the remaining 9 in the oral section.

The values of the individual components are shown in **Table i**. As a conversion rate rule of thumb, 1 long case = 3 short cases = 1 entire oral station.

Strategies for answering questions

As time is extremely limited, especially in the 6-minute short cases, every sentence of your answer must have as many point-scoring opportunities as possible. This requires succinct structure and clarity.

It is inevitable that you will be stronger in some topics than others. Despite the stress of the examination environment, try to avoid making basic errors. The answer to the first question of each case or section will set the tone of the remaining answers. If you answer this incorrectly, you will not be able to achieve a score above 6.

'Front-loading' is the most useful strategy to combat time constraints. This involves stating the main points first, followed by justifications afterwards from the history, examination and investigative findings. This is not limited to diagnoses, and can be used to mention key issues or concerns. This demonstrates higher order thinking, focussed perspective, insight into diagnosis, disease extent and therapy required. It also allows the examiner to cut you off in the least important part of the answer (this happens frequently) as the relevant points will already have been scored.

The strength of your knowledge of a topic may exceed that of the examiner and is one of the criteria to score an 8. This is helped by the fact that examiners are not supposed to examine in their chosen field of subspecialisation.

'End-loading' refers to ending the answer concisely with a relevant topic that you have studied well. The idea is to tempt the examiner to ask you about these topics, as the elaboration may lead to a higher score. Note that such elaboration will not be scored if it has not been specifically asked for, but it will cost valuable time. However, if successful, this strategy is useful to obtain a score of 7 or 8.

Table i Format and mark values of the FRCS(Plast) Section 2 components

Clinical section		Duration (minutes)	Scoring events	Marks on offer	% of total mark
Short-case circuit 1	Short case 1	6	1	16	4
	Short case 2	6	1	16	4
	Short case 3	6	1	16	4
	Short case 4	6	1	16	4
	Short case 5	6	1	16	4
Short-case circuit 2	Short case 1	6	1	16	4
	Short case 2	6	1	16	4
	Short case 3	6	1	16	4
	Short case 4	6	1	16	4
	Short case 5	6	1	16	4
Long-case circuit	Long case 1	15	3	48	12
	Long case 2	15	3	48	12
	Total:	**90**	**16**	**256**	**64**
Oral section					
Station 1					
3 out of the following 5:					
1. Burns	Subtopic 1	10	1	16	4
2. Hand trauma	Subtopic 2	10	1	16	4
3. Maxillofacial trauma	Subtopic 3	10	1	16	4
4. Lower limb trauma					
5. Pressure sores					
Station 2	Head and neck	10	1	16	4
	Cleft	10	1	16	4
	Genitourinary	10	1	16	4
Station 3	Basic sciences	10	1	16	4
	Aesthetics	10	1	16	4
	Ethics and consent	10	1	16	4
	Total:	**90**	**9**	**144**	**36**
	Grand total:	**180**	**25**	**400**	**100%**

In subject areas you are relatively weak in, the balance of power will shift to the examiners. It is far easier to score a 5 than it is to score a compensatory 7. Under pressure, one of the most frequent candidate errors is to end-load with topics they are weak in. Examiners are tasked to uncover weaknesses in the candidate's knowledge. Combined with doubt (body language and factual), this may result in candidates being selectively quizzed on weak topics.

The tenet of cases is to demonstrate the following:

- What is it?
- What is its extent?
- What am I going to do about it?

Stick to mentioning point-scoring items. It is acceptable to not know the diagnosis, but unacceptable to not know the process of arriving at a diagnosis. Lack of knowledge can sometimes be compensated for by identifying the relevant specialists who do. If you have exhausted your knowledge on the topic in question, say so, and the examiners will move on. Do not guess, as you will end-load badly and waste time.

Higher order thinking

The examination is set at a standard expected of a day one consultant plastic surgeon. The candidate's ability to take a full history and examination is already assumed. The expectation is for a contextualised history, examination and investigations tailored to achieve each of the basic tenets (see above). The candidate should also demonstrate the ability to argue and defend his or her choice with a logical process, substantiated by relevant evidence.

Table ii Components of learning skills		
Components of learning	Interpretation	Clinical example (with overlap)
1. Knowing	Recall	Burns can be full-thickness and need treatment
2. Understanding	Meaningful knowledge	If untreated will heal very slowly or may get infected
3. Applying	Using 1 and 2 to produce a useful effect	Excision and reconstruction is a good treatment
4. Analysing	Better understanding achieved by breaking down concept into smaller parts	The methods of reconstruction are full-thickness skin grafts, flaps or Integra with a delayed split skin graft, with pros and cons of each
5. Synthesis	Combine separate ideas to make something new	Slow reepithelialisation is not always a problem, as long as the defect is clean Anaesthesia should be minimised in neonates Neonates are relatively compliant
6. Evaluation	Judgement based on pros and cons	The benefits of debriding an extravasation full-thickness burn in a sick neonate may outweigh the risks of anaesthesia
7. Systems thinking	An appreciation of the workings of complex systems	Using a skin graft creates a donor site, expertise of the staff with skin grafts may be limited, and cosmesis of the recipient site is relatively poor without a dermal substitute
8. Creativity	Using insight and imagination to create something new	The neonate is in a clean and controllable environment with plenty of time for reepithelialisation. Debridement with Integra cover can be made a one-stage procedure by gradually peeling back the silicone layer and allowing reepithelialisation, avoiding a donor site and a skin graft, with better cosmesis overall

The eight components of learning are shown in **Table ii**. The first three items are intuitively recognisable and alone are insufficient to meet the examination requirements. Demonstration of higher order thinking involves items 4–7, with item 8 as a bonus.

Summary

Understand the examination rules, time frames and scoring system. Ensure that you are able to complete each MCQ question in Section 1 within 65 seconds. In Section 2, practice front-loading answers that demonstrate higher-order thinking. Avoid end-loading with topics you are unsure about. Desensitise and condition yourself to the examination format with lots of practice.

Abdominal reconstruction

The most common causes of abdominal wall defects are:

Acquired causes (common)
- Traumatic – road traffic accidents, gunshot wounds
- Neoplastic – post tumour resection
- Infection – necrotising fasciitis

Congenital causes (rare)
- Omphalocoele, gastroschisis, prune belly disease

Aim

The primary goal is wound closure with anatomical reconstruction of the abdominal layers.

Classification

The defect may be classified by:
- Size
- Component
- Location

Size

Classification by size is shown in **Table 1**.

Component

Partial or full thickness defects

Conceptually, the defect may lack support, cover or both. The basic components that contribute to support are muscle and fascia or its synthetic equivalent of mesh or dermal matrices. Skin and soft tissue function only to physiologically partition the wound from the environment. Small defects of either or both cover and support can usually be closed primarily. Component separation may be necessary to facilitate this. From the support perspective, muscle defects should be replaced with innervated functional muscle. However, static support is usually adequate for hernia prevention without the morbidity associated with the former.

The pore-size of the material is key. Macroporous materials such as polypropylene, have a pore-size greater than 75 μm that allows vascular and fibroblastic ingrowth, resulting in greater tissue integration but also adhesion formation. Microporous materials such as PTFE, silastic and Teflon (actually macroporous but has a component that reduces its effective pore-size) are used to minimise adhesion.

The most commonly used static supports are:

- Polypropylene (Prolene, Marlex) meshes are suitable for clean wounds. The porosity permits granulation through it, subsequently transforming it into a graftable bed for cover. A risk of adhesion, fistula formation, extrusion and infection is associated with its use
- Polytetrafluoroethylene (PTFE or Gore-Tex) mesh has a weaker foreign body reaction and reduced tissue ingrowth compared to polypropylene. It forms a weaker tissue interface and minimal

Table 1 Abdominal defects		
Classification	Defect size	Closure method
Small	< 5 cm	Primary closure with simple mobilisation and advancement
Moderate	5–15 cm	• Primary closure with component separation and local advancement (preferred). • Negative pressure wound therapy (NPWT) followed by SSG

Large	> 15 cm	Temporising option for the acute situation
		• Mesh repair, NPWT followed by SSG
		Definitive repair
		• Free tissue transfer or large local flaps
		• Tissue expansion followed by advancement
		  – Expander site options: over the ribs, ilium or between the external and internal oblique muscles in the lumbar region
		  – Carries a 20% complication rate

capsule formation. PTFE has a lower risk of adhesions and fistula formation at the expense of a theoretically higher risk of herniation compared to polypropylene. However, no major differences between the two have been shown in clinical studies. PTFE does not permit sufficient secondary granulation through it to be used as a secondarily graftable bed

- Polyester (Mersilene) is light and conforming but provokes a very strong inflammatory response
- Polyglactin 910 (Vicryl) or polyglycolic acid (Dexon) are both absorbable meshes and thus more suitable for contaminated wounds. While their lifespan in a clean wound is 90 days, this is greatly reduced in a contaminated environment. There may be a higher risk of ulceration, fistula formation and herniation with its use attributable to its strength deterioration with time, but confounded by a more susceptible population that it is used in
- Silastic (silicone) meshes have even lower tissue integration and thus adhesion rate than PTFE but forms a capsule
- Autologous e.g. tensor fascia lata (TFL) fascia has low adhesion rate and good strength. The disadvantages are its limited supply and donor site morbidity. Furthermore, it may take a year to achieve its final strength through remodelling. A TFL graft and pedicled fascial flap differ minimally in strength
- Allogeneic AlloDerm and xenogeneic Permacol are decellularised dermal matrices of human and porcine origin respectively. They act as a tough and resilient avascular structural scaffold when implanted but gradually remodels with time, combining the advantages of a synthetic and autologous material. It is extremely expensive. Alloderm is not available in the UK

The mesh can be placed in the extra or intraperitoneal positions, termed overlay and underlay respectively. Underlay mesh relies on intraabdominal pressure to maintain its position, minimising or avoiding the need for sutures altogether.

By position

Hurwitz and Hollis classified the position of abdominal defects into medial or lateral and upper, middle or lower third defects. This guides management (**Table 2**).

Management

General considerations include maintaining adequate nutrition and wound bed optimisation to reduce inflammation and oedema that may limit tissue advancement.

- Adequate debridement of infected or necrotic tissue is essential
- Immediate vs. delayed closure (also known as staged, temporising or interval closure). Immediate reconstruction is preferable unless contraindicated by significant abdominal distension, acute inflammation and contamination or a defect that is just too large. Attempted primary closure under tension must be avoided as it risks wound breakdown, abdominal compartment syndrome and respiratory compromise

Table 2 Classification of abdominal defects according to position and common reconstructive options	

Medial: upper, middle or lower	• Local flaps are of limited value and can be difficult to advance
	 • Bilateral component separation that can close defects of up to
	   – Upper third: 10 cm
	   – Middle third: 20 cm
	   – Lower third: 6 cm
	 • Fascial relaxation
	 • Staged mesh reconstruction

Lateral: upper, middle or lower	• Local flaps are a better choice • Component separation is of limited use • Prostheses are an option

- Temporising measures are a sensible option in the acute situation to allow resolution of oedema. Visceral manipulation or significant fluid resuscitation is an indicator of high oedema risk. Temporising techniques such as the Bogota bag (a 3L irrigation fluid bag opened out and patched over the defect) or a macroporous mesh may allow primary closure or a reduced defect reconstruction when the oedema is resolved
- The use of local flaps in the acute situation may be complicated by unpredictable flap survival and spreading infection and is thus relatively contraindicated
- NPWT with an intervening mesh layer to cover the bowel can be used to simultaneously accelerate granulation and reduce oedema

Options for definitive closure include:

- Tissue expansion
- Pedicled and free flaps

Flaps for abdominal reconstruction

Flaps provide a vascularised soft tissue cover and support for full thickness wounds and are ideal for contaminated wounds where prosthetic materials are preferentially avoided.

Muscle flaps

Muscle flaps provide intrinsic dynamic support but are inadequate in practice due to factors such as partial denervation. As such, they need to be reinforced with mesh when used. There are more local flap choices available for lateral than medial defects.

- The rectus abdominis (RA) flap is the most versatile workhorse flap as it can be raised on either pedicle with a choice of either a transverse or vertical skin paddle. However, it may be unavailable as it is frequently in the zone of tissue loss. It is less suitable for epigastric defects
- The tensor fascia lata (TFL) is the flap of choice for inferior defects. It is supplied by the lateral circumflex femoral artery (LCFA) that enters the muscle 6 cm below the anterior superior iliac spine (ASIS). The

muscle itself is short but a myocutaneous flap can be raised from the ASIS to a point 6 cm above the knee. However, its distal third is less reliable and thus should not be placed over crucial coverage areas
- The rectus femoris (RF) is also supplied by the LCFA but originates from the anterior inferior iliac spine. The RF flap has a low pivot point that limits its use to defects of the lower abdomen. The overlying skin may be harvested with the flap but may be of variable reliability

Cutaneous flaps

- Thoracoepigastric (TA) flaps can cover the upper third of the abdomen. It is a transverse upper abdominal flap (with the IMF being the upper limit) based on medial perforators from the internal mammary/superior epigastric artery system. Flap delay is recommended if a flap length that exceeds the limit defined by the posterior axillary fold is required
- The iliolumbar bipedicled flap based on both superficial circumflex iliac vessels and perforating cutaneous branches of the lumbar vessels may be used in conjunction with the TFL for lateral abdominal wall defects
- Groin flaps have a wide arc of rotation and can cover the lower abdomen
- The pedicled ALT flap can be used to cover large abdominal defects up the xiphisternum. Most of the anterior thigh can be harvested, with the flap based on both medial and lateral perforators

Summary

- Lower abdomen: TFL, RA, RF and other thigh muscles (gracilis, sartorius), groin, external oblique (EO) turnover flaps
- Middle third: RA, EO, TFL, RF
- Upper abdomen: RA, EO turnover, TA, extended LD

Component separation technique

The basic principle of the technique is that greater mobilisation is achieved with the layers of the abdominal wall moving separately instead of en-bloc. The two main planes of separation lie between the two oblique muscles and behind the rectus. The external oblique contribution to the rectus sheath is divided along its length, leaving the sheath tethered to the internal oblique and transversus abdominis contributions only. Denervation is minimised as the neurovascular plane lies between the latter two muscles.

Bilateral dissection allows advancement of up to 10, 20 and 6 cm at the epigastric, umbilical and suprapubic areas respectively.

Fascial partition release is an alternative that employs bilateral parasagittal relaxing incisions in the external oblique or transversus abdominis fascia to facilitate the coaptation of the linea alba.

Further reading

Leppaniemi A, Tukiainen E. Reconstruction of complex abdominal wall defects. Scand J Surg 2013;102:14–19.

Related topics of interest

- Abdominoplasty
- Tissue expansion
- Vacuum wound closure

Abdominoplasty

Extra-abdominal fat is arranged in the following layers:

- The superficial layer or Camper's layer is uniformly compact with numerous dense fibrous septa. It is continuous with the superficial fascia and fat of the thorax, lower limbs and Dartos fascia in males. The deep layer or Gallaudet's fascia bears less dense fat that is less vascular and more susceptible to fluctuations in weight
- In areas of the trunk that are dilatable such as the lower thorax and abdomen, the interval between the superficial and deep layers condense to form a strong membranous layer known as Scarpa's fascia. It is continuous with Colles' penoscrotal fascia and the fascia lata of the thigh. These characteristics are exploited clinically, with the toughness of Scarpa's fascia useful for dead space closure as well as high lateral tension thigh lifts
- No true deep fascia exists on the trunk, as it would otherwise inhibit expansion and thus respiration

Abdominoplasty is the surgical removal of excess skin and fat from the anterior abdominal wall. The following components should be critically assessed in the abdominoplasty patient:

- Excess skin
- Excess fat
- Muscle diastasis
- Abdominal striae and scars

Surgery is limited to the removal of excess tissue that is unresponsive to exercise and dietary changes. Future pregnancy is a contraindication for abdominoplasty as rectus sheath plication can limit physiological expansion in addition to the cosmetic reversal.

Patients with skin of good elasticity and little excess may benefit more from liposuction alone to address the excess fat.

The pertinent examination findings are the presence or absence of herniae, rectus diastasis, the relative contribution of intra and extra-abdominal fat to the excess abdominal volume, skin quality and its excess.

Procedures

Abdominoplasty. The most common is a full abdominoplasty (Matarasso Type IV). This involves a suprapubic incision from ASIS to ASIS, umbilical repositioning, rectus sheath plication and excision of the pannus.

- Markings: Midline axis, ASISs, a gullwing or W-shaped incision joining the ASISs with the middle portion 5–7 cm cranial to the anterior vulval commissure and a periumbilical incision preserving its deep vascularity. There is considerable variation in scar design both of the lower abdomen and the umbilicus. All the variations in lower abdominal incision design attempt to combat dog ear formation by narrowing the length mismatch between the upper (longer) and lower (shorter) incisions. The classic Regnault open W and the gullwing attempt to lengthen the lower incision, whereas ruching the upper flap attempts to shorten the upper incision. More recent geometric manipulations such as the U-M abdominoplasty and the W-M aim to do the same. Skin excision should be done to maintain minimal tension on closure, with the central part of the upper skin flap being most vulnerable
- The umbilicus is delivered through the flap and positioned at the level of the iliac crests. The shape of the umbilical cut-out is also a subject of furious debate, with the aim to recreate a naturally-shaped umbilicus and periumbilical contour with little or no scar visible
- Drains are frequently used, as are binders or compression garments that are worn for support for two weeks. No heavy lifting is advised for six weeks

Mini-abdominoplasty aims to remove excess tissue that lies predominantly below the umbilicus. It is a less extensive procedure with a shorter scar and it involves only modest undermining and trimming that obviates the need to reposition the umbilicus.

For situations where the umbilicus is tethering the inferior movement of the abdominal flap, a Wilkinson abdominoplasty may be appropriate. This involves the detachment of the umbilicus from its deep blood supply and allowing it to survive by its superficial blood supply alone. This umbilical floating manoeuvre permits a further 2 cm of inferior flap movement. It is useful in patients with upper abdominal laxity and a high positioned umbilicus.

Belt (circumferential) lipectomy is indicated for those with more extensive encircling bulk. In this situation, an abdominoplasty incision will not suffice as the upper/lower flap length mismatch is so great that the dog-ears have to be chased all the way round to the back circumferentially. This typically applies to the massive weight loss (MWL) patient. Belt lipectomy also has the simultaneous advantage of providing a moderate thigh and buttock lift. This procedure requires intraoperative positional change from supine to prone or from supine to both lateral decubitus.

Reverse abdominoplasty may be an option for those with Kocher cholecystectomy scars. It also has the added benefit of providing up to 100 cc of tissue for breast autoaugmentation and a moderate upper body lift, especially useful in the MWL patient.

Umbilicus

The aesthetics of a 'natural looking' umbilicus are subjective, changing with time and fashion, but the general consensus is that a vertically orientated umbilicus with a superior hood and slight surrounding fullness is most desirable. The umbilicus tends to become more hooded and thus appears deeper with age. It takes on a more transverse orientation after childbirth.

During a traditional abdominoplasty, the umbilicus is repositioned through the flap. The stalk may be tacked down to the anterior rectus sheath or Scarpa's fascia to create the illusion of natural contour. De-fatting the midline of the flap to recreate the raphe effect may add to the periumbilical aesthetic in the suitable patient. The incision to deliver the umbilicus through the flap can be of shapes such as the reverse omega or smiley-face with a superiorly based flap. They all have their advocates, but no consensus.

Supplementary procedures

- Plication of the recti may be required for significant muscle diastasis. The aponeurosis is tightened in an elongated diamond pattern with a running No. 0 nylon suture. Strangulation of the umbilicus must be avoided. Bupivacaine instilled into the sheath by single injection or continuous infusion via catheter has been shown to reduce postoperative pain. Transverse plication superiorly and inferiorly ('lying H') has also been attempted. Overzealous plication may cause respiratory or thromboembolic complications. Plication has a correctional effect that lasts at least 6 months, evidenced by current studies with CT scans
- A fleur-de-lys-shaped incision (inverted T) is used to tackle both transverse and caudo-cranial excess at the expense of an additional midline vertical scar. The fleur-de-lys can also be used to revise unsightly paramedian or midline scars. A cranial extension of the fleur-de-lys to the xiphisternum, also termed an anchor-line incision, is especially useful for massive transverse excess after MWL
- High lateral tension abdominoplasty: Flap undermining is limited to the central paramedian area, preserving the perforating blood supply in Huger Zone III (see below) while allowing access for rectus sheath plication. The high lateral skin resection coupled with undermining of the inferior flap laterally permits a lateral thigh lift along this vector. It is important to recognise that this lift is less efficient than a formal thigh lift as mechanical advantage is lost the further away the pull from the target
- Progressive tension sutures are used to distribute tension away from the skin closure and its associated complications such as wound breakdown and scar hypertrophy and stretching. This is achieved by placement of sutures at

regular 1–2 cm intervals between the underside of the superior abdominal flap and the fascia of the abdominal musculature, while progressively advancing the flap inferiorly. The quilting effect that this provides also reduces seroma formation. Note that in principle, the progressive tension and quilting effect are independent. Quilting for seroma reduction is effective even in the absence of the progressive tension manoeuvre

- Liposuction (see below)

Liposuction

Liposuction permits the reduction of subcutaneous fat volume with no effect on any skin excess. Any skin reduction thus depends entirely on the residual skin elasticity for contraction. As such, the prerequisite of liposuction as a sole modality is minimal skin excess and good skin tone. It may be used as an adjunct to abdominoplasty to reduce flank volume and permit a shorter abdominoplasty scar.

Huger classified the vascularity of the abdominal wall into three zones. The first is deep and the latter two superficial.

I. Epigastrium, umbilical and suprapubic areas. This central area extends from xiphisternum to a point halfway between the umbilicus and pubic symphysis, bound laterally by the lateral borders of the recti. Perforating branches of the deep superior (DSEP) and inferior epigastric arteries (DIEP) supply it

II. Branches of the external iliac artery supply the inferior iliac fossae and hypogastrium. These are the superficial circumflex iliac, superficial inferior epigastric (SIEA) and superficial external pudendal arteries

III. The intercostal, subcostal and lumbar arteries that run from lateral to medial supply the flanks and lateral abdominal wall

The abdominoplasty flap is solely reliant on Zone III as the blood supply of Zones I and II are necessarily divided when the flap in raised. Aggressive liposuction in the lateral areas risk damage to Zone III vessels and may lead to necrosis of the most vulnerable area. This is the central inferior portion as it is most distal and subject to the most tension. Liposuction can be safely combined with a full abdominoplasty by observing the following principles outlined by Matarasso:

- Flaps should be undermined no more than enough to permit closure to maximise the preservation of Zone III vessels
- Surgery should be avoided in smokers and those with concurrent comorbidities such as diabetes
- Liposuction use should be judicious and area dependent: restricted (SA4) in the infraumbilical zone, cautious (SA3) in the epigastrium (terrible triangle), limited (SA2) in the lateral areas of the flap, safe (SA1) in the flank and inferior to the abdominoplasty incision
- Stage the liposuction

Saldanha popularised a more modern technique incorporating these principles termed lipoabdominoplasty or Brazilian abdominoplasty. In this technique, liposuction is performed to empty out the fat in the abdominal wall, while preserving the vasculature and increasing skin mobility. The remnant fibrous matrix that previously held fat collapses and the resultant skin excess is drawn inferomedially, where it is excised leaving an extended Pfannenstiel incision. The flap is raised only in the midline and sufficient only to permit rectus plication. This leaves the vasculature in Zones II and III intact with Zone I partially intact. This improved residual vasculature permits a more aggressive liposuction in the beginning and leaves a shorter scar. However, it is limited to patients with no transverse skin excess and minor caudocranial excess. It is unsuitable for the MWL patient.

Complications

Major complications such as thromboembolism are very rare, but more common if liposuction is combined with abdominoplasty. The minor complication rate is 5–10% and more common in smokers, diabetics, those with obesity, and if abdominoplasty is combined with gynaecological procedures. Beware of respiratory compromise from raised intraabdominal pressure due to over-tight closure.

- Seroma (6%): Moderate sized seromas should be drained. Quilting sutures are effective in reducing seroma. Some advocate leaving a layer of subscarpal fat on the abdominal fascia and over the inguinal areas to preserve the lymphatics but robust evidence is lacking. Pitanguy advocates the avoidance of desiccation, meticulous haemostasis and adequate drainage, all of which is good practice but the effect on seroma rates remain unproven
- Infection, dehiscence and necrosis (5–7%): Increased with smoking and tension of closure
- Scar problems: Hypertrophic and stretched scarring is common
- Decreased sensation (10%): Damage to lateral femoral cutaneous nerve (L2–3, found 1–6 cm medial to ASIS)
- Dog-ears: This occurs from the length mismatch between the upper and lower flaps. This can be eliminated at the cost of a longer scar extending into the flanks or the excess distributed along the entire scar by `cheating' it in forming minor folds along its length that even out with time. Alternatively, dog-ear excision can be delayed to allow maximum skin contraction. Since dog-ears are a convex contour deformity, emptying out the fat (but not excising skin) under the dog-ear will flatten out the dog-ear. The resultant skin excess contracts and may form a pucker which may or may not be cosmetically acceptable

Abdominoplasty patients are uncompromising and are associated with a significant rate of postoperative dissatisfaction most commonly associated with dog-ears, residual fullness overhanging the scar and unnatural umbilical appearance.

Contraindications

Smoking, diabetes and morbid obesity in addition to a cardiovascular and/or thromboembolic disease are contraindications due to the high risk of complications and resultant high risk/benefit ratio. Supraumbilical scarring is a relative contraindication as it has a higher complication rate of 23% vs. 7% in the unscarred. Fat necrosis is the most common, implying impaired vascularity as the aetiology. If abdominoplasty is contemplated in such a subgroup, vascularity must be maximised by avoiding wound tension, flap over-dissection and minimising or avoiding liposuction altogether.

Further reading

Hurvitz KA, Olaya WA, Nguyen A, Wells JH. Evidence-based medicine: abdominoplasty. Plast Reconstr Surg 2014;133:1214–21.

Related topic of interest

- Liposuction

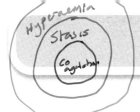

Acute burns

A burn is damage caused by a pathological excess of energy within the tissues. Thermal burns are the most common and are the focus of this section. The threshold temperature for protein denaturation and permanent cell damage is 43°C and 45°C, respectively. Significant burn injuries invoke a systemic response that if left untreated, has a high mortality rate.

Jackson's burn model

This theoretical model divides the tissue damage into 3-dimensional concentric zones around the burn.

- Zone of coagulation: Ground zero. Tissue here is necrotic and has undergone irreversible damage [handwritten: coagulation]
- Zone of stasis: Adjacent tissue that has undergone sublethal damage and is in a precarious condition. It is hypoperfused and oedematous and may progress to necrosis or recover. Improved perfusion from adequate resuscitation and measures such as cooling increase chances of recovery. Continuing inflammation, superimposed infection or ischaemia promotes necrosis of this area. Effective burn management maximises tissue survival in this zone [handwritten: Stasis]
- Zone of hyperaemia: Tissue here is minimally damaged and will recover. Usually in 7-10 days. There is a transient increase in blood supply by vasodilation [handwritten: Hyperaemia]

Types of thermal burn

Burn depth is dependent on the energy transferred, which in turn is related to temperature and contact time. The relationship is not linear but exponential. While thermodynamic subtleties are outside the scope of this discussion, flame burns are more likely to produce deeper burns than scalds.

- Scald: Caused by hot liquids or gases
- Flame burn: Caused by combustion of clothing, flammable liquids on skin or direct contact with naked flames

- Flash burn: Caused by self-limited ignition of gases or plasma. No continuous heat source beyond this
- Radiator burn: Caused by close proximity to a heat source
- Contact burn: Caused by physical contact with a solid heat source
  - Bitumen burns are unique contact burns where the contact is prolonged due to its strong adherence to skin. Bitumen or tarmac is used in road construction and is not to be confused with chemical tar, which is a carcinogenic poly-aromatic hydrocarbon compound used in waterproofing. Molten bitumen has a temperature of 140–200°C but cools rapidly even before it comes into contact with skin. Standard treatment involves cooling but subsequent removal of the hardened bitumen is controversial. Inexperienced removal may worsen the injury. Agents that facilitate removal are:

  - Kerosene, alcohol or acetone act quickly but may be potentially toxic
  - Oil and butter may take 10-15 minutes to work and results are variable
  - Petrolatum-based commercial preparations work but may not be readily available

First aid — [handwritten: stop burning process]

This aims to stop the burning process and involves:

- Removing the source. Burnt clothing (melted or saturated in hot liquid) retains heat, perpetuates the burning process and should be removed
- Cooling the small areas for a minimum of 10 minutes and preferably until pain stops. Cooling large areas risk hypothermia and should be avoided. Cooling reduces protein denaturation and improves survivability in the zone of stasis. This effect is lost if cooling is delayed beyond the first hour. Cooling for analgesic

purposes remains effective regardless. Ice must not be used as it may generate a frostbite injury that worsens the burn

History

Take an 'AMPLE' history:

- Allergies
- Medication
- Past medical history
- Last meal
- Event history
- Cause: This estimates the type and expected general burn depth. Associated injuries are common and the dramatic burn frequently distracts physicians. The lethality of a burn is in the order of hours to days, whereas associated injuries may kill the patient in the order of minutes if unrecognised
- Place: An enclosed space raises suspicion of an airway burn that is both thermal and chemical

Primary survey

Initial treatment should follow standard ATLS algorithms. Burn-specific points are detailed below.

- Airway and cervical spine: Full-blown airway obstruction or late signs such as hoarseness and stridor are easy to spot. However, suspicions of an early asymptomatic airway burn lie in the history. Early anaesthetic assessment is paramount in this situation and if intubation is indicated, ensure that the endotracheal tube is cut long or not at all. Facial swelling around the tube over the next few days will otherwise cause loss of airway security. Circumferential full-thickness neck burns may cause extrinsic compression and escharotomy may be necessary
- Breathing: 100% O_2 is given. Life-threatening injuries such as tension pneumothorax, massive haemothorax and massive flail chest can result from the initial incident. Circumferential full-thickness chest burns may limit ventilatory movements. The chest can

be escharotomised in a breastplate fashion with bilateral anterior axillary line incisions with an inverted-V incision over the rib margin connecting them. This allows independent excursion of the anterior chest wall

- Circulation: Stem bleeding if present and initiate fluid resuscitation

Inhalational injury

Inhalational injury is associated with a >75% mortality in large burns. The presence of concomitant inhalational injury in an otherwise isolated burn increases the mortality risk from 1–2% to 40%, where ARDS is the prime cause of death. It is classified into:

- Supraglottic: Hot gases cause a thermal burn of the upper airway mucosa, resulting in oedema. Symptomatic obstruction may be delayed for up to 2 days and often resolves spontaneously after a few days. Thermal injury to the lower airway is rare due to the high thermal capacity of the upper airway. Superheated steam however, has the potential to cause a thermal burn of the lower airway
- Subglottic: Chemical injury is caused by noxious, irritant gases or chemical compounds. Aldehydes, sulphur dioxide, ammonia and chlorine can form strong acids or alkalis that inhibit mucociliary clearance and cause surfactant loss. Subsequent airway collapse and alveolar damage is exacerbated by airway oedema. Secondary mucosal sloughing and secondary infection exacerbates the damage after 72 hours
- Systemic: Inhaled gases may have metabolic effects.
  - Cyanide poisoning: This is rare but causes irreversible inhibition of cytochrome oxidase and the electron transport chain, causing a global energy crisis at the cellular level. Treatment options carry substantial risk in themselves and while most effective if administered as soon as possible, is frequently not feasible. The safest option is a single dose of hydroxycobalamin. Sodium

Sodium
thiosulphate infusion followed by sodium nitrite is an alternative but risks hypotensive vasodilatation. Fortunately, the inhaled cyanide dose is frequently small and antidote treatment is rarely indicated

- Carbon monoxide (CO) poisoning: CO has 200 times the affinity of oxygen for haemoglobin and thus reduces its oxygen carrying capacity. CO also impedes cellular metabolism by inhibiting cytochrome p450 and may display synergistic toxicity with cyanide
  - Carboxyhaemoglobin levels (COHb) reflect the severity of poisoning. Smokers have up to a 10% baseline level compared to 5% in non-smokers
    - 15–20% : Headache and confusion
    - 20–40% : Hallucinations and ataxia
    - > 60% : Fatal
  - Nomograms can be used to extrapolate levels at the time of exposure
  - The mainstay of treatment is oxygen therapy. The 250 minute half-life of COHb in room air is reduced to 40–60 minutes with 100% oxygen. Hyperbaric oxygen accelerates this process but any additional quantifiable outcomes are unclear. Oxygen should be continued for a further 24–48 hours to combat a secondary release of tissue-bound CO

A high index of suspicion for inhalational injury is paramount. Thermally induced swelling may be delayed but rapidly progressive. In such situations, err on the side of caution, as prophylactic elective intubation is preferable to emergency intubation for overt respiratory distress. Endoscopic examination may reveal direct evidence of upper-airway injury in selected equivocal cases. However, attempts to objectively measure inhalational injury have not been promising. The diagnosis remains solely clinical. Two or more of the following indicate an increased risk of inhalational injury:

- Burn sustained in an enclosed space
- Singed nasal hairs
- Burns or soot in oral cavity or pharynx
- Hoarseness or voice change

The mainstay of treatment is supportive, in combination with intubation and lavage or suction as deemed appropriate. Mucolytics, free-radical scavengers such as acetylcysteine, and chelators such as desferrioxamine and heparin (unknown mechanism of action), have been advocated but their effectiveness is unproven. Steroids are deleterious and should be avoided.

Secondary survey

The secondary survey involves a head-to-toe examination to detect other injuries:

- Remove clothing
- Examine for wounds
- Assess area and depth of burn

The neurological status is assessed by the patient's responses using the Glasgow Coma Scale or the simpler AVPU system (Alert, responsive to Voice, responsive to Pain or Unconscious). Remember to assess the pupillary reflexes.

The wounds are then covered with simple temporary dressings that are clean (not necessarily sterile), moist and cool (to reduce pain). Cling-film or saline-soaked gauze is perfectly adequate. Topical antiseptics or antibiotics are not required.

Specific assessment of burns

Depth

Burn depth assessment determines the short-term treatment (grafting) and long-term outcome (scarring) of the burn wound. The clinical characteristics of the various burn depths are delineated in Table 3. Scalds are more likely to be heterogeneous in depth.

Clinical assessment is subjective (assessor-dependant) and dynamic. The dynamicity is attributed to the potential for burn depth to progress in the first 2–3 days. Peripheral vasoconstrictors such as inotropes may cause zones of stasis to progress to necrosis. However, the balance of systemic support at the expense of burn depth is a judgement call based on priority. While it is easy to distinguish superficial burns that will heal conservatively from deep burns that require surgery, burns of an intermediate depth are more difficult to assess. A watch-and-wait strategy to allow these equivocal areas to declare themselves may be employed.

- Patency of blood vessels: Skin blanching with pressure and subsequent refill demonstrates patency of perfusion. The pinprick-bleeding test may be used to supplement but is frequently unnecessary
- Laser Doppler imaging (LDI): LDI is a non-invasive method of burn depth estimation that measures laser frequency change and relates this to perfusion, displayed on a map. The map is colour coded in red and blue, which signify areas of increased and decreased perfusion respectively. It is expensive, requires training and is rather unwieldy, rendering its use limited to large institutions. It remains the only FDA-approved technique for this purpose at this time. The LDI is 95–97% accurate and yields reliable predictive values to identify burns that will heal within 3 weeks. It is useful for reducing cost and morbidity by minimising unnecessary surgery and also provides an objective measurement that is vital for research
- Thermal imaging or thermography: This technique exploits the fact that full-thickness burns are >2% cooler than unburned skin by assessing the temperature response following a thermal pulse. However, its accuracy is compromised by evaporative heat loss from the burn and works poorly in granulating wounds
- Vital dyes: Dyes are of low clinical utility
  - Non-fluorescent e.g. Evans blue, patent blue V detect surface necrosis only and thus are of low clinical utility
  - Fluorescent dyes e.g. fluorescein and indocyanine green have poor burn penetration

NIRS (near infrared spectroscopy) use is currently limited to research only.

Area

Total burn surface area (TBSA) is used as a crude but practical proxy for the severity of the burn injury. It does not incorporate burn depth or any inhalation burn component and as such, such variables must be separately accounted for. The larger the TBSA, the greater the severity of the burn and subsequent inflammatory response. The increased capillary permeability permits and perpetuates an extravascular fluid shift from the re-equilibration of the oncotic pressure gradient of Starling's forces. This results in intravascular

Table 3 Features associated with different depths of burn					
Description	Colour and texture	Blisters?	Capillary refill	Sensation/pain	Healing
Superficial	Pink and dry	No	Rapid	Sensate, painful	Involves epidermis only Desquamates after a few days and heals without scarring
Superficial partial thickness	Pink/red, wet under blisters, slight oedema	Yes	Present	Sensate, painful	Heals in 7–10 days without scarring
Deep dermal	Pale or red with fixed staining, dense oedema	Possible	Poor or absent	Sensation decreased or absent, may not be painful	Re-epithelializes from residual dermal elements in wound bed Takes >2 weeks to heal and with scar
Full thickness	White, pale or black, leathery	No	No	No	Re-epithelialization occurs only from wound edges Wound bed granulates and autodebrides eschar if left to heal by secondary intention

dehydration that has hypoperfusion and hypovolaemic consequences. The TBSA is thus a risk predictor for the development of hypovolaemic shock and renal failure.

The threshold TBSA for which a burn produces such a significant systemic response is >15% in adults and 10% in children. While somewhat arbitrary, it is a useful rule of thumb to administer formal fluid resuscitation that is clinically validated. In contrast, classifications based on full-thickness burn depth do not directly correlate and are less useful for this purpose. TBSA estimation by digital photography and telemedicine has been shown to be clinically effective.

The following methods are useful in TBSA estimation:

- Wallace's rule of nines: The body is divided into surface area regions of 9% (head and neck, each upper limb), 18% (each lower limb, anterior trunk, posterior trunk). The perineum is a 1% area, as well as the front and back of neck. While it is easily remembered, the rule overestimates the burn size. It is unsuitable for use in children in this form due to their different body proportions. While modifications exist to account for this, the rule becomes unwieldy and loses its main advantage of ease, while maintaining its inaccuracy. The serial halving technique allows rapid estimation in the A&E department
- Hand area: The surface area of the patient's volar palm and fingers in adduction approximates 1% of total body surface area. Its utility lies in quantifying areas of patchy burns. The actual area has been calculated to average 0.89% by 3D scanning and this varies with stature. While total body surface area increases with BMI, the hand area is minimally affected due to its relatively low fat content
- Burn charts: The Lund and Browder chart (**Figure 1** and **Table 4**) accounts for the variation in body proportions with age and provides a permanent and accurate estimation and visual documentation of the burned areas, the TBSA and burn depth. However, it does not account for inhalational injury and is less reliable

in those with altered body proportions such as obesity, pregnancy, macromastia and amputees. The Lund and Browder chart remains the mainstay of burn documentation

- Erythema is not included in the TBSA assessment as it represents reversible intra-epidermal damage only that does not significantly contribute to the systemic response

Burn oedema

The systemic mechanisms for extracellular fluid shifts outlined above result in tissue oedema. Oedema occurs in both burnt and unburned tissue, depending upon the size of the burn. While the timing of peak oedema varies with burn size and the volume of resuscitative fluid administered, the majority of oedema occurs early. Up to 90% of maximal oedema occurs by 4 hours.

Alterations in capillary haemodynamics underpin the development of oedema but exact mechanisms have not been fully elucidated. A simplified explanation utilises the Starling force argument and is as follows:

Starling forces comprise of two sets of opposing forces that act to push fluid between the intra and extravascular spaces. The two components responsible for this are the hydrostatic pressure and oncotic pressure.

- Hydrostatic pressure: The combination of arterial vasodilatation and venoconstriction creates a bottleneck in the capillaries and increases capillary hydrostatic pressure, which is an outward force. As fluid is pushed into the extravascular interstitium, interstitial hydrostatic pressure increases transiently as it attempts to equilibrate
- Oncotic pressure: This force is generated by plasma protein concentration. The higher the relative concentration, the stronger the oncotic pressure for fluid to enter its compartment. At rest, the intravascular space has a high oncotic pressure due to its high plasma protein concentration relative to the interstitium. As capillary permeability increases, the plasma proteins leak into the extravascular space and increase its oncotic pressure. The subsequent equilibration gradually

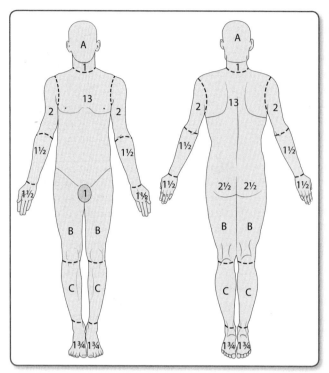

Figure 1 Commonly used burn diagram (Lund and Browder chart, first described in 1944) used to record the burn distribution and assess the surface area involved. Erythema is not included.

Table 4 Lund and Browder age-dependent modifications of body surface area						
	Age (years)					
	0	1	5	10	15	Adult
A—half of head	9.5	8.5	6.5	5.5	4.5	3.5
B—half of thigh	2.75	2.35	4	4.25	4.5	4.75
C—half of leg	2.5	2.5	2.75	3	3.25	3

drives more fluid into the extravascular space. The net result is a intravascular space depleted of fluid and also the ability to retain it. In addition, macromolecular destruction from the burn increases extravascular osmotic load and burn-induced increase in tissue compliance making extravascular water retention and oedema progressively easier

- Capillary permeability is increased, peaking at 3–6 hours, This is reversed usually by the 24-hour mark. Free radical lipid peroxidation and endothelial damage may underlie this phenomenon. The

cessation of capillary permeability and gradual diuresis reverses the oedema as a rough rule of thumb, from day 3 onwards

Resuscitation

Formal intravenous fluid resuscitation is administered when TBSA exceeds 15% in adults and 10% in children. Below this threshold, oral fluids are deemed sufficient but are dependent on the clinical considerations and compliance. There is literature that suggests that oral resuscitation can be adequate in burns of up to 40% TBSA in the carefully selected patient, but this is not routine. Similarly, proctoclysis remains unconventional and largely unnecessary.

There are many resuscitation formulae in use, of which the most common is the Parkland formula. Contrary to popular belief, the formula was described by Charles Baxter. It is named after the Parkland Hospital in Dallas. The formula is only an estimation of the fluid requirement that requires monitoring. More fluids may be required for burn injury invisible from the surface such as inhalational injury, electrical burns and those with concomitant crush injuries.

Early resuscitation is of paramount importance as an increased delay correlates with poorer outcomes. The calculations are made from the time of the burning as the starting point, not the time of presentation. Resuscitation volume V (mL) is calculated as:

$$V \text{ (mL)} = 4 \times \text{TBSA (\%)} \times \text{body weight (kg)}.$$

The calculated volume V is given over the first 24 hours in the following schedule: half over the first 8 hours and the remainder over 16 hours. Hartmann's solution (Ringer's lactate) is the resuscitative fluid of choice. In circumstances where there is a delay in presentation and in the absence of clinical shock, the calculated deficit should be compensated for as soon as practically possible e.g. within 2 hours.

Note that the original development studies that titrated fluid volume to cardiac output did not substantiate a correlation to warrant the 4 times multiplier constant nor rationale for 8- and 16-hour time blocks. There is a tendency for this regime to overestimate fluid requirements and may cause sodium overload.

Fluid regimes in the subsequent 24 hours are far more variable. It is common to give less crystalloid, e.g. 2 ml per TBSA per kg and 0.5 ml/kg of 5% albumin (colloid rescue). Colloid is less useful in the first 24 hour due to the high capillary permeability negating its ability to hold intravascular oncotic pressure. It is thus more effective when given beyond this timeframe.

Maintenance fluids are needed for children (see Paediatric burns).

Alternatives

- Monafo (1970) used hypertonic saline to reduce infused volumes and the risk of abdominal compartment syndrome. This is not to be taken lightly as it carries a risk of central pontine myelinolysis
- Muir and Barclay (1974) used albumin on the basis that it was more physiological. This regime partitions the initial 36-hour period into blocks of 4, 4, 4, 6, 6 and 12 hours. Fluid adjustments are made at the end of each block as needed, most commonly reductions. No advantages have been demonstrated with this regime when compared to crystalloid regimes
  - The Albumin controversy: Colloids have a long track record of use in effective burns resuscitation. The 1998 Cochrane report suggested that the use of colloids was associated with a small but measureable increase in mortality. The report reviewed the use of albumin in the critically ill rather than specifically addressing its use in burns patients. There were only three studies that involved burns patients and they were in the minority. The albumin regimens were highly disparate from regimes used today. Despite increased fluid accumulation, especially in the lung, following colloid use in the first 24 hours, it is now generally accepted that the report overstated this risk. There should thus be no barrier to the proper use of colloids in burns patients

Monitoring

Formulae serve only as guides and require timely titration to the patient response. Over-resuscitation is a common pitfall (fluid creep) due to goal-orientated therapy and reluctance to reduce infusions even when appropriate. The risk of compartment syndrome (CS) increases significantly with infusion in excess of 0.25 L/kg. Measures of adequate resuscitation:

- Blood pressure is insensitive as it remains well maintained in moderate intravascular loss

- Pulse rate is unreliable. Tachycardia is a non-specific symptom. Furthermore, patients with low reserves, such as the elderly, may not be able to produce a tachycardia
- Temperature: The core-peripheral temperature gradient can be used to gauge the peripheral perfusion, but has numerous confounding factors affecting its reliability
- Urine output is the gold-standard measure. The target is a range of 0.5–1.0 ml/kg/h for adults and a minimum of 1 ml/kg/h in children. However, urine output is not a true surrogate for organ perfusion

The central venous pressure (CVP) and PCWP have been used but is invasive and may be inaccurate in the acute phase of a major burn. Haematocrit and haemoglobin concentration are historical guides that underestimate requirements.

A subset of higher risk burn patients may warrant supranormal resuscitation. They are patients with a higher risk of ARDS/SIRS and have elevated serum lactate and base deficits, due to oxygen debt, anaerobic metabolism and lactic acidosis. Urine output targets in these situations may exceed the conventional range. Overall, such regimes of goal-directed hyperdynamic resuscitation towards supraphysiological targets using parameters such as lactate base deficit, oxygen delivery (Do_2), venous oxygen (Vo_2) have not shown any significant improvements in mortality.

Other factors

Decompression

Tissue oedema in combination with loss of soft tissue elasticity may lead to elevated compartment pressures.
- Compartment syndrome with limb burns
- Airway obstruction with neck burns
- Breathing problems with thoracic burns

Decompression is required in established or impending CS. In contrast to classical CS where the pressure is sustained by a tight muscle fascia alone, burn CS may be also be caused by compression of the skin and superficial soft tissue, rendered inelastic and constrictive by the burn or its consequent oedema. Escharotomy alone may thus be adequate, but a fasciotomy may be required when significant muscle swelling is identified. Decompression is best performed under controlled conditions in the operating room under general anaesthesia (GA) and with diathermy. The preferred lines of incision are used and care is taken to avoid iatrogenic nerve damage. The ulnar and common peroneal nerves are most commonly injured. The forearm is may be decompressed with preaxial and postaxial incisions. The alternative single volar forearm S incision adequately decompresses the dorsal compartment in >50% of cases, even if not supplemented by a dorsal longitudinal incision. It is important to evaluate/monitor the adequacy of the decompression. The gold-standard remains clinical assessment but adjuncts that may assist in monitoring include capillary refill, Doppler signalling, pin-prick (looking for bright red capillary blood) and oxygen saturation of the affected part.

Burns nutrition

Adequate feeding is important for wound healing and resistance to infection. The catabolic response is prolonged and more pronounced in major burns and the daily calorific requirement increases by 1.5–1.75 times normal. A resultant weight loss of >10% body weight is associated with a worse outcome whilst a loss in lean mass of >40% carries a high mortality rate.

In major burns, a feeding tube should be inserted immediately to decompress the gut and commence feeding, preferably within 8 hours.
Estimating the required nutrition:

- Formula-based: Formulae calculate the increased calorific requirement. The Harris-Benedict Equation and Curreri Formula are the most well-known, but suffer from numerous caveats. They underestimate by 23% and overestimate by 58% respectively, leading to advocates for an average of the two. The former is validated only in adults, whereas the Curreri works for both adults and children. However, both formulae have not been validated for use in large burns

- Objective measurement: Indirect calorimetry is calculated from inspired and expired oxygen and carbon dioxide (CO_2). It is more accurate but suffers from impracticality and is of limited availability

In principle, the burns diet should be calorie and protein rich. A dedicated burns nutritionist is essential. Monitoring with nitrogen balance studies is uncommon. Overfeeding must be avoided as it increases fat mass and hyperglycaemia, which impair healing.

- The addition of glutamine, arginine and omega 3 fatty acids are of theoretical benefit but remain clinically unproven
  - Glutamine is the preferred fuel for dividing cells, gluconeogenesis and is involved in renal acid-base balance. It is usually abundant but becomes a conditionally essential amino acid after severe trauma, when demand outstrips supply. There is evidence to suggest a reduction of mortality and morbidity in non-burned critically ill patients. It appears to be safe at doses of <0.57 g/kg/day but the optimal treatment duration and dosage are unknown
- There is no evidence for vitamin replacement in the previously healthy
- Anabolic hormone use is controversial. The anabolic response to restore body weight occurs at one tenth of the rate of loss. Anabolic hormones such as hGH (increased mortality in adults and increased scarring), oxandrolone (improves lean body mass, increases protein synthesis and bone mineralisation with fewer complications than hGH), low dose insulin and IGF has been shown to reduce catabolism and loss in muscle mass. Similarly, β-blockers have been used in children to modulate the metabolic response

Total parenteral nutrition is not indicated in acute burns and is associated with a higher mortality rate. Early enteral feeding is preferred as it increases gut perfusion, preserves gut integrity, reduces bacterial translocation and is safer with fewer complications. Nasojejunal tube feeding may be advantageous in patients who require frequent GA, as the feed can be maintained throughout due to the low risk of aspiration.

Pain relief

Adequate pain relief reduces catabolism in addition to improving comfort. Opiates are best given intravenously as absorption from intramuscular administration is unpredictable. Additional analgesia should be given before dressing changes.

- IV opiates
- IV non-opiates such as midazolam should be used with great caution, as they act synergistically with opioids
- Oral morphine: 30–90 minutes required for peak effect. A dose of 0.3 mg/kg in children is recommended, but 0.5–1 mg/kg may be more appropriate. Uncertain bioavailability (15–50%), inability to give additional doses and the long post-procedural sedation may be problematic
- Inhaled nitrous oxide (Entonox) is safe with rapid onset but has limited analgesic properties. It is popular in some units but there is limited evidence for its use in burns

Infection

Burns are sterile at time of infliction, but may undergo the following:

- Contamination: Bacteria are transient and do not affect the wound
- Colonisation: Bacteria multiply but do not cause disease
- Infection: Bacterial growth and invasion into host tissue leads to cellular injury and host reaction. Wound healing is delayed

Regular dressings with physical cleansing of the wound and the use of topical antimicrobials are the mainstay of reducing infection risk. Prophylactic systemic antibiotics are not usually warranted. Antibiotics do not effectively penetrate the eschar and indiscriminate use will promote resistance. Antibiotics are used in treatment only and guided by clinical assessment. Wound swabs are notoriously unreliable when used alone. Sepsis should be suspected if there is a change in temperature, blood glucose or the acute onset of heart failure, pulmonary oedema, ARDS or ileus.

It is important that wound swabs are taken in correct manner to maximise the yield of meaningful results:

- Cleanse wound with sterile saline to remove purulent debris and reduce extraneous micro-organisms

- Moisten swab with sterile saline (will attach bacteria more effectively) and use a zigzag motion whilst rotating the swab to sample the whole wound surface
- It is what is left growing on the burn after cleaning, not what is in the debris, that is most likely to cause infection

Further reading

Cartotto R, Zhou A. Fluid creep: the pendulum hasn't swung back yet! J Burn Care Res 2010;31:551–8.

Related topics of interest

- Burns dressings
- Burns surgery
- Chemical burns
- Paediatric burns

Basal cell carcinoma

Approximately 30 different types of skin cancer exist, of which 99% comprise BCCs, SCCs and melanomas. BCC is the most common malignancy in Caucasians. The incidence ranges from 700 per 100,000 in Australia to 2–3 per 100,000 in Hong Kong. The UK and US share a similar incidence of 100–200 per 100,000. The causes have been attributed to sun exposure, racial predilection and composition, as well as lifestyle. The incidence is increasing by up to 10% per year worldwide. It is more common in males but the proportional incidence in females is rising.

The term basal cell carcinoma is a misnomer. BCCs do not arise from the epidermal basal cells but instead from the pluripotent cells of the pilosebaceous adnexa. This accounts for the occasional appendiceal differentiation in these tumours. BCCs are most common on the face (75% on face, of which 25% are on the nose) where cumulative sun exposure is highest. The lesion is generally slow growing, but is locally destructive. The classical features (of the nodular type or rodent ulcer, see below) are raised pearly edges and telangiectasia with or without central ulceration. The picket fence pattern is the classical histological finding, depicted by undifferentiated cells in nodules with peripheral palisading.

Early BCCs may be mistaken for trichoepitheliomas in appearance. Trichoepitheliomas may be differentiated by their predominant midface location and tend to be <1 cm in diameter, multiple in nature and may display an autosomal dominant inheritance pattern.

Dermatoscopes are magnifying devices that allow an optimal view of skin lesions. They utilise non-polarised or cross-polarised light with an intervening liquid medium (usually oil) to reduce glare, resulting in an improved image. Newer devices do not require an oil medium. The dermatoscopic features of BCCs may include:

- Minor degrees of ulceration that were not obvious on clinical examination
- Arborising telangiectasia

- Spoke-wheel areas

As a rule of thumb, BCCs do not metastasise. While an exceptionally small number that have been documented to do so, it is so rare that the diagnosis must be questioned in the presence of metastasis.

There are a large number of morphological subtypes of BCC. The most clinically relevant are as follows:

- Nodular: This is the most common. A combination of nodular growth and ulceration lead to the classical appearance. Nodular BCCs may be pigmented, often unevenly, and may be misdiagnosed as malignant melanoma. The pigmentation is caused by phagocytosis of apoptotic tumour cells that are laden with melanosomes. Pigmented BCCs are more common in darker-skinned races (>75% in Chinese, <5% in Caucasians)
- Superficial: These are most common on the trunk. The lesions are red, scaly and may bear small ulcers. They are easily mistaken for eczema or psoriasis. Islands of normal-looking skin are common within the affected area but true multifocality is rare
- Infiltrative lesions come in two forms:
  - Morpheaform/sclerosing: An intense fibrotic reaction produces a scar-like lesion with ill-defined margins. They can spread locally without causing elevation. They constitute 5% of all BCCs and have an overall incomplete excision rate of up to a third.
  - Non-morpheaform: There is little fibrosis and these lesions are often difficult to see
- Basosquamous lesions are relatively rare and behave more like SCC in terms of growth rate and metastatic potential

Risk factors

- Sun exposure: UVB causes DNA damage (p53 tumour suppressor gene at 9q22). The strongest association is seen with repeated sunburn in childhood. It causes field effect damage. There is a 50% increased risk of

9q22

developing a further BCC after the initial, in the subsequent 5 years. PUVA treatment for psoriasis is a modest risk factor
- Immunosuppression: There is a 10-fold increased risk for BCC in transplant patients, with 50% occurring in the first 5 years. The highest relative risk increase however, is for Kaposi sarcoma at >200-fold, but the condition has an exceedingly low population incidence
- Carcinogens such as aromatic hydrocarbons and arsenic. While rare, arsenic causes multiple superficial BCCs
- Irradiation
- Genetic conditions such as xeroderma pigmentosum and Gorlin syndrome. The latter is autosomal dominant and is caused by PTCH gene mutation on chromosome 9q, resulting in altered sonic hedgehog (SHH) signalling. SHH inhibition is the subject of current salvage medical therapy for BCC in candidates unsuitable for surgery and radiotherapy. Patients with Gardner syndrome (SOD) have soft tissue tumours such as BCCs, osteomas and dermoids
- Pre-existing sebaceous naevus of Jadassohn. This is a congenital hamartoma that is reported to have a 10–20% risk of malignant change. However, most of the lesions previously attributed to BCC were actually benign trichoblastomas. A recent French series quotes a transformation risk nearer to 1%

Treatment

Surgical excision is the standard curative treatment. The BAD/BAPRAS BCC guidelines quote a cure rate proportional to the margins taken. For non-infiltrative BCCs, the cure rates are:

- 3 mm = 86%
- 4 mm = 94%
- 5 mm = 96%

While following such margins in non-cosmetically sensitive areas are not an issue, the bulk of BCC excisional work of the plastic surgeon will be in areas that are. The crucial factors to consider are:
- The structures sacrificed with a larger margin

- The structures sacrificed with recurrence
- The expected frequency of recurrence

By using the location of the BCC, its potential anatomical extensions, the histological subtype and cosmetic unit understanding, a particular margin can be reasonably justified. It is important to realise that the cosmetic unit principle may actually favour a larger margin than that recommended for cure. In these cases, the higher cure rate is an added bonus. Moh's surgery may be a suitable alternative if tissue conservation is paramount. However, it is equally paramount to consider the need for temporising cover as Moh's surgery may be done at a location without access to your expertise. Extensive eyelid resection for example, risks exposure of the globe.

- Frozen section (FS): Retrospective reviews show that lesions that can be excised with 3–4 mm margins (5 mm for SCC) do not benefit from FS. There is only an 85% concordance between FS and the gold-standard paraffin-fixed sections
- Incomplete excision: Incomplete excision rates range from 2–18% and are most frequent in the danger areas such as the medial canthus, external auditory canal and alar base. Tumours tend to extend deeper at these locations as these are lines of embryonic fusion
  - The risk of incomplete excision in a re-excision of an incomplete excision is 30–50%
  - Of these 30–50%, 40% progress to clinical recurrence
  - Incompletely excised lesions should be re-excised if possible
- Recurrence: BCCs greater than 2 cm in size or of an infiltrative type have a higher recurrence rate. Recurrent lesions tend to be more aggressive in behaviour thus a wider excision margin of 5–10 mm is often suggested. However, there is no evidence for this at present
- Moh's micrographic surgery (MMS): The lesion is excised and the base of the specimen is mapped out with a 2 mm tangential shave of the wound bed. If the tangential shave reveals tumour abutting the deep margin, another tangential shave is taken and the process repeated until

a complete excision is achieved. This minimises the amount of normal tissue removed and is especially useful in areas where maximal tissue preservation is paramount, or where margins are visually indistinct. A 95–99% complete excision rate is reported for primary BCC, and rates in excess of 90% for incompletely excised BCC. However, it is extremely time and labour intensive and is unnecessary for the majority of BCCs, which are small and simple

Other treatments

- Curettage with or without electrodesiccation: The lesion is scooped out piecemeal along its natural plane of cleavage between tumour and normal tissue. In general, tumour tissue is softer than normal dermis and is amenable to curettage, whereas dermis is not. Sclerosing BCCs and previous scars are hard and do not curette well. The base usually cauterised, although there is little evidence that this improves oncological clearance. The recurrence rate is quoted at 10%, but the study subjects are very heterogeneous, lack uniform protocols, and no margin information provided for valid comparison. It is inappropriate for recurrent, morphoeic or high-risk lesions
- Cryotherapy with liquid nitrogen has a comparable 10% recurrence rate. As it is destructive, no histological information is obtained. The treated area needs to exceed the lesion margin by 4–6 mm. Despite this, cryotherapy for BCC has higher recurrence rates than curettage and is unsuitable for recurrent lesions
- Radiotherapy is an effective alternative primary treatment for superficial BCCs with cure rates of up to 94%. It is not recommended for young patients as the risk of carcinogenesis, ulceration, pigmentation, chondritis and long-term cosmetic impairment is significant. The latter may be minimised with the newer fractionated regimes

Newer treatments

- 5% Imiquimod (Aldara, 3M Pharmaceuticals) is an immuno-modulator that acts on Toll-like receptors and stimulates the local production of cytokines, especially the interferons that destroy the tumour. It is applied topically for 6 weeks with an 85% response rate. It recently attained FDA approval for the treatment of superficial BCCs, in addition to actinic keratosis and genital warts. Long-term results are being assessed
- Photodynamic therapy utilises laser or non-laser light energy to activate a chemosensitising agent that has been sequestered by the target cells. One such agent, topical methyl aminolevulinate 16% (Metvix), is taken up by malignant cells and converted to porphyrins that are then activated by red light (570–670 nm) causing selective cellular destruction. Treatment is usually repeated after a week. Due to the limited tissue penetration of light, only superficial lesions are suitable for treatment. The overall response rate is 85% in selected lesions with tumour thickness predicting outcome. While the cosmetic outcome is good, clearance rates are inferior to surgical excision. It is not widely used in UK for this purpose
- Topical 5% fluorouracil can be used to treat multiple superficial BCCs. The prolonged treatment time and higher recurrence rates make it a less favoured option except for low risk, non-facial lesions
- Ablative CO_2 lasers have been used for low-risk lesions but also suffer from lack of histological examination

Others

- Oral retinoids may be useful in preventing or delaying the formation of new tumours. It has been used in conditions such as Gorlin syndrome, XP and in transplant patients, as well as those with widespread severe actinic damage. The protection stops when the medication is discontinued

- Intralesional interferon α2b and BCG vaccine injections have been described. Whilst the use of intralesional bleomycin electrochemotherapy may be effective, long-term follow-up data is lacking. These are unconventional and are should be considered measures of last resort.

Follow-up

There is a 36–50% risk of another BCC in the 5 years after excision. Six-monthly follow-up is recommended for 5 years, but policies are highly variable. GP involvement attenuates the appearance of the true resources required for monitoring such a common tumour in the UK population.

Further reading

Telfer NR, Colver GB, Morton CA, et al. Guidelines for the management of basal cell carcinoma. Br J Dermatol 2008;159:35–48.

Related topics of interest

- Melanoma
- Squamous cell carcinomas
- Ultraviolet light

Blepharoplasty

Eyelid anatomy

The eyelid can be viewed as consisting of layers:

- Skin: Eyelid skin is the thinnest in the body
- Orbicularis oculi: Pretarsal, preseptal and periorbital components
- Orbital septum: This is analogous to the deep fascia of eyelid and lies immediately deep to the preseptal orbicularis. The septum is continuous with the orbital periosteum, pretarsal (conjoint) fascia of orbicularis and levator palpebrae superioris (LPS). It acts as a fat-retaining barrier but fat seldom herniates through unrepaired incisions in it after blepharoplasty. Vertical septa run perpendicular to the septum, partitioning the intra-ocular fat into fat pads
- Tarsal plate, levator aponeurosis and Muller's muscle
    - The LPS acts as an upper lid retractor which arises from the annulus of Zinn, runs superior to the globe to Whitnall's ligament, where it changes direction and courses inferiorly as an aponeurotic sheet (14–20 mm in height). This inserts onto the anterior 7–8 mm of the upper tarsal plate and sends interdigitations to the overlying orbicularis oculi. The analogous lower lid retractor is the capsulopalpebral fascia that arises in two sheets around the inferior oblique muscle (IO), which fuse anteriorly as Lockwood's ligament. From this, the anterior fascial continuation fuses with the lower lid septum 5 mm below the inferior tarsus. Together, this structure retracts the lower lid in synchrony with inferior globe rotation when looking downwards
    - Muller's muscle originates from the under surface of LPS and inserts with a short (0.5–1 mm long) tendon into tarsal plate. It is sympathetically innervated and when paralysed in conditions such as Horner syndrome, manifests as 2–3 mm of ptosis
    - The tarsal plate is non-cartilaginous. It comprises connective tissue that encompasses the Meibomian glands. Along with the glands of Zeiss, the Meibomian glands are holocrine glands that produce the lipid component of the tear film (in contrast to the watery secretions of the lacrimal glands). The upper tarsal plate is 10 mm high in Caucasians and the upper eyelid crease lies 7–12 mm from the lashes
- Conjunctiva
  In simple terms, the skin is closely juxtaposed with the orbicularis muscle whilst the conjunctiva is closely juxtaposed to the tarsal plate (the two lamellae). The muscle and tarsal plate layers are attached in a loosely adherent plane that carries the neurovascular structures to the conjunctiva

Other aspects

- Fat pads: The two fat pads in the upper lid are separated from the lacrimal gland by fibres of the superior oblique muscle. As there is no lacrimal gland in the lower lid, three fat pads exist, partitioned by the IO and its arcuate expansion laterally. The IO muscle lies relatively anterior and is thus vulnerable during fat resection
- Canthal tendons: The lateral canthal tendon arises from the tarsal plate and inserts on Whitnall tubercle, located over the inner aspect of lateral orbital rim, 10 mm below the zygomaticofacial suture. It lies at a more superior level than the medial canthal tendon. The medial canthal tendon is tripartite and inserts on both sides of the lacrimal sac and superior to it

Upper blepharoplasty

Excessive upper eyelid overhang lends a tired appearance. It is rarely severe enough to impair the visual field. It is important to differentiate true dermatochalasis from elements of brow and eyelid ptosis, both of which may occur concurrently or independently. A simple blepharoplasty will only address dermatochalasis.

Assessment

Obtain a comprehensive and relevant eye history that includes problems such as dry eyes, diplopia, contact lens use, previous eye, eyelid and brow surgery and botulinum toxin use. Anticoagulant use should be excluded. The examination should take place in good lighting with the patient sitting upright. It is important to:

- Exclude compensated brow ptosis (CBP): Look at the brow position with eyes open and closed. Brow descent and relaxation of the corrugator frown when the eyes are closed suggest that there is compensatory frontalis contraction to raise brow and upper eyelids when the eyes are open
- While a minor degree of CBP is normal, significant CBP may not manifest as transverse forehead furrows in the young and in Asians who have thicker forehead soft tissue
- After blepharoplasty, the need for CBP is removed and the brow drops to a degree. This drop is exaggerated if significant CBP was present. The medial brow tends to drop more than the lateral as the muscle greater insertions on this side. This may result in an angry look, with furrows due to unopposed corrugator and procerus contraction
- Good results with blepharoplasty generally require proper brow positioning as a first priority
- After the brow is lifted to the optimal position, check for lagophthalmos. A minimum of 30 mm of vertical upper lid height is required and overaggressive surgery may compromise this. Performing blepharoplasty without correcting brow ptosis first may lead to overaggressive resection of skin drawing the heavy brow skin down into upper eyelid area that will be unattractive
- Examine the eyelids for lid ptosis and skin quality
- Gently push on globe to assess the degree of fat pad bulging

In selected cases
- Visual fields and acuity screening

- Bell's phenomenon: The absence of this protective reflex increases risk of corneal damage postoperatively
- Schirmer test: This tests tear production but is an unreliable predictor for postoperative dry eye syndrome (65% have normal preoperative tests). Preoperative abnormal eye function or anatomy is a better indicator, such as scleral show, lagophthalmos or a very lax lower lid
  - Schirmer I: Reflex secretion test. A 5×35 mm strip is folded at 5 mm and placed in lateral third of lower lid. Less than 10 mm of soakage in 5 minutes is low
  - Schirmer II: Baseline secretion test. Repeated with topical local anaesthesia to block reflex secretion

Surgery

The patient should be carefully marked awake and prior to any injections, upright and then supine. Meticulous haemostasis is important. Variables to consider include:

- Skin incisions: Supratarsal incisions are most common. The lower incision should be 8–10 mm above the lid margin and the limit of the upper incision is then determined by pinching the excess gently at several points along the lid, until lagophthalmos just occurs. A minimum of 10–12 mm should be left between the upper incision line and the eyebrow
- Muscle excision: if the underlying orbicularis muscle is overdeveloped or stretched, then the fibres may be trimmed conservatively with the rationale of reducing excess muscle bulk that may obscure folds
  - The skin muscle flap may be sutured to the levator to recreate a precise fold, the rationale being that surgery disrupts the connections between the fold and levator mechanisms. Although many such as Flowers and Fernandez advocate this anchoring, it is not universal
- Fat excision: if orbital fat is clearly bulging, the orbital septum is incised at a high level to avoid LPS injury and only fat that

herniates out without pressure is excised to avoid a 'hollowed out' look. If the fat is not bulging, then the septum can be left intact. The LPS is located below the fat and can be identified as a shiny structure that moves with eye opening. Avoid damage to this

Tissue sparing blepharoplasty is becoming the standard technique and emphasises less aggressive resection.

Postoperative care

- Sutures are removed after 5 days
- Avoid hard contact lenses for a minimum of 3 weeks

Complications

Overall, the rate of complications is low but asymmetry is most common (35%) and may necessitate revision.

- Lagophthalmos for a week is almost inevitable to a certain degree but persistent problems may be due to excessive skin excision or inadvertent incorporation of septum into the incision
- Other lid deformities:
  - Lid retraction from adhesions that may be reduced by interposing orbital fat
  - Excess fat removal may cause hollowing and may require fat replacement
- Chemosis is common and is commonly due to transient oedema-induced disturbance of the lacrimal system or temporary paralysis of the orbicularis oculi. However, persistent epiphora may reflect true damage to the lacrimal system
- Retrobulbar haemorrhage is very rare but serious (see 'Orbital fractures' and 'Zygomatic fractures'). There is rapid onset of pain, proptosis and ecchymosis with or without visual disturbance. If left for more than 90 minutes, permanent visual damage may result. Urgent decompression with lateral cantholysis may be sufficient, although the source of bleeding is frequently not found. Mannitol or acetazolamide may be used to reduce intraocular pressure. Administration of 95% oxygen or 5% CO_2 mix will cause

intracerebral and intraocular vasodilation, reducing the pressure further

Lower eyelid

Anatomy

The Meibomian glands of the lower lid are less well developed than the upper lid and thus the inferior tarsal plate is smaller. The inferior eyelid crease is more prominent in children due to the adherence of the pretarsal orbicularis muscle to the skin.

Assessment

The patient should be assessed sitting up and facing the examiner.

- Assess lid position
- Lid tone: The snap test is used to assess lid laxity, which if excessive may require concomitant lateral canthopexy or canthoplasty
- Tissue looseness and testing with finger traction: Descent of the lateral canthal tendon suggests laxity due to changes in the orbicularis or attenuation of the ligament system. If lid laxity remains after the lateral canthus is elevated to its optimal position, then a lid shortening procedure may be needed. If the canthal tendon descent is not addressed, a negative canthal tilt will persist or be exaggerated post-operatively
- Fat herniation

Transcutaneous lower lid blepharoplasty

The transcutaneous lower blepharoplasty incision lies along the subciliary margin. The dissection plane of lower blepharoplasty incisions has been a subject of debate and is between a skin-only flap versus a composite skin and orbicularis flap. The arguments for the former are a better plane for addressing redundant skin and preserving orbicularis innervation at the expense of greater risks of devascularisation and lymphatic drainage issues of the skin. The latter advocates an avascular plane that is less prone to scarring at the expense of a higher risk of muscle denervation. There is little clinical difference in practice.

- Minimal to no skin excision is the norm. If in doubt, do not resect or under-resect
- Slightly more (2–3 mm) muscle than skin is usually resected to avoid muscle overlap
- Bulging fat is removed through small incisions in the septum

The current trend is to be more conservative with fat resection to avoid the hollowed out look. The incisions usually heal well with a small but significant risk (15–20%) of scleral show, lid retraction and frank ectropion (rare), resulting in dry eyes due to failure of the evaporation seal. The seal is held by surface tension contact between the lid and globe. The aetiology is multifactorial but can be caused by excessive scar-based retraction of the middle lamella and its adjacent structures such as the capsulopalpebral fascia. Note that this can occur in the absence of lower lid skin excision and as such all traumas should be minimised.

Transconjunctival lower blepharoplasty (TCLB)

The conjunctiva is incised 6 mm from the lid margin or 2 mm below the tarsal plate (taking care to stay > 4 mm from the punctum medially). This is the operation of choice if the pathology is limited to excess fat bulging. The main advantage is reduced lower lid trauma and reduced lid retraction but lateral exposure is limited, particularly for lateral fat removal.

- Skin-only flaps do not disturb muscle and excision of a thin strip of subciliary skin can be combined with TCLB
- Excess fat is addressed in either of two ways: Fat excision and fat repositioning
- A retroseptal approach is preferred as it allows better visualisation of the fat. With the fat excision technique, only the fat that prolapses out is excised. With fat repositioning, the arcus marginalis is released and the excess fat redraped over the inferior orbital rim, simultaneously eliminating the fat bulge and improving the contour of the lid-cheek junction
- Laser blepharoplasty is a skin-tightening procedure that is limited to minor skin excess of the lower lid or used as an adjuvant procedure to tweak the postoperative result

Further reading

Pacella SJ, Nahai FR, Nahai F, et al. Transconjunctival blepharoplasty for upper and lower eyelids. Plastic Reconstructive Surg 2010;125:384–94.

Related topics of interest

- Complications
- Eyelid reconstruction
- Orbital fracture
- Sedation
- Zygomatic fracture

Botulinum toxin

Clostridium botulinum is a spore-forming, gram-positive, anaerobic rod. A number of immunologically distinct potent neurotoxins (from A–G) are produced by the different strains. Botulinum toxin A is the most widely studied. The toxin consists of two subunits, a light and heavy chain connected by disulphide bridges. It selectively inhibits acetylcholine release at neuromuscular junctions and cholinergic sweat glands in a dose-dependent manner.

For Botox (Allergan), one unit is the calculated median intraperitoneal LD_{50} in a 20 g Swiss Webster mouse. Assay methods differ for other preparations and thus cannot be directly compared, but roughly 1 U Botox is equivalent to 4 U Dysport or 50-100 U Myobloc. Human LD_{50} has not established but is approximately 3000 U for a 70 kg man. It is approved for use in cervical dystonia (200 U), strabismus (1-2 U per muscle), and blepharospasm (2-3 U). The recommended maximum dose is 400-600 U in 3 months with a maximum single dose of 360 U.

Rhytides

Wrinkles (rhytides) in the skin are partly due to the contraction of underlying muscles (dynamic wrinkles) and partly due to a loss of elasticity from sun damage (static wrinkles). Botulinum toxin will reduce dynamic wrinkles by muscle paralysis but is ineffective against static wrinkles. Static wrinkles are treated with fillers or surgery.

The effect of toxin A on glabellar lines was an incidental finding when used to treat strabismus and torticollis. Botox (Allergan) subsequently attained FDA approval for the treatment of glabellar lines in 2003. It is extensively used off-label in cosmetic surgery for a wide variety of indications and at different sites. The specific licensing is brand-specific for the various botulinum toxins. Botulinum toxin is also used in conditions such as dystonias (blepharospasm and hemifacial spasm) or hyperhidrosis (excess sweating) in the axilla or face (Frey's syndrome).

The most common wrinkle areas treated are shown in **Table 5**.

The toxin (approximately 5 U per site for Botox) is injected directly into muscle with the needle bevel facing down to direct the toxin downwards. Subcutaneous injection is less effective and allows greater diffusion to adjacent muscles. The onset of action is delayed for 1-3 days because the toxin needs to be internalised and cleaved to take effect. The effects peak at 1-2 weeks and last for 8-12 weeks. Booster doses that prolong the effect up to 9 months may be due in part to muscle atrophy. Patients should be reassessed 2 weeks (minimum 7 days) later for effect and need for additional injections.

Other folds and wrinkles include: lower and upper eyelid wrinkles, circumoral lines (orbicularis oris), nasal lines (nasalis), marionette folds or drooping labial commissure, chin folds or cobblestone chin (mentalis), platysmal folds or turkey neck, and décolleté folds.

Botulinum toxin may also be used to:
- Treat gummy smile by using botulinum toxin on the upper lip
- Balance out the face in those with unilateral facial palsy
- Reduce masseter (and calf) hypertrophy
- Reduce sweating in Frey's syndrome and other causes of hyperhidrosis

Mechanism of action

The actual neurotoxin is 150 kDa in size but is complexed to other proteins in the native state making up an average size of 700–900 kDa. The complexing proteins distinguish the various brands of botulinum toxin available.
- The C end of the heavy chain of the toxin molecule has proteolytic activity; it binds with high affinity to a specific receptor on the presynaptic membrane of cholinergic nerve endings (**Figure 2**) – the latest evidence suggests that it comes from the vesicle membrane
- The toxin is internalised by receptor-mediated endocytosis and then cleaved into its constituent chains

Table 5 Common areas treated with botulinum toxin		
Wrinkle	**Underlying muscle**	**Notes**
Glabella (vertical frown lines)	Corrugator supercilii, medial portion of orbicularis oculi, procerus, depressor supercilii	Medial brow elevation through injection of depressor (at the level of medial canthus) may be desirable in females for a younger look but not in males.
Forehead (horizontal frown lines)	Frontal belly of the occipitofrontalis	Keep 1 cm away from eyebrow. Overtreatment may cause brow ptosis especially in those over 60.
Periorbital/lateral canthus (crows' feet)	Lateral part of orbicularis oculi (observe pattern of wrinkling with squinting)	Injection may cause lateral brow elevation due to paralysis of the orbicularis oculi but is often desirable.

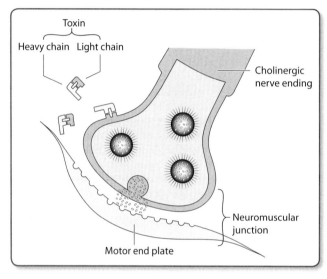

Figure 2 The toxin is internalized into the cholinergic nerve ending after binding to specific receptors through the heavy chain. The light chain then cleaves SNAP-25 to block exocytosis of vesicles containing neurotransmitters.

- The light chain is released into the cytoplasm and cleaves SNAP-25 (synaptosomal-associated protein of 25 kDa, which is on the intracellular surface of plasma membrane) preventing the fusion of acetylcholine vesicles with the plasma membrane. Toxin E also cleaves SNAP-25 but at a different site
- Atonic or flaccid paralysis of skeletal muscle (and also inhibition of parasympathetic end organs) results. This lasts until new synapses are reformed, reactivating the terminals (**Figure 2**)

A variety of commercial products that are currently available are shown in **Table 6**. These have undergone different formulations and processing techniques, which seem to affect action as well as immunogenicity. Prior to 1998, Botox had 25 ng of neurotoxin complex protein per 100 units but the subsequent formulation only had 5 ng. Caution is also required in interpreting animal studies as there is species-specific sensitivity. Rats are relatively insensitive to toxin B while it is as effective as toxin A in mice. Toxin B is less frequently used cosmetically due to greater discomfort on injection (pH 5.6) and shorter duration of action.

Contraindications

The use of botulinum toxin is contraindicated in areas of infection and inflammation or in patients with prior allergic reactions to

Table 6 Commercial preparations of botulinum toxin		
Trade name (manufacturer)	Storage	Notes
Botox (Allergan) toxin A (new generic name: **onabotulinumtoxin A**)	Lyophilised into crystals and reconstituted with saline (preservatives may reduce pain* but make little clinical difference); usage within 4 hour is recommended but effective in practice for at least 1 week (up to 6) when stored at 2–8°C	Four times more potent than Dysport. Reformulated after 1997 to a form that has reduced immunogenicity.
Dysport (Ipsen) toxin A (new generic name: **abobotulinumtoxin A**)	Powder reconstituted with saline, can be stored at 2–8°C	Less potent per unit compared to Botox. More likely to diffuse further from injection site.
NeuroBloc (Eisai, Europe), MYOBLOC (Elan, USA) toxin B (new generic name: **rimabotulinumtoxin B**)	Supplied in solution; does not need reconstituting. Can be stored in refrigerators for up to 20 months or at room temperature for 9 months.	Less potent than toxin A. Faster onset of action (begins as early as 4 hours, peaking at 2 weeks) but lasts half as long as toxin A. Cleaves synaptobrevin (VAMP) in the presynaptic nerve ending (like toxins D, F and G but at different sites) FDA approved in 2000 for use in cervical dystonia. Shares structural homology with tetanus toxin.

*Alam M. Arch Dermatol 2002;138:510–514

the toxin or its other constituents such as albumin. In addition, caution is required in

- Pre-existing neuromuscular disease, e.g. myasthenia gravis, Eaton-Lambert myasthenic syndrome
- Concomitant use of neuromuscular drugs or anticoagulants. Aminoglycosides potentiate the effect of the toxin, whereas chloroquine reduces it

Botulinum toxin (A or B) is not approved for use in children less than 12 years of age, but has been used off-label in this age group for limb spasticity in cerebral palsy patients. It is important to understand that despite their wide use for various conditions, the efficacy, safety and optimal dosage have not been established in most cases. An alert was issued by the FDA in April 2009 regarding reports of deaths related to diffusion of the toxin, mostly in paediatric patients with cerebral palsy being treated for spasticity. Subsequently boxed warnings were included and names were changed to reinforce the differences between the toxins particularly with regard to potency.

Complications

In general, complications are rare with careful use as there is a large safety margin. The most common complication is temporary unwanted paralysis. The transient ptosis rate is quoted at 3% (lasts 1–6 weeks and treatable with Albalon/naphazoline eyedrops). Dysphagia has been reported following platysmal injections. One should expect the toxin to diffuse within a 0.5–1.5 cm radius and patients are advised to avoid massaging the area or lying down for 4 hours after injection. Side effects depend in part on diffusion distances: Myobloc > Dysport > Botox.

- Headaches are common. A flu-like illness is less common
- Bruising is uncommon
- On occasion, there may be a rash (including erythema multiforme), allergy or urticaria
- May trigger an outbreak of cold sores. Treat with aciclovir prophylactically in those with a history of cold sores

As the toxin decreases the range of emotive expression, this may be an issue for actors (or politicians). As always, maximising results and patient satisfaction comes from picking the right treatment for the problem, for example, deeper perioral wrinkles would be better treated with fillers rather than botulinum toxin injections. Treatment of platysmal bands (best in those with good skin elasticity and minimal submental fat) requires higher doses with an attending risk of dysphagia, dysphonia and neck weakness.

Immunity

Antibody-mediated immunity to the toxin may lead to treatment failure, but is rare (3–10%). The light chain contains the well-conserved toxin moiety whilst the heavy chain of different toxins contains dissimilar domains that allow specific binding to the neurone. Neutralising antibodies generally bind to the latter and as such, substituting the toxin serotype is likely to be effective. Non-neutralising antibodies tend to have no effect on the toxin action. There are suggestions that the different manufacturing techniques of toxin B versus A means makes it less immunogenic but long-term studies are required.

Overall, the phenomenon is not well studied. The figures often quoted are based on early products (up to 30% in children treated for spasticity) and newer formulations are claim fewer problems with immunity (less than 5%, 1–2% according to manufacturers) particularly for cosmetic patients. Although the critical factors have not been fully elucidated, immunity is generally accepted to be more common when multiple high doses (cumulative > 200 U) are given, particularly as boosters. Smaller doses should thus be given over sufficiently long intervals.

Further reading

Kopera D. Botulinum toxin historical aspects: from food poisoning to pharmaceutical. Int J Dermatol 2011;50:976–80.

Related areas of interest

- Complications
- Hidradenitis suppurativa and hyperhidrosis
- Facial reanimation
- Tissue fillers

Brachial plexus injuries

The commonest cause of brachial plexus injury (BPI) is high velocity trauma. Five 5% percent of all motorcycle injuries have a BPI. Motorcycle injuries are responsible for 85% of BPI cases. Other causes include falling from a height or birth trauma.

The sensory neuron has its cell body outside of spinal cord in the dorsal root ganglion (DRG). Avulsion injuries often tear the preganglionic afferent axon whilst the postganglionic efferent section is intact. Preganglionic injuries do not cause Wallerian degeneration or neuroma formation because the axons remain in continuity with the neuron in the ganglion. Postganglionic lesions are physiologically similar to other peripheral nerve injuries.

Types of brachial plexus injuries

- Avulsion
- Rupture - the nerve is torn but not at the spinal attachment
- Neuroma - the nerve has torn and healed but scar tissue prevents the injured nerve from conducting signals to the muscles
- Neuropraxia – transient reversible nerve injury and is the most common type of BPI

Leffert classification (NEJM 1974) Leffert

- I Open
- II Closed, subdivided into supraclavicular or infraclavicular injuries:
  - IIa Supraclavicular: Subdivided into preganglionic or postganglionic
    - Preganglionic: Avulsion of nerve roots that is usually due to high-velocity trauma. Associated injuries are common. There are no proximal stumps, neuromas do not form and thus the Tinel's sign is negative. *Pseudomeningoceles* and denervation of deep neck muscles are common. Horner's syndrome (ptosis, miosis, anhidrosis) may be present

- Postganglionic: Usually due to traction injuries and roots remain intact. As there are proximal stumps with neuroma formation, Tinel's sign will be positive. Deep dorsal neck muscles are intact and pseudomeningoceles are not a feature
  - IIb Infraclavicular: Injuries usually involve the trunks. The functional loss is based on trunk involved. Upper (biceps, shoulder muscles), middle (wrist, finger extension) and lower (wrist, finger flexion)
- III Radiation induced
- IV Obstetric
  - IVa Erb–Duchenne (upper root): porter's or waiter's tip hand
  - IVb Dejerine-Klumpke (lower root)

It is important to establish the pattern of injury. In general, preganglionic lesions have little chance of spontaneous recovery (although Carlstedt 1995 obtained promising initial results with the repair of preganglionic lesions by replanting nerve rootlets directly into the spinal cord). Postganglionic lesions that remain in continuity have a chance of spontaneous recovery. Those not in continuity may be reconstructed.

The patient may present with:

- Pain, especially of the neck and shoulder. Persistent pain of greater than 6-month duration is associated with a poor prognosis
- Paraesthesia and dysaesthesia
- Weakness, paralysis or heaviness in the extremity

Differential diagnoses

- Breast cancer (usually lower plexus involvement and painful)
- Radiation therapy (upper plexus and painless)
- Parsonage–Turner syndrome (may first affect suprascapular nerve)
- Pancoast tumour

Evaluation

History

The position of the arm at the time of injury can affect the levels involved.

- When the arm is abducted, the force is directed in line with C7. A lower plexus lesion is more likely as the coracoid process acts as a fulcrum. In addition, C8 and T1 lack the protective transverse radicular ligaments that C5–7 has that resist traction forces
- An upper plexus injury is more likely if the arm is adducted as the first rib acts as a fulcrum to direct the traction forces

Examination

- Colour, trophic changes and limb vascularity
- Check for Horner's syndrome
- Tinel's sign: Its absence suggests a poor prognosis

Motor examination

Significant variations occur in pattern of the spinal nerves within the cord and anomalous patterns of innervation may make identifying the levels involved challenging. In addition, C4 may contribute a branch to the plexus (prefixed) in up to 60% of cases. This may explain recovery in the distribution of a nerve root that is otherwise clinically avulsed. Keep in mind that most individual muscles have contributions from multiple cervical levels.

- Range of joint motion: Passive and active. Check for contractures
- Test muscle power: The British MRC M2 grade (gravity eliminated) is especially relevant. If M1, palpation is key
  - Supraclavicular: Suprascapular (supraspinatus), dorsal scapular (rhomboids), long thoracic (serratus anterior) nerves. Winging of scapula may indicate preganglionic injury
  - Infraclavicular: Medial and lateral pectoral (pectoralis major and minor), subscapular (subscapularis) and thoracodorsal (LD) nerves. Test by asking the patient to cough
- Nerve screening:
  - Shoulder abduction (axillary nerve)
  - Wrist extension (low radial nerve) and elbow extension (high radial nerve)
  - Elbow flexion (musculocutaneous nerve)
  - Finger and wrist flexion (median and ulnar nerve)

Sensory examination

In the acute phase, deep pressure sensation (burning sensation when pinching and pulling nail base outwards) may be the only sign of nerve continuity in the absence of motor function or any other sensation. A negative finding of deep pressure sensation is less helpful as neuropraxia may persist beyond 6 months. Sensation recovers in a fairly consistent sequence delineated as follows:

1. Pain and temperature: Protective sensation
2. Sweating: Check with the ninhydrin test. The affected hand is placed on bond paper for 15 seconds. The paper is then sprayed with the ninhydrin reagent that turns the amino acids in sweat purple
3. Low frequency vibrations (30 kHz): Tests the fast adapting receptors
4. Moving two-point discrimination (2pd): Tests the innervation density of quick receptors
5. Constant touch: Tests the slow adapting receptors
6. Static 2pd: Tests the innervation density of slow receptors that are dependent on cortical integration and may be normal in nerve compression syndromes (NCS)
7. High frequency vibration (256 kHz): This is a threshold test that is more sensitive for NCS (other threshold tests include light touch, Semmes–Weinstein monofilament and vibrometry)

Initial treatment

Imaging

- X-ray: Exclude fractures of cervical spine, clavicle, scapula, first rib and proximal humerus. Keep cervical support until cervical spine fractures have been excluded
  - A chest X-ray (CXR) may show scapulothoracic dissociation (increased distance between the spinous processes

of the thoracic spine and the scapula on AP view). CXR may also show rib fractures (affecting intercostal nerve availability as donors) or elevated hemidiaphragm (suggestive of phrenic nerve injury and should be investigated further with inspiratory/expiratory X-rays or fluoroscopy)

- CT scanning may be indicated if there is doubt about the neck, particularly the odontoid and the cervicothoracic junction. CT of the chest may reveal subclavian vessel injuries or fractures of scapula, humerus and thoracic spine
- Angiography is valuable in evaluating any suspected vascular disruption. The incidence of axillary artery avulsion may be as high as 20%
- The utility of plain MRI in acute BPI is sparse due to its poor level of contrast between nerve tissue and subarachnoid space. Furthermore, this is compromised by the low resolution of the root sleeves due to thick slicing. However, it is the only technique for visualisation of the postganglionic brachial plexus. Its use is increasing although the impact on surgical decision-making is yet to be defined

Myelograms

Myelograms are rarely needed.
- Plain film: A large diverticulum or meningocele is diagnostic of preganglionic root avulsion (as opposed to postganglionic extraforaminal rupture). The most reliable indicator of root avulsion is an absent root shadow. This investigation should be delayed for 6–12 weeks as blood clots may occlude the opening of a pseudomeningocele
- CT myelogram: The sensitivity and specificity is not well delineated. The slices are too thick (5 mm thickness when 0.5 mm would be ideal). The current multidetector CT cuts at 1 mm and may be better. It can detect lower concentrations of contrast medium than standard myelography and thus may demonstrate small meningoceles. However, it suffers from artefact problems

- MRI myelogram: This is done with T2 weighting that accentuates the contrast between nerve tissue and cerebral spinal fluid

Electrophysiologic

- Lamina test: Electrical stimulation is applied to exiting roots to test patient perception as a screening test for avulsion
- Nerve conduction tests:
  - Compound action potentials (APs) only appear if the nerve is functioning and is absent in crush injuries and entrapment syndromes. It is important to gauge their size (related to number of functioning axons), velocity and shape (injured nerves demonstrate broader, irregular and smaller APs)
    - Mainly used to examine the main branches, e.g. median and ulnar. A demyelinating conduction block is detectable in the first few weeks unless the axons are severed. Its presence indicates a reasonably good prognosis
  - Sensory nerve action potentials (SNAPs) may help to differentiate preganglionic from postganglionic injuries. If the injury is proximal to the DRG, there is no Wallerian degeneration and thus a SNAP in a nerve with an anaesthetic dermatome confirms a preganglionic lesion. C5 is the exception, as it does not contribute significantly to a major peripheral sensory nerve
    - Somatosensory evoked potentials are less useful than SNAPs
- Electromyography (EMG): Traditionally, EMG is performed at 3 weeks. An F wave is sought, which is a later response and has a lesser magnitude than the main compound muscle action potential. A discharge is detectable from denervated muscle after 10–21 days due to its intrinsic pacemaker activity. In preganglionic injuries, denervating potentials may be seen in segmental paraspinal muscles innervated by the posterior primary rami. In the absence of denervation signs in a paralysed muscle 3 weeks after injury, EMG can be used to confirm neuropraxia

Surgery

The treatment of BPI is not confined to surgery. It is complex and is best addressed by a multidisciplinary team with an orthotist, occupational therapists, physical therapists and physicians.

Indications

In the past, most BPIs were treated conservatively and any residual deficit 12–18 months later was then pronounced permanent. Limb amputations were not uncommon. Although the shoulder deficit can be considered permanent at 9–12 months, the recovery of more distal function may be occasionally observed more than a year after the injury.

Patient co-operation, motivation, and understanding of the operative goals are vital to successful treatment. Significant recovery after nerve grafting can take more than 18 months, and maintaining joint mobility, minimising oedema, and treating deafferentation pain is challenging. This may improve with nerve reconstruction.

- Contraindications to surgery include unfavourable patient factors such as advanced age (adversely affects the functional results after nerve transfers) or unmotivated patients with lack of understanding of surgical goals, or severe limb changes such as joint contractures or severe oedema
- The timing of surgery is not universally agreed upon. Whilst the trend is towards early surgery, (such as if biceps function has not returned after 3 months), it does depend on other factors. Early surgery on a complete flail limb is more appropriate than on a partial injury that may recover significantly if surgery is delayed for a few months
- Intraoperative diagnosis: Even with preoperative testing, the exact lesion (level, type and extent) can only be accurately determined at the time of surgery. Helpful signs include the following:
  - Nerves may feel empty or look pale
  - Biopsies of root with immunohistochemistry may help
  - Vital signs rising during resection of neuroma indicate continuity with spinal cord
  - Intraoperative action potentials may be elicited

In general, the surgical options consist of nerve transfers, nerve grafting, muscle transfers, free muscle transfers, and scar neurolysis. The latter may help in incomplete lesions. The primary surgical concerns are the availability of proximal intraplexus donors and adequate nerve graft material (great distances are involved).

- Donors
  - The best donors are the intraplexus, ipsilateral C5–7 roots that have escaped injury. Distal nerve-to-nerve transfers close to the target muscle, such as the medial pectoral nerve, avoid the need for grafting and reduce the distance for nerve regeneration.
    - Contralateral donors: e.g. C7 root
    - Extraplexus donors: e.g. spinal accessory nerve for the shoulder and intercostals for the elbow (T3–11). Nerve harvest can be challenging and provide relatively fewer fibres. Only 40% of the 1200 fibres in these nerves are motor
- Grafts
  - Sural nerve graft (45 cm) can usually be harvested through three or four small incisions
  - Bilateral saphenous nerve
  - The vascularised ulnar nerve is reported to have faster nerve regeneration and better final outcome

Postganglionic injuries have the best prognosis and are best treated with interpositional grafts to bridge the motor donor and distal target.

- Those with avulsion of a few roots, e.g. C5/6, should have reconstruction of shoulder and elbow as a priority. Shoulder reconstruction, e.g. distal spinal accessory nerve (recipient) to suprascapular nerve (donor)
- Intraplexus neurotisation of the biceps and deltoids with nerves such as the ulnar or medial pectoral is possible

- The subgroup with the best prognosis is patients with an upper plexus injury only as the hand is spared and only short grafts are needed. As more roots are injured, fewer potential donors are available. Global avulsion carries the worst prognosis, and typically requires extraplexus or contralateral donors such as:
  - Accessory nerve to suprascapular nerve
  - Intercostal nerves to shoulder/elbow
  - Contralateral C7

The management of neuroma-in-continuity is challenging and depends heavily on the integrity of the perineurium.

- Microneurolysis to relieve pressure may be effective in releasing bulging of entrapped fascicles
- Neuroma excision with interpositional grafting is possible, but caution is required in partial lesions

Other procedures include:

- Muscle transfer: Either free (e.g. LD, RF, gracilis-adductor longus usually anastomosed to intercostals or accessory nerve) or pedicled (e.g. LD, sternoclavicular part of PM, pectoralis minor)
- Rotational osteotomy of humerus to improve the external rotation of arm
- Arthrodesis: for example, wrist fusion before tendon transfer to hand

Postoperative care

- It is important to maintain the position of head, neck and shoulder with a brace. The shoulder should be kept in 45° of abduction for up to 6–8 weeks
- Physiotherapy, ultrasound and massage are useful to reduce adhesions
- Regular evaluation with the Tinel test (3–4 cm advancement per month. Recovery rates of 5–14 cm/month have been reported with vascularised grafts

Further reading

Kozin SH. The evaluation and treatment of children with brachial plexus birth injury. J Hand Surg 2011;36:1360–9.

Related topic of interest

- Facial reanimation

Breast augmentation

Breast augmentation is a common surgical procedure and is on the rise worldwide. One percent of all women in the United States have had breast augmentation. The most common indication is cosmetic enhancement.

Preoperative planning

Several key measurements on which key decisions are made when planning a breast augmentation.

The following five measurements are advocated by Tebbetts and known as the High 5 process:

1. • Breast base width (BBW): The distance between the lateral and medial borders of visible mound. The width of the breast determines the maximum width of the implant. The ideal implant width should match the BBW
2. • Superior pole pinch thickness (measure in cm with calliper). This estimates the amount of soft tissue cover in the thinnest part of the breast. Soft tissue cover is key in maintaining the longevity of the augmented breast. If >2 cm, the subglandular plane is possible, and if <2 cm, consider a subpectoral plane for additional coverage
3. • Measure nipple to IMF on stretch (N-IMF). This determines whether or not the IMF needs to be lowered and by how much. If the fold cannot be lowered, the implant chosen should have a lower ventral curvature that matches this dimension so that the point of maximal projection is behind the nipple. Alternatively, alter the nipple position with a mastopexy. Some of all of these measures may be used depending on the architecture of the breast presented
4. • Breast envelope (tight, normal or loose, with or without ptosis) higher profile implants may be better for looser envelopes. This can be estimated by pulling the areolar forwards as an anterior skin stretch test

• Percentage contribution of existing breast volume to maximally augmented volume. This measurement is estimated by eye

Determine if the patient's preference is for a natural concavity in the upper pole, known as a natural look, or a convex upper pole, which is an augmented look. Patients do not adhere to these definitions and it is essential to ascertain what a natural or augmented look for the individual means.

General warnings to patients

Patient counselling is key. The basic choices to make are implant type, incision and plane of insertion.

• A perfectly natural breast in both visual and tactile dimensions cannot be achieved with implant-based augmentation. An implant will always be palpable and is more pronounced in those with thin tissues. If a palpable implant is to be avoided, the patient should not get an implant
• In terms of the visual and tactile result:
  – The larger the implant (particularly >350 cc), the worse the breast will look with time as the pressure effect will cause gradual parenchymal atrophy of the native breast and possibly cartilage modelling. The thinner the soft tissue cover, the worse the cosmetic result
  – Adequately filled saline implants will feel firmer than normal breast tissue. Saline implants are rarely used in the UK. However, silicone implants come in various degrees of filling. The more underfilled the implant, the softer it will feel, at the expense of greater traction rippling

Types of implants

Cosmetic breast augmentation in the UK is performed almost exclusively with silicone implants. Due to the previous FDA moratorium issues with silicone implants in the US from 1992 to 2006, saline implants retain a significant proportion of the US market.

Filling

- Silicone (dimethylsiloxane) is inert but elicits a mild inflammatory reaction. The viscosity or cohesiveness is determined by the degree of crosslinkage between the silicone molecules. The first generation of implants designed and used by Cronin and Gerow in the 1960s were firm and teardrop shaped. The thick-walled silicone sac contained a thick gel and had a Dacron back-wall. In response to demand for a softer feel, second generation implants (1979–1987) had thinner shells and silicone gels that were non-cohesive. Problems with silicone bleed and leakage led in 1987 to development of implants with cohesive gels that were thicker and retained their shape even when cut. Cohesive gel implants require a longer incision as excessive pressure will cause gel fracture
  - The large numbers of product modifications render implant comparison difficult and this should be borne in mind when reviewing the literature
  - Saline implants retain a silicone elastomer shell, despite the US silicone controversy. The feel is inferior to silicone in mimicking a natural breast but this effect is diminished with a substantial volume of tissue in front of the implant. They run a risk of deflation with rupture but do not suffer from silicone gel bleed nor silicone granulomas. Deliberate deflation can be exploited to more accurately estimate the residual breast dimensions and true nipple position in the secondary case, such as in capsular contracture. Intraoperative inflation (as opposed to fixed volume) allows the use of smaller incisions and distant insertion sites such as the trans-umbilical. Saline implants are frequently used as breast tissue expanders in the UK
  - Dual lumen implants consist of a fixed volume gel chamber and a variable volume saline chamber that combines the benefits of the two. The early double lumen implants had an outer saline shell to theoretically combat gel bleed from the inner silicone core. Modern double lumen devices such as the Becker (Mentor) reverse this arrangement to harness the natural feel of the silicone. These implants come marked by the ratio of gel to saline. For example, a Becker 35 comprises 35% gel and 65% saline if fully filled to the recommended volume
  - The saline component necessitates a filling port. Ports are either distant (connected via a tube to a port buried subcutaneously) or integral (built into the implant usually at the anterior upper pole). Permanent double lumen implants such as the Becker, have a removable port that when pulled out, the remaining implant acts as a fixed volume implant. All integral port devices at this time are licensed as temporary implants only, limiting their use to tissue expansion
  - Dual lumen implants are very expensive (two to three times the cost of fixed volume gel implants) and the ports palpable. Distant ports are vulnerable to flipping and may occasionally leak if the tube does not break off at the correct point when pulled out
- Soy implants (Trilucent) were introduced in 1994 and have since been withdrawn. The gradual oxidation of the soy oil into a malodorous rancid material was unacceptable and had a high deflation rate. The capsular contracture that developed was lumpy and was abnormally high at 10%
- Hydrogel implants have also been withdrawn. The high water affinity of the gel caused problems of osmotic enlargement and was associated with a high rate of capsular contracture in the long term

Shell

- Smooth implants refer to the outer surface of the shell. They have been shown to have a higher rate of capsule contracture in the subglandular plane. Their use as a permanent implant is uncommon in the UK. There have been arguments for placing them in the submuscular plane but the majority of these studies suffer from confounding factors such as variation in the implant filler used, technique and use of antimicrobial irrigation that makes direct comparison difficult

- Textured implants have, as its name suggests, a textured grainy surface that is designed to reduce capsule contracture. The exact mechanism of action is unknown but thought to be a contributed to by altered lines of tension in the resulting capsule resulting in non-concentric contraction. It was initially designed to mimic the texture of polyurethane foam-covered implants, with the current texturing created by negative polyurethane foam imprint or by salt dissolution. Polyurethane foam created an intense inflammatory reaction with incorporation of the foam into the fibrous capsule. This does not occur with textured implants
  - There are studies in the literature that both support and negate the anti-capsular contracture effect of texturing
  - Textured implants are more expensive and may be more palpable due to the thicker shells
- Polyurethane implants are making resurgence. The capsular contracture rate is less than 2% at the 10-year mark; with some studies suggesting the early capsular contracture reduction rate diminishes by year 7. A small modification of implant technique is required, as these implants remain fixed in the position they are inserted. The original concern with polyurethane implants (Bristol-Myers Squibb) was that the renally excreted breakdown product, 2,4 toluene diamine (2,4 TDA) was carcinogenic in rats. Subsequent studies have shown that this was an artefact of the laboratory process

and not cause for concern. The current generation of polyurethane implants (Silimed) remain unavailable in the US but remain available in Europe, Australia and South America

Shape

- Round implants have an identical base width and height. The point of maximal projection is at the centre, halfway from the bottom only when placed horizontally. When in the vertical position, gravity causes inferior displacement of the volume and results in a pseudo-anatomical shape. This causes a degree of inferior displacement of the point of maximal projection. However in general, they retain a higher fill volume in the upper pole compared to anatomical implants and are useful in creating upper pole convexity
- Anatomical implants have a base width that differs from its height. In addition, the point of maximal projection is one third of the height from the bottom. The height is referred to as low, moderate or full, depending on whether or not the height exceeds the base width. They are useful to restore breast height and restore a natural upper pole slope which is either straight or bears a slight concavity. In addition, they are invaluable in producing differentially greater lower pole projection. As these implants do not have rotational symmetry by design, they are prone to rotational displacement if the pocket is not a snug fit
  - There is roughly 25% more projection with an anatomical implant for an equivalent volume of a round one
  - Round saline implants can be made more anatomical by under filling and placement in a loose pocket, at the risk of greater rippling and implant failure

Placement

Submuscular

The rate of capsular contracture is reduced from 30% to 12% when placed in the submuscular plane. This effect is more consistent than that of texturing but applies to both smooth and textured implants. However, there is less of a difference with saline implants.

- There is less visible and/or palpable rippling. The muscle smooths the transition of the upper pole
- The sensory nerves are less vulnerable to damage as they are more mobile in this plane
- There is less hindrance to mammography
- Muscle cover reduces theoretical contamination from the glandular or ductal tissue

However, disadvantages include:

- Potentially increased bleeding due to the plane of dissection
- More initial postoperative discomfort (related to amount of muscle dissection)
- Muscle contraction may distort implant shape and cause shifting particularly superiorly. IMF control is less precise
- A deep cleavage may not be possible as this is entirely dependent on the point of pectoralis major insertion on the individual's sternum
- A double-bubble or Snoopy deformity may result in those with pre-existing glandular ptosis as the parenchyma slides off the pectoralis   Snoopy.

Total submuscular (below pectoralis major, serratus anterior laterally and the RA fascia inferiorly) primary augmentation is uncommon, but is frequently used in the reconstruction setting. There is reduced lower pole fullness and an increased rate of superior migration with this approach.

Subpectoral augmentation is the commonest method in the US. It involves placement under the pectoralis major only, leaving the inferior pole uncovered to varying degrees.

Tebbetts' dual plane placement attempts to quantify the degree of lower pole exposure to the gland, by varying the amount of release of the inferior pectoralis major insertion and the attachment of the gland to the muscle.

The endpoint is the relationship of the inferior pectoral border relative to the nipple areolar complex. The technique reduces double-bubbling by promoting adherence to the gland, while retaining the muscle cover in the most crucial area, the upper pole

Subglandular/submammary

Implants placed under the breast gland and above the muscle tend to fill the skin envelope better and, by occupying the more anatomical position of the breast, produces a better aesthetic result. However, the main disadvantages are:

- Higher rate of capsular contracture
- Greater hindrance to mammography (but not prohibitive)
- As the implant is closer to the skin, rippling of the implant surface that may be palpable/visible particularly in those with a thinner soft tissue envelope. Subglandular augmentation is not recommended in those with <2 cm upper pole thickness for this reason

The subfascial plane has been described but has not been shown to offer any benefits over the subglandular plane. The implant is inserted under the pectoralis fascia, over the pectoralis muscle. This fascia is less than 1 mm thick.

Access

The clinical features of various types of access are given in **Table 7**. Smaller incisions of only 2–3 cm in length are required for saline implants as they are inserted in their deflated form.

Postoperative care

Most patients can expect to return to work after a week.

- Drains are not necessary but are still used widely
- Support with a brassiere (sports) is recommended for 3–6 weeks

Table 7 Clinical features of different types of access. The best is one which offers the best access and control but with least trauma to normal tissues		
Type of access	Comments	Disadvantages
Inframammary	Simplest with good exposure allowing accurate placement without violation of parenchyma. Good for patients with obvious IMF crease and scar is hidden under most circumstances.	Potentially bigger scar. Not to be used if the IMF is poorly formed and likely to be displaced, particularly onto chest wall.
Periareolar incision Semicircular	Scarring is usually well disguised except in those with a lightly coloured areola. Versatile approach: Can reach all parts and allows accurate positioning including lower pole. Especially if mastopexy or parenchymal alteration, e.g. tuberous breasts, is also required.	Minimum areolar size of 25 mm for incision of 40 mm. Insertion of larger implants may not be possible due to the limited exposure. Risk of nipple paraesthesia may be increased. The incision necessarily traverses the parenchyma. Risk of bacterial contamination.
Axillary	Scar in axilla behind edge of PM and does not violate breast tissue. Useful when above routes are contraindicated (e.g. small areola or poor IMF). Difficult to position implant precisely, particularly lower pole thus not used in complex cases, e.g. tuberous breast. This is a blind dissection of subpectoral plane unless facilitated by endoscope. Divide PM 5–10 mm above marked IMF.	Difficult to accurately place implants, especially subglandularly. Risk of haematoma, malposition, asymmetry and poor IMF with need for revision. Risk of injury to intercostal brachii nerve and subclavian vein. Limited to saline or small silicone implants. Less popular now than in the 1990s.
Transumbilical – [transumbilical breast augmentation (TUBA)]	Expander is tunnelled up to the breast to develop the pocket and then is replaced by the definitive saline implant. Accurate placement (especially subpectoral) is difficult. Scar is less noticeable but caution needed in the very thin patient.	Contraindicated in those with abdominal scars or herniae. Longer operative time and may need conversion to open technique for bleeding control. Limited to saline or small silicone implants. Implants inserted this way are not FDA approved and off-label.

Further reading

Spear S, ed. Breast Augmentation. Clin Plast Surg 2009; 36 (Jan).

Related topic of interest

- Breast augmentation – complications and safety

Breast augmentation – complications and safety

Breast augmentation carries an overall 20% revision rate, which is among the highest in PRS. These historical figures may not accurately reflect the outcomes of current generation implants as their design and insertion technique have changed considerably in the last few decades.

Local complications

Local complications occur with a significant frequency that accumulates over time.

- 1 in 4 implant patients will need a second operation within 5 years (1 in 3 reconstructive patients and 1 in 8 augmentation patients)
- The FDA prospective study in 2000 showed removal rates for aesthetic saline implants to be 8% and 12–14% at 3 and 5 years respectively. The corresponding rates for reconstructive implants were 2–3 times higher. These figures are higher than those reported in more recent prospective studies
- Irradiation increases most of the risk of implant complications

Early complications

Infection occurs in 2–3% of cases, where *Staphylococcus aureus* is five times more common as the causative agent than *S. epidermidis*. The use of prophylactic antibiotics against perioperative contamination, especially from the ducts, is almost universal. Some advocate covering the nipple and the incision site with adhesive film to further reduce contamination. Infected implants may be salvaged in rare cases

Haematomas (also about 2–3%) should be evacuated, as they are associated with an increased risk of infection and contracture, in addition to the shape distortion. Seromas may be more common with the use of cautery or concentrated irrigating solutions but most are resorbed within 4–5 days. In January 2011, the FDA issued a report on the rare occurrence of anaplastic large cell lymphoma (ALCL) in implant patients (34 cases from 1997–2010). ALCL is associated with late onset, persistent peri-implant seromas.

Position/size

- The implant may be asymmetric or otherwise displaced
  - Symmastia is the apparent merging of the two breasts in the midline. This is caused by violation of the midline resulting in medial migration of one or both implants. It is difficult to treat and thus is best avoided. Risk factors include multiple operations, large implants (> 400 ml or wider than hemithorax) and excessive medial dissection
- Implants may be palpable and/or visible especially in very thin patients. Rippling is a common cause of dissatisfaction and may be due to traction or edge rippling. It may be improved by increasing coverage over the implant, increasing the fill, choosing an implant with a thicker shell or more cohesive gel or increasing the implant support from below. The only way of eliminating rippling altogether is explantation

Late complications

- Capsular contracture formation (above grade III) occurs at a rate of approximately 10% in saline versus 20% in silicone in 5 years, with an overall reoperation rate of 15%. The exact cause(s) are unclear, but theories include a foreign body reaction (hypertrophic scar theory) and the more recently popular low-level bacterial infection (biofilm theory)
  - The assessment is still rather subjective (see **Table 8**) as Baker's criteria remain subjective. There are no universally accepted objective and validated measures
  - Prophylactic intravenous antibiotics do not seem to influence the contracture rate but the effect

Baker

Table 8 Baker classification of capsular contracture
I. Normal implant
II. Palpable capsule
III. Visible distortion of implant
IV. Painful implant

of irrigation (e.g. bacitracin, cephalosporin/gentamicin) is inconsistent
- Povidone-iodine has a consistent beneficial effect (12% vs 28% using saline irrigation) that is independent of the effect of texturing (largely unpredictable). The FDA has banned povidone-iodine irrigation due to reports of saline implant deflation (related to intraluminal povidone-iodine causing valve patch delamination). Even though intraluminal povidone-iodine is neither the norm nor practised anymore and extraluminal povidone-iodine shown to be safe, the ban persists
- Other strategies include strict asepsis and haemostasis, and use of lint-free gauze and powder-free gloves
- Exercises and massage to move the implant within the pocket is controversial and largely unproven though there may be psychological benefits
- Capsules are generally treated with open capsulectomy/capsulotomy and implant exchange. Closed capsulotomy is not recommended as the forces involved exceed the breaking strength of the implant and several studies have demonstrated increase in MRI detected ruptures in those with previously closed capsulotomies. Patients with one episode of capsular contracture are more likely to develop capsules with further operations
- Rupture. The rupture of saline implants is easily detected and is estimated at 3% at 3 years and 10% at 5 years for saline. Cohesive silicone implants do not extrude and thus ruptures are usually asymptomatic and underreported.

Estimated 6 year rupture rates are less than 1% (compared to 15–30 % in older implants). Most ruptures are intracapsular and even though the dangers are unproven, the FDA recommends removal
- The accuracy of clinical detection including squeeze testing is poor. MMG is unreliable whilst conventional MMG (not Eklund views) may actually cause rupture. Silicone levels in the blood are not indicative of rupture. Endoscopic examination has been suggested but this is impractical particularly for outpatient screening
- Silicone implant ruptures are best detected using MRI (linguine sign on T2, 99% positive predictive value) or ultrasound (snowstorm appearance, 80% sensitivity and specificity with experienced ultrasonographer). The FDA recommends routine MRI screening for rupture 5 years after insertion, and then after every 2 years but adoption of this policy varies widely. Some have suggested an algorithm for investigation based on the symptoms and age of implants
  - Asymptomatic (6.5% rupture rate/ risk) – screen with USG
  - Symptomatic and age less than 10 years (31% risk)
  - Symptomatic and age more than 10 years (64% risk) – USG not useful as even patients with negative scans have 37% risk thus use MRI
- Microscopic gel bleed (leakage of silicone oil) may occur and elevated silicone levels can be detected around intact implants (silicone > saline > controls). Silicone is not detectable more than 2 mm beyond the implant due to the scar tissue that forms around it. Newer implants with much thicker shells claim to have a lower bleed rate. The foreign body reaction to implants is not an immune response to silicone. No specific antibodies against silicone have been detected to date
- Exposure of implants is uncommon (2%) but is increased in those with thin skin envelopes and smokers. Although removal of the implant and delayed replacement (particularly under muscle or additional

soft tissue) produces the most predictable results, salvage by conservative means may be successful in those without overt signs of infection. Published studies involve small numbers of patients and management needs to be individualised

- Others
  - Skin numbness is usually temporary but may persist in 10–15% of patients. Nipple insensitivity is more common if the implant is placed subglandularly or via periareolar route
  - Breast pain of varying degrees is experienced by 10–20% of patients. 5% of patients may experience nipple hypersensitivity
    - Mondor's disease (Henri Mondor 1939) is a painful venous thrombosis on chest wall or breast. It is usually benign and may follow local trauma but has been associated with breast cancer
  - Galactorrhoea (~ 1–2 weeks after surgery) is rare and may be related to nerve irritation causing prolactin release. Treatment includes bromocriptine or intercostal blocks

The safety of silicone breast implants

Silicone is a silicon-carbon-based polymer and differs from elemental silicon (Si). By the time it was first used in breast implants in 1963, it had already been in use for many years in various medical devices, tubes and syringes. In 1992, in response to reports that silicone implants cause cancer and autoimmune disease, the FDA ordered a moratorium on their cosmetic use (their use in reconstruction was still allowed as part of an approved study). Updated large-scale studies have shown that silicone implants do not cause cancer, autoimmune or connective tissue diseases and there is no issue with pregnancy or breast-feeding. The moratorium was lifted in November 2006 but mandatory monitoring as part of ongoing studies remains in place.

Patients with silicone implants seem to have a reduced rate of breast cancer. Early reports suggested that breast tumours in augmented patients were more advanced but this was not been confirmed by subsequent studies (including Silverstein's own follow-up paper, which in fact suggest that the risk of breast cancer is actually reduced). This may be related to smaller amounts of breast tissue or increased immunity. Studies in rats suggest that this may be related to tissue expander effects on blood flow and blood from implant patients has been shown to kill cancer cells in situ. The large Alberta study with over 13,000 patients found no difference in 5 and 10-year survival rates in patients with or without implants.

Other issues
Mammography

The concern is that the radio-opaque silicone of the implant and any associated capsule or microcalcification may hinder breast screening by MMG. Augmenting the breast reduces the amount it can be compressed (to 7.5 cm vs 4.5 cm in non-augmented) which decreases the detail visualised. The general consensus is that MMG can still be satisfactory with an experienced radiologist and some technique modification

- The Eklund technique pushes the implant posteriorly out of the way and involves a larger number of views (mediolateral oblique, craniocaudal and 90% lateral) to increase the amount of breast tissue visualised from 56% to 64% for patients with subglandular implants and from 75% to 85% for submuscular implants. There is a theoretical risk of causing rupture with MMG/ Eklund but it is unlikely with proper techniques

Some recommend preoperative mammograms for patients over 35 years of age, and/or with a positive family history. The relative problems with subsequent breast screening should be part of the informed consent; otherwise screening should be the same

- MRI is a better modality, although lacking in specificity and is not a routine screening tool yet
- Ultrasound cannot detect microcalcification reliably

Breastfeeding

A study found similar levels of silicone in breast milk in patients with (n = 6) or without implants, demonstrating the ubiquitous presence of silicone in the modern environment. In fact, cow's milk and infant formula contain more silicone than breast milk from women with implants.

Other methods of breast augmentation

Injectables

Early attempts at breast augmentation with injections of liquid silicone, paraffin, petroleum jelly, etc. were fraught with complications and have been largely abandoned in most countries (silicone injections are legal in some parts of South America).

Injections of more biocompatible materials such as polyacrylamide hydrogels have been used more recently in various countries, although concerns about significant complications with displacement, infection and possible neurotoxicity limit their wider approval. More recent developments include the use of autologous fat or large particle hyaluronic acid (HA) (Macrolane VRF, Q Med) for temporary breast augmentation.

- Primary breast augmentation with fat grafting has been performed. The current concerns are fat necrosis with palpable lumps, microcalcification that may hinder breast screening and the introduction of fat stem cells may have unknown effects on carcinogenesis. Despite these concerns, fat grafting to the breast is an invaluable tool for augmentation and treatment of breast deformities and has gained widespread use in the UK, Europe and US. Fat grafting should not be done into the parenchyma itself
- Reports from Sweden demonstrate that the effects of Macrolane last for approximately 2 years. There have been reports of capsule formation and concerns over breast screening. The company have since voluntarily withdrawn the product for use in breast augmentation

Suction devices

Devices that apply 200 mmHg pressure and worn 12 hours a day for 10 weeks have been used. One study with 17 patients found modest increases (100 ml) with recoil in the first week. There was no significant further reduction thereafter at 30 weeks with a stable volume increase of 55%. MRI supposedly showed an increase in tissue and not oedema, and a mechanism similar to tissue expansion is proposed. Side effects, such as blistering and skin abrasions, have been reported.

Suction supplemented by adjuvant fat grafting has been used for breast volume increase, as part of proprietary systems such as the BRAVA.

Further reading

Joint guidelines from Association of Breast Surgery, British Association of Plastic, Reconstruction and Aesthetic Surgeons and British Association of Aesthetic Plastic Surgeons. Lipomodelling guidelines for breast surgery. August 2012.

Related topic of interest

- Breast reconstruction

Breast reconstruction

The majority of reconstructions are a result of oncological breast surgery. The goal is to reconstruct a breast that symmetrically matches the normal contralateral breast in size, shape, texture and nipple position with little or no scarring. In practice, mimicking natural ptosis and a good IMF are the most difficult aspects to achieve. Reconstruction is usually a multistage procedure that may involve surgery on the contralateral breast. High revision rates are to be expected.

It is important to distinguish between a reconstruction for salvage (recurrence) and that for cosmesis (primary reconstruction). Speed, simplicity and robust cover may be prioritized at the expense of suboptimal cosmesis with the former, but not the latter.

Breast conserving surgery (BCS) is oncologically safe in the long-term and provides a superior aesthetic result if performed in the correct patient. Up to 40% of breast cancer patients still require mastectomy due to factors such as multifocality (invasive or DCIS), unfavourable size or site, salvage recurrence after BCS or informed patient choice. The evidence for the oncological safety of BCS does not extend to tumours of >4 cm diameter.

Breast conserving surgery

The principle of BCS is that in certain circumstances, local disease control can be achieved by wide local excision and radiotherapy, while preserving the natural breast shape and appearance. Similar survival rates to MRM can be achieved. Adjuvant radiation decreases recurrence rates from 40% to 8% and thus essential. Reconstruction of the defect is of paramount importance in maintaining the aesthetic appearance. While small defects may be adequately closed primarily, it should be less than acceptable to leave larger parenchymal defects unreconstructed. Such defects will invariably produce breast distortion that negates the very aim of BCS. This is avoided with oncoplastic surgery techniques of partial breast reconstruction.

Oncoplastic surgery

Oncoplastic surgery conceptually unites the ablative and reconstructive aspects of breast cancer surgery. This is frequently a cooperative effort between a breast and plastic surgeon with a common goal of maximising the aesthetic outcome without compromising the oncological resection. This cooperation extends from total breast reconstructions to partial breast reconstructions. Optimal placements of incisions are a particular advantage with this, permitting a variety of local flaps for defect reconstruction. These are cases that may have otherwise resulted in reconstructions of poorer cosmesis or greater magnitude.

Partial breast reconstructive techniques are divided into volume displacement and volume replacement techniques. The former involves redistributes the volume loss to restore shape at the expense of size and is termed therapeutic mammoplasty. The latter involves importation of tissue (local, regional or distant) to restore volume and preserve size. The exact techniques used depend on the defect size relative to the breast and its position. When a skin defect is present over the excised area, the tissue may be imported with a corresponding skin paddle.

In the presence of oncological suitability, the ideal candidates for BCS are women with medium to large breasts (or smaller breasted women with ptosis) requiring excision of <10-20% breast volume, who also require a breast reduction for quality of life issues.

Volume displacement

Therapeutic mammoplasty techniques are based extensively on breast reduction and mastopexy techniques for managing skin incisions (access), nipple pedicle vascularity (nipple position and viability) and parenchymal reshaping post-excision. It is important to note that the technique for skin access should be separated from that of glandular manipulation when considering this. Wise patterns do not necessitate inferior pedicles and vertical scar techniques do not rigidly prescribe a superior pedicle.

- The easiest defects to reconstruct are cancers that fall within the predicted excision areas for a breast reduction. This includes all areas within the Wise-pattern keyhole (retroareolar, lower pole, inferomedial and inferolateral). This is termed Scenario A in the Nottingham approach. A standard breast reduction is performed if the nipple can be preserved. Otherwise, the skin and parenchyma within the keyhole pattern is excised and closed as a closing wedge mammoplasty. Bat-wing (tennis-ball) excisions of skin and parenchyma may be suitable for tumours immediately superior to the nipple-areolar complex in the large, ptotic breast
- Defects that fall outside of this require reconstruction with local parenchymal flaps, (termed Scenario B in the Nottingham approach) or regional/distant flaps (volume replacement). The two general local choices are extended pedicles and secondary pedicles
  - Extended pedicles: These are distal parenchymal extensions of the nipple pedicle such as a superior pedicle with an inferior extension. The extension is transposed, folded or rotated into the adjacent defect and secured, simultaneously positioning the nipple in the correct position on the mound, and the parenchyma then re-coned into shape
  - Secondary pedicles: These are pedicled flaps that are created from tissue that is normally excised and transposed or rotated into the defect
  - The choice is dictated by pre-existing scars, propensity for the extended pedicle to kink, size of secondary pedicle and location of the defect relative to the proposed extended or secondary pedicles
- Contralateral symmetrising mammoplasty can be performed simultaneously and with a standard breast reduction technique
- Defects in the upper medial quadrant are the most difficult to reconstruct with volume displacement, but are the least common

Volume replacement

- Volume replacement techniques are dictated by site, volume and whether skin is required
- LICAP, TAP and partial LD flaps are local and regional options that are limited by reach to the lateral two thirds of the breast. IMAPs will cover the lower pole and inferomedial quadrants. Superomedial defects may require free-tissue transfer with flaps such as the TUG
- Flaps involving the thoracodorsal pedicle may sacrifice a future LD flap for salvage

Some patients subsequently have a mastectomy for aesthetic or oncological reasons.

- Approximately one third will have deformities requiring further correction, such as completion mastectomy and formal reconstruction for improved aesthetics
- Formal reconstruction may also be needed if marginal involvement or recurrence requires more radical excision such as MRM

Mastectomy

Skin-sparing mastectomies (SSM) aim to remove all breast tissue including the nipple-areolar complex (NAC) while preserving the 3-dimensional skin envelope. This facilitates precise restoration of the preoperative breast shape with immediate reconstruction. This advantage is lost in the delayed reconstruction.

The mastectomy skin flap is most vulnerable in SSM and its survival is a major factor in the success or failure of a reconstruction. The commonest problems are buttonholing of the skin, diathermy burns on the skin under surface, excessively thin skin flaps (subdermal instead of a suprafascial mastectomy) and unnecessary sacrifice of the internal mammary perforators. This is most crucial in implant-based reconstructions. Terminology clarification:

- Nipple-sparing mastectomy (NSM): SSM with preservation of the NAC. Has been confusingly used interchangeably with SSM. NSM does not eliminate ductal epithelium within the nipple and has an oncological risk. The remaining NAC may be insensate, dyspigmented and lose projection, but there is no reconstructed NAC that matches the original. There is a trend towards more NSM for prophylactic and therapeutic indications for small tumours that are far from the nipple. Negative intraoperative NAC biopsies for tumour are required for sparing

- Subcutaneous mastectomy: SSM with preservation of significant amounts of breast tissue. Has also been confusingly used interchangeably with SSM or NSM. The term is redundant
- Simple mastectomy: Removal of breast skin, NAC and all breast tissue
- Radical mastectomy (Halsted): Simple mastectomy with removal of pectoralis muscles and axillary lymph nodes
- Modified radical mastectomy: Radical mastectomy that spares the pectoralis muscles

Timing

Immediate reconstruction is regarded as the gold standard as it improves body image and quality of life with minimal interruption. The main surgical advantages are preservation of the skin flaps in their original state, IMF and 3-dimensional breast envelope. The overall aesthetic result tends to be superior, with better ptosis creation (to match) and superior fullness compared with delayed reconstruction.

Irradiation of the reconstructed breast will result in a worse aesthetic result and halt the development of signs of breast aging. The arguments against the oncological concerns of immediate reconstruction with radiotherapy are:

- Immediate reconstruction does not interfere with adjuvant therapy that includes radiotherapy, chemotherapy and hormonal therapy
- General wound complications are not significantly more frequent than if mastectomy alone were performed. This does not delay adjuvant therapy. However, this analysis excludes specific

complications such as implant failure and increased need for blood transfusion after flap surgery. The deleterious immunosuppressive effect of allogeneic blood transfusions in cancer patients has not been fully elucidated but a 3-unit threshold may be significant

- There is no delay in diagnosis of recurrent tumours in reconstructed breasts
- Immediate reconstruction is not only oncologically safe, but may be theoretically safer. Further surgical trauma from delayed reconstruction may cause immunosuppression and stimulate previously dormant tumour cells

In reality the need for radiotherapy may only be clear after histological examination. It is more appropriate to think of the likelihood for radiotherapy in the pre-operative period to guide the choice of reconstructive technique (implant-based vs. autologous).

If the decision has been made for delayed reconstruction, then it is prudent to wait until both patient and tissues have recovered. In general,

- Chemotherapy (CMF): 6 weeks after last dose and with normal haematology
- Radiotherapy: Sufficiently supple soft tissue is achieved at minimum of 3 months, but frequently a 6-month threshold is used

While a significant proportion of mastectomy patients may not want reconstruction, it is the duty of the surgeon to advise of its availability (frequently neglected aspect).

Reconstructive options

No reconstruction

A simple external prosthesis or padded bra may be sufficient. The acceptance rate is highly variable.

Implant-based reconstruction

Implant-based reconstruction sacrifices longevity of the reconstruction for simplicity of the individual procedure, even in the ideal patient.

Implants are usually placed in the subpectoral plane with serratus anterior cover in the inferolateral corner. While the procedure may be similar in the immediate and delayed scenario, the rationale differs.

- Immediate: The mastectomy flap is at greatest risk of breakdown and implant exposure. Total submuscular coverage acts as a second barrier if this occurs. Thickness of the cover is secondary
- Delayed: The mastectomy flap is reliable and not of concern. Thickness of the cover is of prime importance as tissue expansion will thin it and risk exposure. The mastectomy flap acts as a second barrier to expansion-induced breaches of the pectoralis cover. Patients with sufficiently thick inferior pole tissue (or augmented with thoracoabdominal advancement) may permit subcutaneous implants (dual-plane). As the total submuscular coverage may limit expansion, this may be desirable for differential lower pole expansion, such as to create symmetrising ptosis. In general, the aesthetic result of an implant-based reconstruction is better the more tissue there is in front of it

Tissue expansion is required when there is insufficient skin cover to accommodate the implant desired. While almost universal in the delayed scenario, this is still an issue in immediate reconstruction unless only a very small amount of skin is excised or a greatly reduced implant size is accepted. In addition, the total volume a total submuscular plane can accommodate is limited without expansion.

Expansion aims to gradually enlarge the pocket over several months by serial percutaneous instillation of saline. They may be achieved using single (saline only) or dual-lumen implants (gel and saline) (**Table 9**). Over-expansion of approximately 25–30% may be performed and maintained for 6–12 weeks to allow for capsular maturation. Overexpansion of anatomically shaped dual-lumen implant pockets in planned one-stage reconstructions may result in implant rotation. For one-stage reconstructions, the port is pulled or plugged and removed and the residual implant left as a fixed volume device. For two-stage reconstructions, the expander is then exchanged for a smaller prosthesis to recreate a degree of ptosis.

- Although overexpansion is safe due to the generous safety margin of implants and data shows no increase in leakage, it may increase muscle spasm and upward migration
- Using expander implants makes matching other side easier
- For distant port expanders, the normal sized port (tolerates 20 expansions vs. 10 expansions for miniports) is often a better choice, particularly in obese patients to allow easier palpation. If the filling port is never removed, it carries a risk of leakage
- Implant-based reconstruction is relatively contraindicated if radiotherapy is required. Irradiation of the implant-based reconstruction carries a 75% risk of capsular contracture, and is never first choice in this scenario. This can be somewhat circumvented by insertion of temporary single-lumen expanders at the

Table 9 Types of dual-lumen expanders	
Implant type	**Characteristics**
Becker expander implant (Hilton Becker 1984) (Mentor Inc.)	• 25%, 50% (round) or 35% (anatomical) silicone by final volume. • Distant filling port can be pulled out converting it into a permanent fixed volume implant.
Allergan Style 150 dual-lumen implant	• 50% (anatomical) silicone by final volume, otherwise similar to Becker.
Allergan Natrelle Style 133 expander Mentor Siltex Contour Profile Styles 6100, 6200 & 6300	• Integrated filling port over implant located by magnet. • Licensed for temporary use only and not beyond 6 months.
Sientra ACX double-chamber expander	• These are the only dual-saline lumen expanders with an anterior and posterior chamber to allow differential expansion. • Like the Allergan 133, they have integrated filling ports and licensed for temporary use only.

time of reconstruction. If radiotherapy is not required, the second stage is substitution of the expander for a fixed volume device. If radiotherapy is required, the expander is deflated prior to it and the second stage is an autologous tissue-based reconstruction. This is the approach currently adopted at the Memorial Sloan Kettering Center. However, this necessarily consigns every patient to a two-stage reconstruction

Autologous reconstruction

Flap orientation provides the basic shape. Flap tailoring and shaping allows fine-tuning to achieve optimal aesthetic results.

- An oblique flap orientation may provide more lateral fullness
- A vertical flap orientation provides better infraclavicular fill. The inferior-most zone may be folded under to augment projection at the expense of breast height
- Large, broad and ptotic breasts are better reconstructed with transversely orientated flaps. This carries more central tissue and less infraclavicular fill
- Suturing a transverse island into a U-shape, creating central projection is a useful manoeuvre to cone flaps. Care must be taken not to compromise flap vascularity when this is done

Pedicled flaps

- Latissimus dorsi (LD): This is a versatile and reliable flap with a necrosis rate of <1% and may be preferable to the TRAM/DIEP in higher-risk patients such as the overweight, smokers and diabetics
- Donor site seromas are common although the incidence may be reduced by the use of quilting sutures
- If raised conventionally, the LD lacks sufficient volume to reconstruct anything other than small breasts. The extended LD flap modification that incorporates adjacent zones of fat may allow the omission of an implant (see Latissimus dorsi flap)
- If the thoracodorsal vessels are damaged during axillary dissection, the flap may still be raised on the serratus anterior branch. However, the arc of rotation is reduced

- LD tendon division is a variable practice. Complete division allows its reorientation along the anterior axillary fold, recreating its aesthetic appearance. However, division risks direct pedicle damage and inadvertent traction on it afterwards. Partial tendon section is a compromise that retains most benefits
- Thoracodorsal nerve sectioning is variable practice. Arguments for it are the elimination of unwanted contractions at the expense of muscle atrophy. Proponents of nerve preservation argue the opposite. A MRI comparative study showed no difference in volume in consistency whether or not sectioning was performed
- pTRAM (pedicled transverse rectus abdominis myocutaneous): This has an increased risk of necrosis (12% in some series), frequently due to venous insufficiency. It can be supercharged and turbocharged by anastomosing DIEA and DIEV to the thoracodorsal pedicle respectively
- The flap is usually pedicled on the contralateral superior epigastric artery as the less acute angle kinks less thereby improving venous drainage. There has been a recent revival of the ipsilateral pTRAM where the pedicle is draped in a curve rather than folded to reduce compression
- The reconstructed breast tends to have a less distinct IMF due to migration and bulge of the pedicle at the medial end (may be reduced by cutting its innervation, particularly up to T8)
- The abdominal flap has greater donor bulk are the better choice for reconstructing the larger breast without an implant. If further volume is required, the pTRAM can be combined with an implants or a larger bipedicled flap, although a free flap may be a better choice if this is the case
- Donor site morbidity is an issue, as the recti are needed for first 40° of abdominal flexion. Between 10 and 20% of these patients do not return to their jobs or hobbies. One study did not find any functional or satisfaction difference between bilateral DIEPs and bilateral TRAMs (Chun PRS 2010) but these findings have been disputed

Free flaps

As well as improved vascularity, free flaps offer better control of breast shape in projection and ptosis. However, there is a 1-6% risk of complete flap loss and requires microsurgical expertise. The longer operating times and greater anaesthetic risk render it unsuitable for patients with significant co-morbidities.

The abdominal flaps cannot be reliably used in those who have had previous abdominoplasty or liposuction. The presence of a Pfannenstiel scar (usually low and muscle splitting) does not preclude use of the flap.

- fTRAM: The entire rectus muscle is taken with the overlying flap and deep inferior epigastric vessels
- DIEP flaps have the advantage of leaving the muscle mass and fascia behind, thus resulting in less donor site morbidity and shorter hospital stay compared to pTRAMs (Garvey, PRS 2006)
  - The main perforators lie within an 8 cm radius from the umbilicus. The pedicle is longer (average 10 cm) than the fTRAM. The use of MR angiography or 64-slice CT helps identify the perforator of choice and its course. Cases with small multiple perforators can be identified pre-operatively and a fTRAM planned instead
  - The SIEV should be preserved as an option to turbo-charge (strictly 'turbo-drain') the flap if required. The venous drainage may either be deep or superficial dominant. Useful recipient vessels are the turndown cephalic and external jugular veins
- msTRAM: The muscle-sparing TRAM offers a compromise by taking the lateral and medial rows with the intervening muscle up to about 2 inches below the umbilicus. The arguments against this are that the remaining muscle is poorly innervated and non-functional

When considering abdominal flaps for breast reconstruction, one suggested strategy is:

- Elevate lateral row of perforators and release the fascial collars to allow vessel expansion. If the vessel size is < 1.5 mm then explore the medial row. If these perforators are also small (< 1.5 mm) then a msTRAM is preferable to a DIEP, but if the medial row vessels are larger, then a DIEP is possible
  - If size of medial row vessel is 1.5–3 mm, then a DIEP should be raised on more than one perforator
  - If size of medial row vessel is > 3 mm, then a single perforator DIEP is feasible

Less common free flaps can be used when TRAM/DIEP flaps are not available. Note that non-central donor sites may need a contralateral procedure to balance the donor-site deformity.

- Superficial inferior epigastric artery (SIEA) is present only 65% of the time, and may be inadequate to support the flap alone. The artery arises from the (common) femoral artery 1–3 cm below the inguinal ligament halfway between the ASIS and the pubis and may have common origin with the superficial circumflex artery. The pedicle is shorter and the vessels are small. The skin paddle lies at a lower level than the TRAM/DIEP
- Superior gluteal artery perforator (SGAP) flaps (Allen, 1995) provide reasonable shape due to reasonable amounts of fat and muscle (13 × 30 cm for direct closure) but has a relatively short central pedicle (thus more suited for anastomosis to the internal thoracic arteries). It is commonly harvested as a horizontal ellipse on the upper buttock centred on the pedicle (one third of the distance from posterior superior iliac spine (PSIS) to greater trochanter). The scar axis runs from the PSIS to apex of greater trochanter, and although well hidden, the resultant contour defect may not be
- Inferior gluteal artery perforator (IGAP) flaps have longer pedicles and leave a less obvious scar than SGAPs. It lies along a more vertical axis halfway between the greater trochanter and ischial tuberosity. Direct closure is possible if the harvest is limited to 12 × 25 cm. As the sciatic nerve is exposed during the dissection, it is theoretically at risk particularly from the effects of postoperative scarring. There is an additional variable functional loss

associated with division of the inferior gluteal nerve

- The DCIA (Rubens) flap uses the soft tissue around the iliac crest. Closure of the abdominal wall must be meticulous and donor site pain can be a problem. It is an uncommon choice but may be useful for patients who have previously had abdominoplasty
- TUG and PAP flaps have been described

Reconstruction and the irradiated breast

The possible scenarios involving reconstruction of a previously irradiated breast are:

- Immediate reconstruction (addressed above)
- After MRM and RT (delayed reconstruction)
- Unacceptable deformities following BCS and RT
- Recurrence after BCS/MRM and RT

Autologous reconstruction is preferred. Any RT-induced redness must have subsided and the soft tissue suppleness restored prior to undertaking delayed reconstruction.

The primary issue is lack of skin. The commonest choices for total breast reconstruction are the DIEP or TRAM flaps that usually provide skin in abundance. Gluteal flaps (IGAP, SGAP) are alternatives although preference is variable from unit to unit. The extended LD is a suitable alternative if the demand for skin is limited. In addition, patient culture, race and individual variation may alter the preference considerably.

Further reading

Macmillan RD, James R, Gale KL, McCulley SJ. Therapeutic mammaplasty. J Surg Oncol 2014;110:90–95.

Related topics of interest

- Breast augmentation
- Microsurgery
- Nipple areolar reconstruction
- Pressure sores
- Tissue expansion

Breast reduction

The aim of breast reduction is to reduce breast size while maintaining aesthetics (symmetry with minimal scarring) and function (nipple sensation, ability to breast feed).

The 5 main causes of breast hypertrophy are:

1. Idiopathic: Most common
2. Virginal breast hypertrophy (juvenile gigantomastia): Rapid acceleration of breast growth at puberty in a very short space of time either from a baseline of negligible growth or constant growth
3. Gestational hypertrophy: Occurs in pregnancy between gestational week 16–20 and increases with subsequent pregnancies
4. Drug-induced: Oestrogens including HRT; it is a rare side effect of penicillamine
5. Obesity: Breast growth tends to be in proportion to the rest of the body

There is no direct correlation between symptoms and weight or breast size. Symptoms are of greater clinical relevance than absolute breast size. The most common indication for surgery is back pain. Other common symptoms include intertrigo, bra-strap grooving of the shoulders, difficulty with sports and being unable to find suitably fitting clothes. Psychological symptoms include significant embarrassment.

Patient satisfaction from breast reduction is extremely high (95%) and among the highest of any plastic surgery procedure (abdominoplasty 77%). The common causes of dissatisfaction are those of size, shape and symmetry.

Cup size is affected primarily with reduction, with minimal effect on band size unless liposuction is used to alter thoracic girth. Most reduction techniques will sacrifice base width for projection to varying degrees. This combined with the unscientific methods of band and cup size calculation, and brand variability in bra sizes renders any estimation of post-operative cup size a futile exercise.

Reduction mammoplasty considerations

The prime surgical considerations are:

- Pedicle type: The nipple areolar complex (NAC) is raised on a vascular pedicle, which is eventually transposed or rotated into its final position. It is designed to allow accurate positioning on the final mound while preserving the NAC blood supply and sensation. The latter is sacrificed if the NAC cannot be preserved on a pedicle, or as a salvage procedure, where it is excised and inset as a full-thickness graft. While the majority of the pedicles were random pattern when described, they have been subsequently shown to be reliably predictable axial pattern flaps. The excellent vascularity of the breast permits significant leeway with random pattern extensions to either the pedicle or the remaining parenchyma. The pedicle may be raised in a glandular or dermoglandular fashion. The theoretically improved venous return of the latter has not materialised in practice. The pedicle choice influences the manner of parenchymal resection, which in turn determines the aesthetic result
- Skin incision pattern: All skin incision patterns offer good parenchymal access but differ in the resultant scar and ability to deal with skin excess. Wise-pattern incisions allow direct excision of both caudo-cranial and mediolateral excess at the expense of long scars in both dimensions. Vertical incisions deal with mediolateral excess directly but caudo-cranial excess management is addressed through a combination of the following that minimise or eliminate the transverse scar component
  - Dog-ear excision: The cranial dog-ear is hidden in the NAC. The caudal dog-ear is excised in 3 common ways:
    1. Caudal extension, leaving a longer vertical scar that crosses the IMF
    2. Lateral extension, leaving a J-shaped scar
    3. Mediolateral extension, leaving a small inverted-T
  - Bunching-up the closure: This creates numerous transverse folds in the vertical scar that take up the caudo-cranial slack. This is shortening is not sustained over time (Hall-Findlay, 2010)

- Exploiting tissue elasticity: The dog-ear is both a convex contour deformity and a skin-excess phenomenon. The former is addressed by subcutaneous defatting (direct or liposuction), that allows the unsupported dog-ear skin to retract. Any residual is excised as a secondary procedure after allowing maximal contraction. (Note that the liposuction-only reduction mammoplasty utilises the principle of skin retraction alone to address the skin excess.)

All patterns incorporate a periareolar component. Periareolar-only patterns allow skin removal in a concentric pattern only. The disparity between desired NAC circumference and the post-excisional hole circumference of the skin flap delimit the amount of skin excess removal. They tend to flatten the breast in the antero-posterior dimension. Closure results in a puckered periareolar scar.

Skin should not be the sole supporting structure for gland shape, as it is very elastic. Glandular rearrangement and in particular, elimination of inferior pole weight is key to minimising glandular ptosis.

Skin incision patterns and pedicle type are independent and should be viewed that way (**Table 10**). The confusion stems from inappropriate terminology. Inverted-T scar reductions do not automatically equate to inferior pedicle reductions. Similarly, vertical scar reductions are not exclusively superior-pedicle Lejour-type reductions. While this may be true in some or even the majority of cases, both the Wise-pattern and vertical incisions allow the development of any pedicle of choice.

- Moderate ptosis and hypertrophy requiring less than 6–8 cm of NAC elevation: vertical incisions that employ a pedicles in the superior half of the breast are good choices. The Lejour, Lassus and Hall-Findlay are popular choices
- Larger breasts requiring more than 8 cm NAC elevation: Inferior pedicles allow direct superior advancement without kinking and are regarded as safer. However, the heavy inferior pole weight remains and is at risk of bottoming out
- NAC >12–15 cm elevation: Consider free-nipple grafting. Also consider this in the elderly, those at poor anaesthetic risk, the very obese and those requiring a resection of more than 1.5 kg per breast. Complications include unpredictable nipple graft survival, loss of sensation, irregular pigmentation and graft

Table 10 Correlations between pedicle, skin incision and technique		
Pedicle	**Skin incision**	**Technique**
Superior	Vertical	Lejour (liposuction and undermining), Lassus
	Wise	Wise-pattern superior pedicle
Medial	Vertical	Hall-Findlay
Supero-medial	Vertical	Hall-Findlay
Inferior	Wise	Wise-pattern inferior pedicle[1]
	Vertical	SPAIR (Short scar PeriAreolar Inferior pedicle Reduction)[2]
Lateral	Any	Skoog
Central	Periareolar	Benelli
	Wise/vertical	Central mound (Balch)
Vertical bipedicle	Any	McKissock
Horizontal bipedicle	Any	Strombeck
Wuringer septum-based	Any	Hamdi[3]
None (free nipple graft)	Any	Thorek

[1] Although described by Robert Wise (1956), this terminology avoids confusion.
[2] Described by Dennis Hammond
[3] Popularised by Hamdi

tethering. In those with significant ptosis, consider the modified Robertson technique that also eliminates the vertical scar

- Other techniques such as Regnault B or periareolar are less commonly used
- The use of liposuction alone is controversial. A 20% reduction in volume is achieved on average, which may be inadequate. The skin envelope may require >6 months to shrink down

Clinical experience has shown the different types of pedicles (**Table 11**) to be safe when properly designed and executed. The choice is also geographically biased. Wise pattern inferior pedicles are more common in the US (75% of surgeons) and UK, whereas vertical incision superior pedicles are more prevalent in continental Europe.

- Vertical bipedicle: The McKissock technique uses a superior dermal bridge (thus keeping the subdermal plexus) in addition to an inferior dermoglandular pedicle and is regarded as a belts and braces approach with good safety. This tends to result in breasts with too much fullness superiorly with the nipples inclining downwards
- Elimination of the redundant superior pedicle portion led to inferior pedicle techniques that have proved to be versatile and remain widely used (**Figure 3**).
  - The effect of gravity on a heavy lower pole leads to bottoming out of greater magnitude than other techniques
  - Attempts to combat bottoming out with a shortened vertical component (<6 cm) contributes to a boxy-breast as descent is differentially limited centrally.
- Superior pedicles are reliable but have limited mobility as elevating the NAC involves folding the pedicle on itself. The pedicle must be sufficiently thin (axial vessel is at 1–2 cm depth, allowing significant thinning)
- Medial pedicles are rotated and advanced into place after resection of predominantly lower pole tissue. The inferior edge of the pedicle becomes the medial pillar, as the breast is re-coned. Superomedial pedicles are treated in a similar fashion but need to rotate further
- Lateral pedicles (Skoog technique) use a dermal pedicle based on a lateral limb. Alternatively, a mirror-imaged equivalent of the medial pedicle technique may be used
- Central mound techniques (Balch) dispense with the dermal pedicle and rely entirely on the parenchymal mound

Glandular reshaping (re-coning) is best achieved when the Wise-pattern is applied to the parenchyma.

The ability to breastfeed depends more on encouragement and support rather than surgical technique. There is no significant difference in breastfeeding ability between post-operative reduction patients and those with untreated macromastia, as long as the subareolar tissue is sufficiently maintained.

	Nerve	Artery
Table 11 The neurovascular supply to the NAC pedicles		
Inferior, central and lateral pedicles	Lateral fourth intercostal nerve. It splits at the lateral breast border into a superficial and deep branch. The superficial runs in the superficial plane towards the NAC. The deep branch above pectoralis fascia to the mid-breast where turns superficially towards the NAC. Preserving either branch will preserve sensation. Short-term sensation is best with inferior pedicles but this advantage is lost beyond 12 months.	Inferior and central: Deep perforators at the fourth IC space. Lateral: Lateral thoracic artery.
Superior pedicles	Infraclavicular contribution.	Second IC perforator that runs superficially (1–2 cm depth) to enter the NAC superiorly.
Medial pedicles		Third to Fifth IC perforators that run superficially

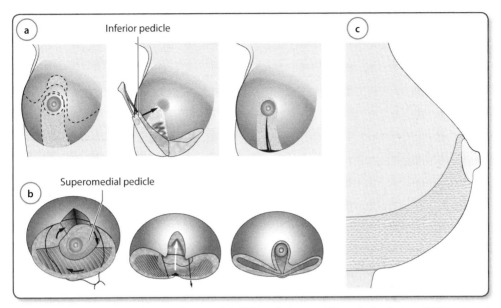

Figure 3 Comparison of (a) inferior T inferior pedicle (ITIP) technique and (b) vertical technique. (c) Side view of the ITIP.

Operative technique

Patients are marked standing. Some use a fixed pattern with extensive preoperative markings, whilst others favour intraoperative tailoring with fewer fixed markings. The primary aim of preoperative marking and measurements is primarily to ensure nipple symmetry rather than to make breasts to a specific formula. Wise-pattern inferior pedicle technique (IMF static)

- Breast axis: from midclavicular line to nipple at IMF
- New nipple placement at the IMF level along the desired breast meridian (Pitanguy's point) and 10–12 cm from midline. The NAC diameter varies from 3.5–5.0 cm depending on patient stature. Placing the nipples too high leads to a deformity that is very difficult to correct. If in doubt, place nipples lower than anticipated. Some degree of nipple medialisation is often necessary
- The central vertical limbs of the excision pattern should be limited to less than 6 cm to combat bottoming out. A pinch-rotation test is used to estimate the excess and thus the angle between the limbs of the keyhole. Maintaining this angle at < 60° may reduce T-junction tension and ischaemia
- Most of the volume reduction should be in the lateral quadrant. Adequate extension of the incision laterally is required to sufficiently mobilise the lateral pillar or else a boxy breast may result
- The pedicle base should be about 8–10 cm. Wider pedicles may impede circulation by increasing tension while contributing little to perfusion

Vertical pattern superior/superomedial/medial pedicle techniques (IMF elevated)
- The IMF is no longer a static structure, but the upper breast border is. Nipple position is based on the latter, 8–10 cm inferior to it in the desired meridian
- The skin excision pattern is bowling-pin shaped. The resultant reduction tends to elevate the IMF
- The Lejour vertical mammaplasty uses a superior pedicle (like Lassus) and became popular due to elimination of the inferior transverse scar that simultaneously provided a longer-lasting attractive breast shape with good projection achieved by re-coning of the gland (by suturing medial and lateral parenchymal pillars with 3-0 PDS)

- It is often combined with liposuction, particularly laterally to reduce breast tail volume and define the lateral breast border
- Skin undermining inferiorly is used to allow skin gathering and promote skin retraction
- The nipple position is marked lower than with the inferior pedicle technique in anticipation of glandular drop
  - The simplified vertical technique (Hall-Findlay technique, **Figure 3**) included several important modifications with the aim of shortening the learning curve. The procedure time is shorter and the incidence of nipple necrosis and numbness is reduced
  - The medial pedicle used is easier to rotate up, while allowing resection of the heavier lateral and inferior breast tissue
  - Less emphasis is placed on shortening the vertical scar by gathering (which may lead to delayed healing). The redundant skin is excised by extending the incision as a J, L or short T
  - The skin flaps are not significantly undermined and less liposuction is used, although it can be useful at the IMF to fine-tune the result (**Figure 3**)

Perioperative care

- The use of local infiltration with adrenaline-containing solutions has been shown to decrease blood loss and the need for blood transfusion. The ASPS MOC data supports this, demonstrating no difference in haematoma rates with its use (Kerrigan, 2013)
- The evidence shows that drains are unnecessary in breast reduction and do not reduce haematoma rates. However, they may be useful in women >50 years or >500 g resection weight to tackle increased drainage
- Current evidence supports a single preoperative dose of antibiotic, in line with evidence in other types of breast surgery. The data is conflicting with reductions specifically (Ahmadi, PRS 2005 = no difference; Veiga-Filho, APS 2010 = lower in antibiotic group)

- Surgical tips:
  - Nipple congestion (some monitor with laser Doppler or indocyanine fluorescence, but is not routine)
    - Remove sutures. Delayed primary closure several days later if decongested
    - Operative exploration to exclude pedicle torsion, compression or haematoma
    - If unsuccessful, consider free nipple graft onto a vascularised bed. If the pedicle was compromised, it is unlikely to support a graft. In addition, the bed is at risk of fat necrosis
  - Difficult closure
    - Remove more parenchyma
    - Consider skin graft (excised secondarily)
    - Partial closure: Leave to heal secondarily or delayed primary closure if oedema resolved

Postoperative care

- A surgical bra is worn for comfort. A typical regime is wearing of a sports bra for 6 weeks and avoiding underwired bras during this period
- Pain with the first menstruation is not uncommon
- Lactation is still possible in 50–70% of patients with the inferior pedicle technique, although it may not be sufficient and supplementation may be required. Patients who become pregnant after reduction surgery tend to be less satisfied, possibly due to increased ptosis

Complications

Most are minor but there is a 4% nipple necrosis rate quoted in the literature
- Obesity: There is conflicting data on the impact of obesity on breast reduction complications. 4 retrospective studies (Zubowski, PRS 2000; Wagner, PRS 2000; Roehl, PRS 2008; Setala JPRAS 2009) show an increased rate (N=1033), whereas another 4 (Stevens, ASJ 2008; Gamboa-Bobadilla, APS 2007; Shah,

JPRAS, 2011; Chun, PRS 2012) show no difference (N=1514). The ASPS MOC data shows increased complications predicted (logistic regression) with BMI >30, smoking, resection weights >1300 g, surgery time of >210 minutes, age >50 years and a history of breast surgery

- Haematoma: usually requires exploration and evacuation
- Wound infection, dehiscence and skin necrosis, especially at T-junction
- Fat necrosis is probably more common than recognised as minor areas resolve spontaneously, but may leave calcifications
- Nipple numbness occurs in around 5% of patients and is more frequent with more radical reductions and superior pedicle techniques. There is some evidence that breast sensation may actually improve, possibly due to relief of chronic nerve traction
- Nipple position that is excessively high
- Shape: Asymmetry, bottoming out, a boxy breast appearance and residual dog-ears may require subsequent revision The IMF-nipple distance may increase postoperatively by up to 30% especially in inferior pedicle techniques, with a loss of projection

- Scar hypertrophy is not uncommon but can be reduced with standard treatments such as silicone and steroid therapy

Oncology

A small percentage of breast reductions will turn out to harbour breast cancer (0.5–4 %). The rate of abnormal findings is dependent on the extent of pathological examination in patients of >40 years.

- Preoperative screening in excess of standard screening mammography guidelines is controversial. The risk of false-positives and unnecessary invasive investigation must be balanced against the risk of detecting malignancy. National screening guidelines vary with country
- The American College of Pathologists recommend that all breast tissue be submitted for pathological examination
- Excised breast tissue is marked prior to being sent for histological examination
- Postoperative changes may include calcification of breast tissue, but the mammographic appearance can usually be distinguished from malignant microcalcification
- Breast reduction itself reduces the long-term risk of developing breast cancer

Further reading

Srinivasaiah N, Iwuchukwu OC, Stanley PR, et al. Risk factors for complications following breast reduction: results from a randomized control trial. Breast J. 2014;20:274–8.

Related topic of interest

- Liposuction

Brow lift

In women, the eyebrow level lies at or just above the supraorbital rim. It curves convexly superior and forms a peak between lateral limbus and lateral canthus of eye. In men, the brow is flatter and parallel with or slightly below superior orbital rim. With ageing, laxity of the forehead leads to brow ptosis and a combination of tissue thinning and a compensatory frontalis contraction leads to transverse static and dynamic wrinkling.

Brow ptosis must be distinguished from upper lid laxity and ptosis. Blepharoplasty in a unrecognised compensatory brow ptosis patient will result in frontalis relaxation post-operatively, resulting in a further drop of the brow, causing a tired and aged look.

If the brow is truly low, it can be lifted with upward traction and suspension. There is some empirical evidence to suggest that lifts will last longer if done earlier, although the skin and soft tissue laxity progresses with age.

Planes of lift

Different planes of lift have been described, though they are often are combined in individual techniques.

- Subcutaneous: This is, theoretically, the most direct approach to remove transverse wrinkles and preserve posterior scalp sensation. However, it is time consuming and may compromise flap vascularity that is reflected in increased complications rates
- Subgaleal: Dissection in this plane is rapid, safe and relatively bloodless, but may stretch more with time. Many surgeons who use this plane will convert to a subperiosteal plane 2 cm above the orbital rim to reduce trauma to the supraorbital neurovascular bundle
- Subperiosteal: This allows more effective traction and anchorage by lifting the inelastic pericranium. Release at the arcus marginalis is required and there is a theoretical loss of nutrient supply to the bones

Open surgery

In the classic technique, this involves a bicoronal incision (7 cm behind the hairline at the midline curving to the apex of the ear). The incision may be moved posteriorly for men with receding hairlines at the expense of a further mechanical disadvantage to the lift. A further side effect is elevation of the hairline (1.5 mm posterior hairline displacement for every 1 mm of brow lift). Caution is required in those with a hairline that is already high or receding. The brow may remain at a similar level postoperatively but may have a more relaxed appearance with fewer (forehead/ glabella) wrinkles.

- The flap is raised and turned over; this may press on the eyes, thus it is important to protect them
- The corrugator muscles are carefully debulked to spare the nerves and to avoid excessive excision that may cause depressions. The frontalis muscle is generally not modified to avoid deformity and to maintain its function. A browlift will tend to relax a hypertrophied muscle
- Although part of the lift is from skin resection, the majority comes from fixation of the flap to the bone or immobile fascia. This is achieved with a variety of methods such as micro-screws and suture bone tunnelling. Postoperative compression is often used to maximise adherence. The elastic band principle, described by Flowers, states that further away the lift/suspension from the brow, the less effective it is
- The open browlift is a reliable procedure but potential complications include infection, necrosis, haematoma, anaesthesia, facial and trigeminal nerve damage, alopecia, asymmetry and overcorrection. Resecting less skin medially will help to avoid the surprised look that can be difficult to subsequently correct

Endoscopic lift

Endoscopic methods use three to five smaller incisions at or behind the hairline to allow development of the dissection plane and resection of over-active depressors. The main advantages are fewer complications (less paraesthesia, scar alopecia and blood loss) and faster recovery but the surgery takes longer and requires specialised instruments with a significant learning curve. Following an early phase of popularity, endoscopic brow lifts are not used as often as they were as its limitations became clearer. In general, it offers a lesser degree of lift (<5 mm) with unconfirmed longevity. The most common complaints are undercorrection and relapse. It is less useful for older patients with deep lines, thicker flaccid skin, significant ptosis and skin excess. It more suitable for younger patients (<40 years) with glabellar frown lines, good skin tone and only moderate brow ptosis. Endoscopic corrugator sectioning may be substituted with botulinum toxin to avoid the potential neurovascular damage in this area.

- The numbers of incisions vary but there are usually two parasagittal and two temporal sites. The central dissection is raised in the subperiosteal plane whilst dissection in the lateral zones is immediately deep to the temporoparietal fascia. Dividing the periosteal layer at their junction joins the two zones

Direct brow lift

This is a useful technique (superciliary excision) in certain circumstances such as patient refusal for more extensive surgery or in conditions where there is localised lateral brow hooding such as established facial palsy in the elderly. It is simple, effective and allows good control of the degree of lift. Scar cosmesis is the major drawback. A direct brow lift will not address the problem of glabellar creases.

- Mark the patient in the sitting position. First, mark the upper border of the brow, then raise the brow to the intended height, holding the marker pen steady at this point. Let the brow drop and mark the forehead at this point. Usually, more skin is excised laterally than medially
- Be aware of position of the supraorbital neurovascular bundle medially. Dissection

here should remain subcutaneous before transitioning deeper laterally
- In patients with facial nerve palsy, the tissues can be anchored to the periosteum (although this may cause some discomfort and accentuate lagophthalmos)

Other less commonly used options include:

- Endotine lift: These are absorbable plates with hooks that are fixed onto the cranium in the subperiosteal plane. The periosteum is hooked on at the appropriate level, providing strong fixation. They come in versions for the lateral brow that are introduced through a upper blepharoplasty incision and versions for the anterior hairline designed for use in a full browlift. They may suffer from palpability, slippage and are expensive
- Gull wing lift
- Midforehead: Only considered if the patient has very deep forehead creases, otherwise the scar is very obvious. It shifts the hairline down that may be a desirable side effect in selected cases
- Temporal lift: This lateral eyebrow lift gives a typical feline look. An incision in the hairy temple allows limited access to the midface sufficient to provide an element of a cheek lift. It cannot be used to correct frown lines
- Limited incision: Lateral hairline incisions are used to access the subperiosteal plane to the lateral brow. It can be combined with blepharoplasty incisions for muscle resection

Postoperative

Some swelling, numbness and headache are to be expected. Endoscopic lifts have fewer symptoms and faster recovery times that is usually a week. A head-up sleeping position aids swelling.

- Infection and bleeding are uncommon complications
- Hair may not grow at the scar site. Peri-incisional hair loss is temporary if it occurs. Scar stretching may occur
- Loss of sensation is common but temporary. Itchiness may be a problem

Further reading

Codner MA, Kikkawa DO, Korn BS, et al.
Blepharoplasty and brow lift. Plast Reconstr Surg
2010; 126:e1–17.

Related topic of interest

- Blepharoplasty

Burn dressings

Much has been written about the desirable properties for the 'perfect dressing', but unfortunately this does not exist. A good dressing should offer:

1. • Protection from further harm, such as from desiccation, infection or mechanical trauma
2. • Promotion of healing
   - Promotes natural autolysis of the eschar (proteolysis and phagocytosis)
   - Provides an optimally moist environment that simultaneously avoids desiccation while capable with absorbing excess exudate to avoid maceration
3. • Pain relief

First aid and dressings

Cooling a burn for at least 10 minutes is beneficial if performed within the first hour of injury. It has been demonstrated to reduce acidosis (lactate production), oedema (histamine release), vascular occlusion (thromboxane release) and pain. Outside of the 1-hour time window, only analgesic benefit persists and cooling may be continued for this sole reason.

Cooling should be restricted in the patient with large burns due to the risk of hypothermia. The traditional adage of cooling the burn while warming the patient applies. First aid dressings need only to be clean (and not necessarily sterile) and moist (primarily to reduce pain). Cling film is a useful and readily available temporary dressing in the assessment phase. Antiseptics or antimicrobials should be avoided at this stage.

Although the heat has a sterilisation effect (Table 12), burn wounds are susceptible to infection due to:

- Compromise to the skin barrier function
- The presence of necrotic tissue in the eschar
- Use of invasive devices and procedures in burn management
- Immunosuppression (both cellular and humoral)

The most common organisms involved are *Pseudomonas aeruginosa* and *Staphylococcus aureus*. Toxic shock syndrome (TSS), a consequence of TSS toxin-producing S. aureus, is rare but severe, especially in children. MRSA infection complicates antimicrobial therapy and poses additional risks to adjacent patients if not isolated. There is little role for prophylactic antibiotics as they do not reduce mortality and promote resistance in this situation. Antibiotics should be restricted to therapeutic indications only.

The onset of severe infection may manifest in atypical and subtle ways. Signs include sudden tachypnoea, hypotension, spiking fevers, tachycardia, ileus, thrombocytopaenia, hypothermia and low leukocyte counts. Local wound changes such as a boggy eschar, cellulitis or the formation of unhealthy granulations should be sought.

A biofilm is an aggregate of microorganisms that are both adherent to each other and to a surface. They are frequently embedded in a self-produced extracellular polymeric substance (EPS) matrix. Biofilms are ubiquitous and may form on living or dead surfaces. Biofilms are an adaptive phenotypical expression that confers greater survivability for microorganisms in adverse conditions, working together as a group. Biofilms are emerging as an important cause of resistance to treatment, and thus are an important target.

Blisters

The management of burn blisters is somewhat open to debate. The only consensus is that ruptured blisters, blisters in which rupture is imminent and functionally compromising blisters are universally debrided. The proponents for preserving intact blisters argue that they provide a naturally moist wound environment for healing and that wound exposure to air is painful. The arguments for debridement include accurate assessment of burn depth, minimisation of non-viable tissue, and prevention of further blister fluid hydrodissection thus limiting the size of the blister. The literature is equivocal and contradictory for the benefits of blister fluid. It is common practice is most burn units for blisters to be debrided.

Definitive dressings

Regimes are very variable and dictated largely by local preferences as high-quality comparative studies are lacking. The two basic aims of burns dressing are to reduce the risk of infection and to optimise healing. To achieve this, the dressing protocol can be adjusted in terms of following:

- Reducing infection by regular thorough cleaning balanced against maximising healing by minimal disturbance to the delicate re-epithelialising wound
  - Analgesia, including opiates, should be given before dressing changes
  - Warm tap water and soap can be used in simple burns. Sterility is not essential. Sterile saline for irrigation or chlorhexidine can be used for larger, deeper burns
- The type of dressing material used

Types of dressings

There is an extremely wide choice of dressings available for burns including:

- Basic dressings such as gauze and tulle
- Occlusive dressings
- Antimicrobials
- Biological dressings

Basic dressings

These absorb exudate and keep the wound dry. The earliest dressings were made of plain cloth. Cotton wool in its native state is non-absorbent due to surface oils. Bleaching increases its absorbency. Gamgee is cotton wool sandwiched in gauze (after Dr. Joseph Sampson Gamgee, Birmingham).

The biggest problem with simple dressings is their propensity to adhere to the wound. When gauze is impregnated with paraffin oil, this adherence is reduced. Dressings such as *tulle gras* are an example (named after Tulle, France, famous for nets). There are a variety of tulle preparations with impregnated antiseptics and antibacterials that are in common use:

- Bactigras (0.5% chlorhexidine)
- Sofra Tulle (framycetin)
- Fucidin Intertulle (fusidic acid)
- Xeroform (3% bismuth tribromophenate)

Types of antiseptic

- Chlorhexidine is a good antiseptic (destroys or inhibits the growth of micro-organisms in/on living tissue) that acts by membrane disruption (rather than ATPase inhibition which was an alternate theory). It is onset of action is quick (20 seconds) but short lasting (about 6 hours) and is inactivated by organic matter. It is less useful as an antimicrobial agent but has wide activity against both gram negative and positive organisms and some fungi. It is ineffective against AFB and spores
- Povidone-iodine
- EUSOL (Edinburgh University solution) is sodium hypochlorite buffered to neutral pH with boric acid. It is no longer available due to concerns with toxicity and is historical

Occlusive dressings

Moist wounds were found to heal quicker (George Winter) and with less inflammation in 1962. Occlusive dressings maintain wound moisture and are less painful than non-occlusive dressings. They are popular with patients, as they need not be changed daily and are comfortable. This is a heterogeneous group of materials with their own advantages and disadvantages:

- Hydrocolloids
- Alginates (derived from seaweed) form a gel when moistened and also have haemostatic properties that make it useful as a dressing for skin graft donor sites
- Hydrofibres such as Aquacel
- Gels and foams

Antimicrobials

- Non-silver: e.g. Bactroban (mupirocin), neomycin and bacitracin. Sulfamylon (mafenide acetate) is formulated as a cream with a broad-spectrum action. Its excellent tissue penetration, especially cartilage, makes it useful for burns of the ear and nose. It has relatively poor activity against gram negatives and has limited activity against *Staphylococci,* including MRSA. Its short duration of action necessitates twice daily application and it can be painful (attributed to the high osmolarity). Its inhibition of carbonic anhydrase may cause alkaline diuresis and a hyperchloraemic metabolic acidosis. The 5% solution formulation is less painful than the 10% cream and can be used to wet gauze soaks every 6–8 hours. Five per cent of patients using Sulfamylon will develop a rash

- Silver: Silver nitrate was found to significantly reduce infection rates in burns patients, in particular *Pseudomonas aeruginosa,* since the 1950s. Silver ions have a proven broad-spectrum antimicrobial action but it is also cytotoxic to keratinocytes and fibroblasts. The low silver concentrations in therapeutic preparations are selectively taken up by microorganisms and concentrated, resulting in protein, nucleic acid and mitochondrial disruption. There have been no descriptions of resistance to silver reported to date. Agyria (the permanent grey discolouration of tissues including the skin due to silver deposition) used to be a complication of silver treatment particularly ingested health remedies (Rosemary Jacobs is the archetypal case) but it is certainly much less common with modern silver products

Silver nitrate

Silver nitrate (0.5%) is cheap but its application is labour-intensive as

reapplication or rewetting needs to be performed every 2 hours to maintain adequate therapeutic concentrations. It also stains tissues a troublesome black colour, which if washed off, shortens the duration of action. As it needs to be made up with distilled water, it may cause electrolyte loss due to its hypotonicity. Methaemoglobinaemia due to the nitrate moiety has been reported in rare cases

Silver sulphadiazine (Flamazine)

Silver sulphadiazine was developed in the 1960s (Fox) and remains the standard burn dressing. It has a good action against gram negatives (better than silver nitrate) and gram positives including *Pseudomonas aeruginosa* and *Staphylococci,* although sporadic resistance to *Pseudomonas* and *Enterobacter* has been reported. There is minimal pain when applied.

Silver sulphadiazine forms a pseudoeschar over the wound bed that may hinder depth assessment. It is thus used only after the treatment decision is made. It is also an option when excision is unsuitable. Its burn eschar penetration is poor and may exacerbate scarring by promoting inflammation at the eschar interface. The increase in vascularity associated with its use increases surgical blood loss. There has been a movement away from SSD recently.

- Systemic absorption of SSD may lead to toxicity and leukopaenia (5–15%). The latter is rarely profound and usually resolves in a few days despite its continued use
- Five per cent of patients develop a rash

Table 12 Typical bacteria present in a burn wound vary according to the timing in relation to the injury	
Stage of burn wound	**Bacteria present**
Preburn	*Staphylococcus epidermis* and some *Staphylococcus aureus* Diphtheroids
Burn	Sterile or normal flora in smaller numbers
Days after	Gram positive especially *S aureus*
Weeks after	Gram negative: *Proteus, Escherichia coli, Klebsiella* *Pseudomonas* less common Anaerobes uncommon

- Methaemoglobinaemia is rare acute haemolytic anaemia that has been reported after SSD use in patients with G6PDH deficiency. It is relatively contraindicated in infants (particularly premature) due to risk of kernicterus from the sulphonamide moiety

SSD is unsuitable for the face but is useful for awkward areas such as the perineum or the hands. Alternative antimicrobials such as Bactroban can be used but are significantly more costly and breed resistance. A recent Cochrane review concluded that SSD has no role in superficial or partial thickness burns and recommend other dressings, e.g. hydrocolloid, silicon nylon, antimicrobial, polyurethane and biosynthetic dressings.

- Flammacerium is SSD with cerium nitrate and its perceived advantage over SSD comes from its ability to form a firm eschar with less inflammation. Cerium is a rare earth metal that displaces calcium ions. However, how this action relates to its activity is unclear. It is bacteriostatic. Flammacerium hardens the burn to a green-yellow eschar with a leathery consistency that is adherent to the underlying wound (as opposed to SSD which tends to macerate the wound)
  - Severe side effects are rare, although a stinging sensation is reported with its use. Toxicity is low but like SSD, there is a risk of methaemoglobinaemia
- Silvazine (Smith and Nephew) consists of SSD with 0.2% chlorhexidine added to improve its antimicrobial action. It works against MRSA but the chlorhexidine may be cytotoxic and carries a risk of sensitisation

A wide variety of silver dressings are available. A Cochrane review in 2010 found insufficient evidence to recommend the use of silver dressings for infected or chronic contaminated wounds.

- Acticoat is a nanocrystalline (greater surface area) silver-impregnated dressing that aims to deliver silver ions continuously to the wound. The dressing needs to be kept moist by sterile water. The frequency of dressing changes can be reduced to once every 3 days, but it is expensive

- Aquacel silver is a hydrofibre dressing that aims to reduce silver toxicity by absorbing bacteria along with wound exudate into the dressing where the silver ions act, instead of releasing silver ions into the wound

Biological dressings

The term "biological dressings' is preferable to 'skin substitutes' as in most cases, they are not incorporated into the wound and are thus temporary. Cadaveric skin is regarded as the gold standard but its wider use is hampered by the general lack of donors. The rejection response is delayed by burn-mediated in major burns patients.

- In viable cadaveric skin, rejection occurs as the graft perfuses and the graft antigens and graft Langerhans cells are exposed to the recipient that activates the immune response that destroys the graft over a period of 7–14 days. Long-term graft survival requires life-long immunosuppression

Xenograft dressings are readily available reasonable substitutes and porcine skin is most biocompatible due to the highest homology with human skin. Amniotic membranes and dressings made from plant material, e.g. banana leaf and potato skin, have also been described in the developing world.

- Porcine skin tends to adhere (related to fibrin-collagen interaction) rather than take and does not revascularise to a significant extent (there may be some ingrowth). Ejection rather than rejection occurs as there are no second set reactions. Thus they are most accurately described as collagen dressings instead of true xenografts. Such dressings are good at relieving pain and have a nonspecific antibacterial action that is related to adherence. Non-viable cadaveric skin behaves similarly. Small portions of biological dressings may be incorporated into wounds but will remodel rapidly

The uses of biological dressings include:

- Coverage of partial-thickness wounds to promote natural healing

- Coverage of debrided wounds while waiting for autograft
- Coverage of widely meshed autografts to keep interstices moist (sandwich grafting or Alexander technique)

Enzymatic dressings

These are a separate class of burns dressings in that they offer a chemical debridement of the burn wound. It is not a novel idea but early enzymatic dressings worked slowly and required frequent changes (e.g. Varidase needs twice daily application, Iruxol Mono – clostridial collagenase is used daily). Newer dressings act more quickly, e.g. Debridase/ Nexobrid (Bromelain derived from pineapples) removes 90% of the burns eschar in 4 hours, but it is not widely available.

'Typical' dressing regimes

- Superficial partial thickness burns will heal quickly regardless and hence there is little to choose from between the different dressing types. Whilst tulle gras (Jelonet) is the simplest and cheapest option, moist wound healing provided by occlusive dressings and biological dressings are more comfortable and less cumbersome. Antimicrobials are not necessary
- The burn wound is exudative in the first 48 hours, thus tulle gras with an absorbent dressing may be used first, followed by either occlusive dressings or skin substitutes
- Mixed/intermediate-depth wounds with significant eschar require dressing regimes that balance the risk of infection against the risk of desiccation. The common options are either an occlusive dressing with non-silver antimicrobial or a silver-based cream or dressing
- Full-thickness burns require excision and grafting, but can be dressed with antimicrobials (silver or non-silver) until surgery

Further reading

Leon-Villapalos J. The use of human deceased donor skin allograft in burn care. Cell and Tissue Banking 2010; 11:99–104.

Related topics of interest

- Acute burns
- Burns surgery

Burns surgery

The surgical management of the burn patient is determined to a large extent by the depth of the burn wound.

- A full thickness burn requires excision and skin replacement unless very small
- A superficial partial thickness burn or less will heal spontaneously within 7–10 days

The challenge arises in burns of intermediate depth. On one hand early excision may sacrifice tissue areas that may otherwise have healed spontaneously. If left to heal with a prolonged period, the risk of infection, hypertrophic scarring and contracture may outweigh the former. A balance must thus be struck between the two. Waiting for intermediate areas to declare its final depth may be weighed against any additional systemic, functional and cosmetic impairment, compared to early surgery. An assessment based on the individual patient must be made.

In general, surgery is considered to expedite healing if the anticipated healing time exceeds 3 weeks. Skin graft healing is achieved in 5–7 days on average.

Early surgery

The arguments for early surgery are:

- Removal of the source of inflammatory mediators in the burn eschar. A burn toxin was shown to exist by injecting sterile burnt skin into the abdomens of healthy mice resulting in an 80% mortality rate
- Removal of a potential site of infection by early wound closure

Zora Janzekovic pioneered early tangential burn excision in the 1950s resulting in a mortality reduction and less bleeding. In addition, reduced sepsis, a shorter hospital stay and reduced costs have been demonstrated since. There is however, no consensus on the exact definition of 'early', although 3–5 days is the accepted norm. In general, one should aim to operate:

- As soon as the patient is stable enough
- Before the wound is colonised (prior to day 5). Excision prior to the 48-hour mark has been shown to reduce wound colonisation and infection
- Before the hyperaemic stage (haemorrhage reduction)

A slight delay to surgery may be indicated in cases of intermediate or mixed depth burns, especially in children.

Surgery

Heat loss during surgery is a potential problem as burnt skin loses its thermoregulatory function and operative exposure increases evaporative losses. The patient temperature must be monitored and the ambient temperature increased. Warming blankets and additional heaters may be necessary.

Blood loss is affected by the method of excision.

- Tangential excision of eschar. The aim is to gradually shave off only the non-viable layers and maximise the preservation of viable skin. The end-point is punctate bleeding of the residual tissue. Bleeding may be significant but can be reduced by:
  - Selective cautery and adrenaline-soaked gauzes (1 in 1-2,000,000)
  - Preoperative tissue infiltration with adrenaline solution
  - Excision under tourniquet control. This may however hinder judgement of the burn depth
  - Pressure bandaging and elevation
  - If skin grafting is to be used, rapid application of the skin grafts. The skin graft is haemostatic
- Fascial excision: Full-thickness or infected wounds can be excised along with subcutaneous tissue down to the fascia. Blood loss is greatly reduced and graft take is good at the expense of poor cosmesis and an increased risk of lymphoedema
- Chemical debridement (see 'Burns Dressings')
- Versajet hydrosurgery (Smith and Nephew) is a recent innovation that utilises pressurised saline to debride wounds. The adjustable pressure settings allow depth control. The handpiece is passed across the surface of the burn in a back and forth motion until the desired depth is achieved. The debris is sucked

back into the handpiece simultaneously by the Venturi effect

Total burn excision should be performed where possible and particularly in young and fit adults without inhalational injury as there are psychological benefits in addition to the physiological. However, excision may be staged depending on local logistical support and the burn depth and size. Herndon (Texas) advocates excising a maximum of 20% surface area per sitting on days 1, 3 and 5 to limit blood loss and anaesthetic time. If burn excision is staged, the general order in a stable patient is:

- Hands and upper limbs
- Lower limbs
- Chest and back
- The face is usually left until last, except for the eyelids, which are a priority

These are not rigid rules and may be altered for logistical and physiological reasons. In large burns, the first priority is to eliminate the maximal amount of necrotic tissue with early wound coverage, thus wide areas such as the lower limb and trunk may be treated first. If limiting anaesthetic time is a priority, operating on areas that do not require turning the patient intraoperatively may be favourable. The number of surgeons available to operate simultaneously may also alter the sequence.

Hand burns

The hands are important for function (prehension and expressing emotions) and cosmesis. Hand burns may warrant aggressive surgery to maximise functional preservation. However, studies comparing early surgery to conservative treatment combined with vigorous physiotherapy have demonstrated similar functional results. More aggressive therapy may reduce scarring particularly in those with pigmented skin.

- Palmar skin is thick and is usually protected by reflex closure, thus rarely needing grafting. Burn oedema on the dorsum can limit MCPJ flexion and thumb adduction, as this is the position of comfort. This not the position of function and is at high risk of developing stiffness
- As such, it is vital to splint the hand in the position of function with the MCPJ in 70°

of flexion, the interphalangeal joints (IPJs) extended, the thumb abducted and wrist in 20° of extension

- When surgery is required, wider sheet grafts (reducing the number of seams) are preferred. Early inspection is performed on Day 4 and early mobilisation initiated to reduce oedema
  - Decompression may be necessary to treat vascular compromise caused by circumferential burn eschars or excessive fluid resuscitation
  - Very small areas of exposed tendon or bone may be allowed to granulate, while maintaining motion. Larger defects should be covered formally with flaps, buried or temporised

Wound closure

The mainstay of large area wound closure is split thickness skin grafting. The increasing problem of finding sufficient donor sites for coverage is a measure of the improvement in major burn survival.

Meshing

Meshing a SSG places holes at regular intervals, which does the following:

- Increases the surface area that can be covered, and thus reduces the donor area required.
- Allows drainage of exudate and trapped air bubbles that may otherwise collect and reduce graft take.
- Improves graft conformity to the contours of the wound, especially on concavities.

The mesh pattern persists after healing and thus sheet grafts are preferred for areas where cosmesis is paramount. Wide mesh ratio (>1:6) SSGs expose the interstices between the skin bridges and may desiccate before re-epithelialisation from the sides can occur. Such widely meshed skin grafts may be covered with a sheet allograft onlay (sandwich technique) with or without cultured keratinocytes to protect the interstices from desiccation.

When there are insufficient donor sites,

- Temporary dressings may be used for the debrided wound whilst waiting for the donor to heal before recropping. Recropping is limited by the residual dermal thickness, as the dermis does not regenerate. Dressing choices include cadaveric skin, porcine skin or Biobrane (silicone covering a nylon mesh with porcine collagen)

- Skin substitutes may be used where skin is in short supply and aims to replace or substitute skin permanently. They may be epidermal, dermal or composite (types I, II and III respectively). The term skin substitute is often misused and incorrectly applied to biological dressings that are temporary
  - Type II (collagen prostheses)
    - Integra is a bilaminate skin substitute that consists of a bovine collagen matrix that is cross-linked with bovine (no longer shark) chondroitin-6-sulphate (pseudodermis) and a silicone covering (pseudoepidermis). The matrix degrades slowly and acts as a template for neodermis formation following the ingrowth of fibroblasts and endothelial cells. The silicone covering is substituted with an ultrathin SSG when the matrix has taken. It is susceptible to infection prior to this and must be monitored closely, with areas of early infection deroofed to permit drainage. Integra is expensive and there is no evidence of survival benefit with its use in burns. The potential for slow revascularisation allows Integra usage over small portions of avascular structures such as bone, cartilage and irradiated structures
  - Type III
    - Apligraf is neonatal dermal (foreskin) fibroblast and keratinocyte seeded onto bovine Type 1 collagen. In contrast to in vitro experiments, its in vivo role is more of a wound modulator with a proven role in healing venous ulcers
- Cultured keratinocytes: Patient keratinocytes can be cultured (Type I, Rheinwald and Green 1975) from a 2×2 cm skin biopsy sample. Cultured epidermal autograft (CEA) can be used in sheet form or as cellular suspensions (faster and most commonly used). The take of CEA is unpredictable (50–70% in burns) due to susceptibility to infection and collagenase digestion. Even when successful, the resultant skin is fragile and prone to blistering as it lacks rete pegs found in mature dermal-epidermal junctions

Other specific areas

- Ear: Chondritis should be treated aggressively with debridement to minimise deformity. Mafenide is particularly useful in this area. Avoid bulky dressings and use soft pillows
- Eyelids: Skin grafts may be used but further functional surgery often needed
- Perineal burns: Usually managed conservatively
- Lower limb: Foot burns are treated aggressively due to the high risk of infection

The postoperative care and rehabilitation is as important, if not more so, than the actual surgery in determining the final patient outcome.

Further reading

Robert N. The scalp as a donor site for split thickness skin graft: a rare complication case report. J Plast Reconstr Aesthet Surg 2011; 64:e118–20.

Related topics of interest

- Acute burns
- Burns dressings
- Burn reconstruction
- Leg ulcers
- Skin grafts
- Tissue expansion
- Vacuum wound closure

Burn reconstruction

The population demand for burns reconstruction is inversely related to the quality of the acute burn care services.

Timing

A sensible approach is crucial. The opposing factors of allowing scar maturation must be weighed against the likelihood of functional compromise if surgery is delayed. Emergency and essential cases require rapid access to surgery and do not pose timing dilemmas. A useful approach for the non-clear-cut cases is a trial of conservative treatment with failure to progress or reaching a plateau in benefit as potential points to consider surgery, if suitable.

- Emergency: Waiting for scar maturation is not appropriate when vital structures such as the eyes are exposed, or when patient's health is compromised such as in entrapment of major nerves or severe microstomia
- Essential: These comprise procedures that if performed early, will improve the patient's final appearance and rehabilitation. Examples include progressive contractures that fail to respond to therapy, or those that prevent performance of activities of daily living
- Elective: This is the largest category and most often related to uncomfortable or aesthetically unpleasant scarring

Prevention/reduction of scar

- Optimise healing with appropriate dressings and timely surgery
- Use medium thickness sheet grafts for cosmetic units in face or hands, with seams across tension lines and transversely over joints
- Avoid crossing joints in a straight line. Use darts to break up the linear edge with grafts and in escharotomies
- Early pressure garment therapy, appropriate use of splints and silicone. Encourage early ambulation and physiotherapy to maximise range of movement

Acute rehabilitation

Joint capsular contracture and tendon shortening will occur if joints are kept immobile for a prolonged period.

- Even in the critically ill, passive ranging should be done twice daily if possible, coinciding with dressing changes with additional analgesia as required. Preserving the existing range with splints that are regularly inspected for fit and potential pressure injury prevents contractures and deformities
- During recovery, rehabilitation consists of passive and active ranging, muscle strengthening exercises and oedema minimisation (with elastic garments, elevation and massage). Activities of daily living (ADL) exercises are focused on a return to one's normal functioning state at work, school or play. If possible, coordinate surgery to allow passive ranging under GA. Continued motivation and encouragement is paramount in the post-discharge period to maintain the progress already achieved

Scar management

Hypertrophic scarring is more likely to occur in wounds that exceed a healing time of 2–3 weeks. Areas with thin elastic skin such as the neck, chest and lower face are prone to distortion, as are areas over joints where constant stretching occurs. Ethnic predisposition compounds this. Helpful strategies include

- Massage: This also helps to reduce dryness when emollients are used
- Pressure garments: Compliance is crucial and adjustments are made to maintain good fit
- Silicone: Available in a sheet (Cica-care) or gel form (Dermatix). Silicone works by reducing transepidermal water loss (TEWL). It seems that keratinocyte dehydration induces the release of pro-fibrotic cytokines such as IL-1beta that [IL 1B] stimulate TGF-beta and fibroblast activity [TGF β]

as well as downregulation of antifibrotic TNF-alpha. The gel form benefits from increased patient compliance/tolerance with fewer side effects such as irritation from occlusion

- Steroid injection
- Surgery: For functional restoration only with adjuvant measures to reduce its recurrence

Burns contracture

Contractures may be subdivided as follows:

- Intrinsic contracture: Contracture of the involved structure itself. Examples include lid shortening from an eyelid contracture. Intrinsic contractures may require release of the intrinsic structure involved or its formal reconstruction
- Extrinsic contracture: Contracture of an adjacent structure that pulls indirectly on the affected structure. Examples include cheek scarring causing ectropion of the lower eyelid. Extrinsic contractures may be treated with surgical release of the contracted structure

Management

Serial casting may be useful for a subset of contractures but the mainstay of treatment remains surgery. Upon release, the resultant tissue deficiency may be treated with local tissue import techniques, (Z-plasties and their variations), skin grafting with or without skin substitutes, tissue expansion or free tissue transfer. When patients are assessed, formulate an inventory of potential donor sites for these techniques in anticipation of reconstruction.

Specific areas

Neck contractures Neck contractures pose a functional and cosmetic deformity. The functional disability is proportional to the degree of neck extension present and can be graded as follows:

- E1: Unable to see objects above the level of the head
- E2: The patient needs to tilt body backwards to make eye contact
- E3: The patient adopts a stooped posture and persistent upward gaze due to severe mentosternal synechiae

Anatomical classifications of neck contracture describe its location (superior/inferior, left/right, complete/incomplete). The upper neck contributes most to neck extension and priority should be given to this area with contracture release when limited tissue is available for reconstruction. Reconstructive options include:

- Full thickness skin grafts from abdomen, which may be pre-expanded depending on the amount of tissue needed
- Flaps: While not first choice, previously burnt skin can be incorporated into the flap. Assumptions of increased complication rates have not been borne out in studies and clinical experience
  - Pedicled flaps
  - The transverse cervical artery flap is based on branches of the transverse cervical artery that originate in the triangle formed by the posterior edge of sternomastoid, external jugular vein (EJV) and clavicle. The flap territory runs from its origin to the shoulder tip and is sufficient to reach the chin.
  - The trapezius flap is based on the descending branch of transverse cervical artery that runs between sternomastoid and levator scapulae and descends between the scapula and midline, along the trapezial undersurface. The flap is raised with part of the muscle. Adequate length is achieved by designing the flap markings to the iliac crest that yields flap dimensions of 40×10 cm
  - Thin free flaps of adequate size are required. Perforator based flaps such as the ALT are commonly used but may require thinning in selected patients

Axillary contractures Contractures of the axilla typically cause an adduction deformity and can be classified by the extent of involvement:

- IA Anterior axillary fold
- IB Posterior axillary fold
- II Both folds
- III Both folds and the axillary dome

Type I and II contractures can usually be dealt with by release and skin grafting. Type III contractures require large amounts of tissue in the form of local parascapular (including bilobed), LD or free flaps.

Hands The reconstructive goal in the burnt hand is to restore basic prehension, especially tip and key pinch, grasp and opposition.

Late complications of deep burns of the hand, particularly those involving significant amounts of soft tissue and joint damage, are difficult to treat. The most common hand late deformities are syndactyly, volar digital contracture, Boutonnière deformity and dorsal skin deficiency. Its treatment requires adequate assessment of the skeleton, joints, tendons and overlying tissue cover. However, extensive scarring frequently makes it difficult to distinguish the source of the pathology encountered. In these situations, the full assessment may only be completed intra-operatively.

Stiffness is the commonest problem in the burnt hand and is most commonly joint-related.

- Early phase stiffness (before 6 weeks) may be treated non-surgically with aggressive mobilisation
- Late stiffness is stiffness that persists (after 6 weeks) despite vigorous regime of joint mobilisation. Surgical joint treatment may be considered only if the intrinsic muscles are working
  - For functional joints, tenolysis is performed and the joints held in the position of function with K-wires
  - In the presence of an intrinsically immobile joint, tenolysis and skin release is futile
  - Thin flaps may be considered when there is a reasonable expectation of improved function. Flaps with a fascial base, such as the lateral arm flap, may have a theoretical advantage in facilitating tendon gliding

Burn syndactyly most commonly affects the first web. There is usually web reversal with the dorsal web being more distal than the volar web. Thumb abduction is limited. Treatment options typically include flaps that incorporate multiple Z-plasties, such as the jumping man and four-flap plasty. Contractures may occur in other areas:

- Elbow: Flexion contractures of the elbow may be associated with heterotropic ossification in the triceps tendon
- Foot: Dorsum involvement may lift the toes off the ground, causing a change in gait
- Popliteal: These may interfere with walking
- Hip contractures are more common in infants and the young

Burn itch

Pruritus or itch is a common complaint that is poorly understood but is often used as a marker of scar maturation. It is more common in burns of the lower limbs and burns that have a healing time that exceeds 3 weeks. Pruritus starts at the time of healing, peaks at the 2–6 month point and may be persistent (29% at 4 years and 5% at 12 years). C fibres that may be functionally distinct from the traditional C-pain fibres transmit itch. The pruritogenic substances involved are not limited to histamine. They include serotonin, proteases, kinins and neuropeptides.

Pruritis is difficult to consistently treat and this is reflected in the myriad therapeutic options. The overall evidence base for its treatment is scanty.

- Clinical psychologists may help by imparting coping strategies to patients
- The commonest first line treatment is an antihistamine in combination with:
  - Emollients: For example, simple moisturisers and aloe vera
  - Pressure garments (thought to decrease histamine release)
  - Opioids and sedatives, as required
- A typical regime is a non-sedative antihistamine during day and a sedative one at night, such as chlorpheniramine

Second line strategies have a less predictable effect. As such, a prudent choice would be one that is simple and has few side effects. These include massage, silicone, transcutaneous electrical neural stimulation (TENS) and capsaicin cream. There is evidence to suggest pulsed dye lasers (PDL) may improve itching when used to address scar redness.

Third line strategies have a greater potential effect at the price of greater potential side effects. These include:

- Topical anaesthetics (EMLA), antihistamines or steroids (skin thins due to inhibition of collagen production)
- H1 and H2 antagonists: Some synergy between the two has been reported. Doxepin or dothiepin, both tricyclic antidepressants, may exert an effect due to their affinity for both H1 and H2 receptors in addition to muscarinic receptors
- Gabapentin may be effective but may cause behavioural problems in children

Further reading

Gheita A, Moftah A, Hosny H. Strategies in the management of post-burn breast deformities. Eur J Plast Surg 2014;37:85–94.

Related topics of interest

- Eyelid reconstruction
- Scalp reconstruction

Chemical burns

Chemical burns account for <5% of burn unit admissions. They are usually either accidental or victims of assault. The severity of a burn depends on:

- Nature and concentration of the agent
- Contact time *Contact time*

In the Western world, industrial exposure frequently involves high concentrations of chemical agents but the injuries tend to be relatively minor due to the greater awareness and the availability of appropriate first-aid. In contrast, accidental exposure at home or post-assault exposure tends to lead to prolonged contact and severe damage, due to under appreciation of the condition. Chemical burns can be categorised as follows:

- Acid
- Alkali
- Organic compounds such as hydrocarbons
- Extravasation injuries

First aid

Always take care to protect yourself.
- Remove the chemical from the patient including contaminated clothing. Immediately irrigate with cool water to dilute the chemical. There is no upper limit on irrigation as long as body temperature is maintained. Running water, as opposed to soaks, are preferred as it dissipates the thermochemical gradient more efficiently. Be aware of the potential damage that the run-off can cause. Wound pain and pH can be used to guide the adequacy of treatment
- Neutralisation of an acid or alkali is not recommended as the exothermic reaction of neutralisation may add or exacerbate a thermal component to the chemical burn. There are animal studies that do not support this. The 5% acetic acid neutralisation of sodium hydroxide burns has been shown in animal studies to reduce dermal damage without an increase in skin temperature. In practice, however, the identity of the chemical is not always known nor is it likely to be pure. Studies with amphoteric polyvalent chemical structures such as Diphoterine show rapid effects without exothermic

reactions; although such products are rather costly but are being used in the industrial sector.

There are certain situations in which water should be avoided:
- Reactive metals such as sodium and potassium undergo violent exothermic reactions when in contact with water, forming highly concentrated alkalis. Such burns should be covered with oil and gently wiped away *oil*
- The penetration of phenol may increase when irrigated with water. Polyethylene glycol wipes are a better alternative *Carbolic acid*
- White phosphorous is the least stable allotrope of phosphorous. It is used in the manufacture of fireworks, ammunition and fertiliser. It is pyrophoric (self-igniting) when in contact with air and produces a characteristic garlic smell when ignited this way, leaving a phosphoric acid residue and a resultant thermochemical burn. White phosphorous rapidly turns yellow when exposed to light and fluoresces green in the dark. A 2% copper sulphate irrigation solution neutralises the phosphorous and turns them black, facilitating their removal. However, copper sulphate causes intravascular haemolysis, renal and cerebral toxicity and is no longer recommended in the US. Instead, a bicarbonate neutralisation of phosphoric acid followed by debridement of residual white phosphorous identified by fluorescence in the dark or emission of smoke in air is recommended (US Navy Manual FM8-285 Conventional Military Chemical Injuries). The burn is treated as a regular thermal burn afterwards

Further management

- Remove jewellery and trim fingernails
- Ophthalmological assessment for eye injuries. Thorough irrigation is required
- Monitor for local and systemic effects such as renal and liver failure. Arterial blood gas analysis may quickly reveal a metabolic acid-base disturbance. If necessary, contact the local poisons service for advice *ABG*

Acids

Coagulative necrosis

Acid burns generally cause coagulative necrosis by protein denaturation. This eschar limits penetration of the acid.

- Hydrochloric and sulphuric acids are found in toilet cleaners
- Formic acid is found in descalers and leaves a burn with a typical green colour
- Hydrofluoric acid is found in cleaning agents and is used in glass etching

Hydrofluoric acid

The toxicity of HF arises predominantly from the fluoride ion instead of the acidic proton. There is intense pain with progressive destruction of soft tissue by liquefactive necrosis (an acid that behaves like an alkali) that allows progressive penetration of the lipid-rich skin and subcutaneous tissue. Skin changes may be delayed by up to 24 hours with more dilute solutions (0–20%).

The systemic effects are caused by the calcium (and magnesium) ion chelation by the fluoride ion causing decalcification of bone, acidosis, hypocalcaemia and arrhythmias (with long QT interval). The classical symptoms of hypocalcaemia (tetany, Chvostek and Trousseau signs) are typically absent. As such, even small burns can be fatal. The ion also has direct effects including inhibition of cellular enzymes, vasodilatation and cardiac depression.

Treatment: The mainstay of treatment of HF burns is chelation of the fluoride ion with calcium administered in various forms. Pain is an important guide to the effectiveness of treatment.

- The risk of systemic toxicity increases with size of the burn (> 5% BSA, any concentration) and concentration (> 1% BSA if > 50% concentration). Due to a delay in symptom presentation, a decision to treat based on burn size and concentration alone is made.

IV
20 ml
Ca gluconate

- Intravenous bolus calcium gluconate (20 ml in 1 litre of crystalloid) can be given. Supplemental intravenous fluids may be required as calcium administration causes polyuria
  - ECG monitoring
  - Inhalation or ingestion is rare but can be treated by nebulised and oral calcium respectively. Inhalation of

fumes is a hazard if the concentration exceeds 60%

- Topical calcium gluconate gel (pre-packaged or made by mixing lubricating jelly with 10% calcium gluconate solution in a 4:1 ratio). Reapply every 30 minutes till pain is relieved
- Injection of the burn with 5% calcium gluconate at a dose of 0.5 ml/cm^2 using a fine needle. Note that calcium solutions themselves can cause extravasation injuries, although the risk is lower with the gluconate than the chloride
- **Infusion** of calcium gluconate intra-arterially or intravenously (in a Bier-type block) up to every 4 hours. Infusion is generally reserved for severe hand burns due to the high risk of complications

Alkali

Alkalis are the most common chemicals found in the home. They cause less immediate damage than acids but tend to cause more eventual destruction. The saponification of fat and protein denaturation with progressive liquefactive necrosis facilitates penetration.

- Sodium and potassium hydroxide are most common chemicals in domestic use and are present in many cleaning agents (oven cleaner, drain cleaner and bleach). They also generate significant heat of dilution (releases heat when diluted)
- Cement burns arise typically in the construction worker who ignores cement entering their boots. Cement is caustic (pH 12–13), but acts slowly, and thus presentation tends to be delayed. Calcium oxide (lime) reacts with water (sweat) generating significant heat of dissolution (releases heat when changing from one state to another) and also reacts chemically to form calcium hydroxide (slaked lime). The latter causes an alkali burn that is responsible for most of the damage

Miscellaneous

- Hydrocarbons: Some of these chemicals dissolve plasma membranes, causing superficial blistering. Systemic absorption of material may lead to respiratory depression, liver and renal failure. Phenol is a typical example

Surgery

A major problem in the management of chemical burns is the continued damage that can result in deep burns. When optimal irrigation is complete, allow demarcation to occur prior to surgery. Early excision and grafting in the presence of continuing chemical burns, may lead to graft failure. Serial debridement with grafting delayed until no further damage is seen is also a viable alternative.

Extravasation injuries

The vast majority (> 99%) recover without serious sequelae. Most damage is limited to the skin and functional deficits are very rare. Neonates are most commonly affected due to a combination of their immature skin, prolonged infusion requirements and inability to report pain. They typically occur on the extremities corresponding to the infusion sites. Types of agents:

- Hyperosmolar agents: E.g. 10% dextrose, contrast media, calcium solutions and TPN
- Cytotoxic agents: These can be hyperosmolar or vesicants
- Vasopressor agents

The incidence may be reduced by:

- Avoiding multiple punctures of the same vein
- Avoiding perfusion under pressure.
- Siting puncture sites in clearly visible areas and inspecting them regularly
- Consider central venous access if more than 5 days of infusion is required

Management

There are few controlled studies in humans, but RCT animal studies have demonstrated the efficacy of hyaluronidase injection (but efficacious only within 12 hours, and ideally within 1 hour) and saline irrigation (but only if performed before necrosis is evident). A typical management protocol is:

First aid: Stop infusion immediately, and with the cannula in place, aspirate fluid if possible. Remove cannula, cover with occlusive dressing and elevate the limb. Consult plastic surgeons urgently. There is no consistency regarding cooling or warming of extravasation injuries. Vasoconstrictive cooling increases the toxicity of vinca-alkaloids while vasodilatory warming increases the toxicity of doxorubicin.

It is difficult to predict which injuries will proceed to necrosis and subsequent functional and cosmetic deficit. Pain, erythema and blanching are poor predictors, although induration persisting for > 24 hours is a marginally better predictor. Early debridement and skin grafting is thus not generally recommended.

Early saline irrigation of the extravasated wound with or without liposuction decreases the complication rate compared to conservative treatment.

- Extensive soft tissue destruction reduced from 52% to 0%
- Minor blistering with delayed healing reduced from 33% to 11.5%
- No complication rate increased from 15% to 88.5%

This is a retrospective study (N=96). Almost all other studies are similarly retrospective with single digit study numbers. There are no randomised controlled trials that address this to date.

The irrigation protocol is:

- Infiltrate 500–1000 units of hyaluronidase subcutaneously
- Puncture skin at the four cardinal clock positions, directing blade towards the centre and in the subcutaneous plane
- Use a 22G cannula to infuse 200–500 ml normal saline through each puncture site, allowing outflow through the others
- Insert passive drains, cover with Jelonet, Betadine gauze and elevate
- Reassess 24 hours later. The incision sites are left to heal secondarily

For established necrosis, treatment consists of dressings with or without debridement.

Further reading

Donoghue AM. Diphoterine for alkali chemical splashes to the skin at alumina refineries. Int J Dermatol 2010;49:894–900.

Chest reconstruction

The commonest problems are fistulae, empyemas and chest wall defects. The general aims of chest reconstruction are

- Adequate resection with wide debridement and control of infection
- Obliteration of cavities
- Restoration of rigidity to reduce physiological flail
- Restoration of the pleural seal

Fistula

Treat this early before infection becomes established. The highest priority is establishing an airtight seal with vascularised tissue.

- Miller approach (1984): Use appropriate antibiotics and debride thoroughly via the original incision. The fistula is covered with muscle with the aim of filling the pleural space, using as many flaps as necessary
- Arnold and Pairolero approach (1996): Introduce a flap through second smaller thoracotomy, aiming only to only cover the fistula and not to completely obliterate the space. The space is left to close secondarily, aided with antibiotic instillation and chest drains

Empyema

The collection is evacuated either by a wide bore chest drain or open drainage followed by packing and dressings to achieve cavity closure by granulation. The general consensus is that the cavity does not need to be filled (actually very difficult to do) if it is clean.

- Space filling: The cavity dead-space is obliterated after it is sealed from the external environment. Choices are flaps of sufficient bulk that include pedicled LD, free contralateral LD or de-epithelialised TRAM flaps
- Space sterilising
  - Eloesser procedure (originally used to treat TB empyema): Marsupialise the cavity using a U-shaped skin flap folded into the pleural cavity to create

tract for drainage and packing. The bronchopleural fistula is thus converted to a bronchocutaneous one. Irrigation is performed through this open window for 8–10 months until the cavity is clean. It has an approximately 60% success rate. It was originally intended as a permanent one-stage procedure for patients unfit for a muscle flap but can be used with secondary closure in mind
  - Clagett procedure (3-stages): Open pleural drainage through an inferolateral window to allow continuous irrigation. Muscle flaps are used to cover bronchopleural fistulae. When the cavity is clean, it is filled with antibiotic solution and closed
- Space collapsing: A thoracoplasty is performed by removing the second to seventh ribs and the intercostal muscles are used to cover the fistulae. The resultant deformity is a problem

Chest wall defects

Reconstruction of a chest wall defect may be considered in its separate components, i.e. rigid support and vascularised soft tissue coverage. To a certain extent, the size of the defect guides the type of reconstruction, although there is no consensus:

- Absolute size: A defect of >5 cm is a commonly used threshold for reconstruction with support in the absence of symptoms
- Number of ribs: Two adjacent ribs can be resected without significant impact on the mechanics
- Symptomatic: Flail chest, pulmonary herniation, severe chest deformity

Smaller defects can usually be repaired with soft tissue alone but larger defects have the potential to cause inefficient ventilation through a large flail segment effect and thus require rigid support. Modifying factors include radiation that makes the chest tissues stiffer and thus more tolerant of larger defects.

Rigid support

Autologous

Bone grafts are an uncommon choice but the options are ribs, iliac crest and rarely tibia or fibula. They require good trabecular contact, otherwise little bone regrowth occurs and the resultant fibrous union provides insufficient support. Fascia has been used but it stretches over time, loses stability and is even less tolerant of infection.

Alloplastic

The successful use of Marlex and Prolene mesh has been demonstrated in large series with a low infection rate and adequate vascularised tissue mesh cover.

- Meshes
  - Marlex (polypropylene) is available in coarse or fine mesh. It may fragment
  - Prolene (polypropylene): A fine, double-weave mesh that is stiff in both planar directions, but tends to wrinkle more
  - Vicryl: A single weave absorbable mesh that is stiff in one planar direction and flexible in the other. Arguments for it are its absorbability avoids long-term mesh biofilm formation especially in infected wounds. Arguments against it are that the lack of permanence weakens the final construct and that meshes should not be placed into an infected cavity in the first place
  - Gore Tex (PTFE): These are relatively thick 2 mm sheets that do not conform easily. It is smoother and there is less tissue ingrowth and hence less incorporation. This also makes it more watertight and can be used to separate cavities. A variation of this is the Gore Dualmesh that has a textured surface on one side and a smooth surface on the other
- Metal: There is a significant of risk of erosion and extrusion that may be movement related
- MMA (methyl methacrylate) sandwich: MMA is a self-curing acrylic resin commonly available in paste form. On exposure to air, it solidifies with a strong exothermic reaction. It is commonly reinforced by combination with Marlex mesh. While the sandwich can be left implanted permanently, adequate strength from its capsule is achieved at 6–8 weeks if mesh removal is required. Preformed MMA implants are also available if intraoperative plasticity is not required.

Muscle cover

Muscle flaps (**Table 13**) alone are often satisfactory for small skeletal defects. There are many choices for local flaps, although availability will depend on previous incisions. A posterolateral scar may signal LD pedicle division whilst a subcostal incision may compromise the superior epigastric supply to RA.

- Pectoralis major (PM) is useful for sternal wounds, anterior chest defects and intrathoracic cover (with rib removal). It can be based on either thoracoacromial (transposition flap) or IMA perforators (turnover flap). The reach and volume of the latter may be limited. Bilateral PMs can be used for larger defects

Table 13 Types of muscle flaps available for chest reconstruction	
Type of muscle flap	**Muscle involved**
Anterior/anterolateral	Latissimus dorsi (LD), rectus abdominis (RA)
Sternal	Pectoralis major (PM), RA, LD, omentum
Posterior (uncommon)—upper	Trapezius
Posterior lower/lateral	LD turnover on intercostal and lumbar perforators Paraspinous LD with vein graft to elongate pedicle
Intrathoracic: Fistula, persistent air-leaks Great vessels, oesophagus	SA, LD, PM RA, omentum Thoracoplasty is rarely used

- Latissimus dorsi (LD) flaps can be used to reconstruct anterior and anterolateral chest defects. It has an extensive arc of rotation with a further 5 cm of length available after tendon division. The flap can also be turned over on the posterior intercostal and lumbar vessels to cover low paraspinal defects. If the thoracodorsal vessels have been transected, the proximal muscle may still be raised on the serratus anterior branches that perfuse the flap through retrograde flow. Pedicle exploration is necessary for this. Alternatively, the LD can be incorporated in a combination flap raised on the subscapular axis
- Serratus anterior (SA) is useful for intrathoracic defects but is rarely used alone for chest wall reconstruction due to its thinness. It can be combined with the LD for greater bulk. Only the inferior three muscle slips should be used to minimise donor morbidity

RA type III
- Rectus abdominis (RA) provides a long type III muscle flap with an option of an overlying large skin island either as a VRAM or TRAM. It has a wide arc of rotation and when pedicled superiorly it can reach the sternal notch. The distal end is least reliable when used in this way. The superior pedicle can still be used even after the internal mammary artery has been divided. The lower intercostal arteries (especially the 8th) will still support a VRAM provided it goes no lower than the umbilicus. The RA flap is not as robust as the LD or PM and provides relatively little muscle by comparison. The inferior epigastric pedicle (and SIEA/SIEV if TRAM) can be kept, as a lifeboat for conversion to a free flap should its vascular adequacy become a problem

Type II
- Trapezius flap: The muscle is supplied superiorly by the descending branch of the TCA and inferiorly by the dorsal scapular, with functional anastomoses between the two systems
  - The trapezius flap is a type II muscle flap based on the TCA (major pedicle which may be divided during neck lymphadenectomy; minor pedicles are branches of the occipital and posterior

intercostal arteries) and is suitable for covering posterosuperior midline defects. It is common to harvest the flap up to 5 cm below the scapula, but an extra long flap may be raised to cover the opposite neck. Larger flaps can also be raised with microvascular augmentation. It is commonly reserved as a salvage option to cover defects of the neck and midface. Its harvest may cause shoulder weakness and it has a 7% failure rate
- Others:
  - External oblique can be used for inferior chest defects up to the level of the IMF. The donor site may be closed in a V-Y fashion
  - Omentum provides a very vascular and large (40 × 60 cm) flap that can be covered with a skin graft. The rich lymphatics are postulated to combat infection well. It is mobilised on the gastroepiploic arteries and is harvested either trans-abdominally or trans-diaphragmatically. With the former, a laparotomy or laparoscopic approach may be used. There is a risk of subphrenic abscesses and an almost inevitable incisional hernia. It is contraindicated in the presence of adhesions
  - Paraspinous flap is supplied by segmental perforators from dorsal aorta that limits the arc of rotation

Other options

- Tissue expansion is usually not a good option due to the common contexts of radiation or infection
- A brief period of temporising negative wound pressure therapy may be beneficial in some cases
- Free flaps are not commonly used due to the numerous pedicled local options. Pedicled flaps can be vascularly augmented as required by anastomoses to vessels such as the thoracodorsal, IMA stump, intercostals and innominate veins

The treatment of postirradiation chest wounds is particularly challenging as these wounds typically have indistinct borders with fibrosis and a larger surrounding zone of radiation damage.

- Ulcers due to radiation tend to deteriorate
- Local reconstructive options particularly vessels as donors or recipients are limited
- The use of alloplastic materials is more likely to fail

On the other hand, these wounds tend to need less support due to the stiffness of irradiated tissues. The aim is to debride aggressively to remove all infected and ischaemic tissue and to reconstruct with well-vascularised tissue.

Sternotomy wounds

There is a 0.4–0.5% incidence of sternotomy wound infections after surgery, although rates as high as 8% have been reported.

- Early dehiscence is often minor, due to superficial infection and can usually be treated with dressings
- Late problems are often major

Pairolero classification

1. Serosanguinous discharge without cellulitis, costochondritis or osteomyelitis (OM). It occurs in first few days postoperatively. Cultures are usually negative. Wounds are explored and can be closed primarily after minimal debridement, without need for reconstruction
2. Purulent mediastinitis with costochondritis and OM. It usually occurs 2–3 weeks after surgery
3. Chronic wound infection with costochondritis and OM, occurring months to years after surgery

In the past, major sternotomy wounds had mortality rates of up to 70%. Sternotomy wounds impact pulmonary function through paradoxical movement and increases energy requirements as efficiency is decreased.

- The development of closed system irrigation decreased mortality rates to 20%
- The use of flaps (omentum and then pectoralis major) was described in 1976, with better healing rates and shorter hospital stays

Current management can be summarised as debridement and vascular cover, with or without NPWT that can improve cardiorespiratory function by splinting the sternal defect. Although the bony edges of a sternal dehiscence do not need to be approximated, the risk of recurrent infection is high if the overlying tissue is simply closed. Inflammation stiffens the mediastinal tissues and impairs collapse of dead space, which must thus be filled. Flaps are used for both cover and filling dead-space.

- Pectoralis major: The muscle can reliably cover the upper two thirds of the sternal defect when pedicled on the thoracoacromial trunk. The humeral insertion can be divided via an incision in deltopectoral groove to increase movement. It is less suited to defects with significant dead space when used this way. A turnover flap based on the IMA perforators may provide more central bulk but some length is sacrificed in the turnover process. The latter may not be reliable after a coronary artery bypass graft (CABG)
- Rectus abdominis can reliably cover the lower two thirds of the sternal defect but the distal portion is least reliable. This can be tackled by flap delay if the extra length is required

The PM and RA have become flaps of first choice for superior and inferior defects respectively. Studies have shown a similar rate of success and complications (haematoma/seroma vs. abdominal dehiscence). While the PM tends to be vulnerable in the inferior end, the RA is the opposite. The two flaps complement each other by being the salvage option for the other. Second choice flaps include the LD and omentum.

Negative pressure wound therapy (NPWT) *can ↑ cardio pulmonary function by splinting*

NPWT has changed the management of chronic wounds. Its primary role in chest reconstruction is as an adjunct and cannot usually be used to close complex wounds alone. It is commonly used to temporise an acute wound in many facets that include allowing serial debridement, patient optimisation, a minor size reduction of the defect and acting as an efficient wound management system until elective definitive cover can be provided under more favourable conditions. Typically:

- Several layers of paraffin gauze or proprietary polyurethane foam is used to line the cavity, stacked appropriately to fill the contour defect
- Start at 50 mm Hg of pressure and increase up to 125 mm Hg as tolerated
- Dressing changes are performed 2–3 times weekly. GA is commonly required if debridement is planned or a strong possibility, especially in the early acute situation

The issues around NPWT are:

- Reduction of cardiac function: Sonometric studies suggest a significant decrease in cardiac output (30%) but subsequent fMRI studies show a much lower decrease (10%). Patients adapt to this and ultimately, flap interposition may attenuate this reduction further
- Respiratory effects: NPWT aids sternal wound stabilisation, improves lung function and reduces the need for mechanical ventilation

Congenital chest deformities

Chest wall deformities are mostly asymptomatic and usually present in adolescence with secondary problems such as scoliosis, back pain from poor posture or psychological upset. Some have lung function problems whilst a few have congenital cardiovascular problems.

- Pectus excavatum: A caved-in deformity of the sternum that is usually worse inferiorly and on the right (i.e. usually asymmetrical) and is the most common congenital chest deformity (1 in 3–400 live births, 90% excavatum vs. 5% carinatum). It is three times more common in males and displays some familial inheritance traits. Ninety per cent of cases are idiopathic but it is associated with Marfan syndrome.

Although most patients are diagnosed before 1 year of age, the condition may not become obvious until adolescence. As it is rarely a functional problem, the indications for reconstruction are not well defined. The inner chest diameter to sternum to spine ratio >3 (normal = 2) has been suggested but it not commonly used. There are several options:

- Ravitch procedure: Osteotomies are performed to raise sternum as a bone flap pedicled superiorly on an IMA, which is then turned over. Deformed cartilages are resected while preserving the periosteal and perichondral sleeves, the sternum restabilised and covered with bilateral PM flaps sutured in the midline. The modified Ravitch repair reduces the amount of resection and adds the use of support bars (Adkins struts that are removed 6 months later). There is a risk of necrosis with sternal turnover procedures but good results are possible with a success rate of up to 97%
- Nuss procedure (1998) is an alternative that exploits tissue malleability in the young to achieve remodelling. It is less suitable for older patients or those with marked asymmetry. The operation involves insertion of a concave stainless steel bar under the sternum via lateral incisions under thoracoscopic guidance. This is then gradually flipped out and stabilised. The bar is removed after 2 years but this depends on the age of the patient. Pneumothorax and bar displacement are the most common complications and postoperative pain greater than with the open procedure. Detailed long-term results are not available, although recurrence rates are quoted at 8%
- Silicone implant designed by 3D CT or mould/impression
- Lipofilling: This is becoming a more frequent option due to its low morbidity. However, excavatum is more prominent (and consequently present more frequently) in the thin who frequently lack sufficient donor volumes for lipofilling

- Pectus carinatum: This is a pigeon or barrel chest deformity. Heart and lung development is usually normal but pain, while rare, can lead to suboptimal pulmonary function. Treatment is usually cosmetic. In women, breast augmentation may be used to camouflage the deformity but risks accentuation of nipple deviation that is frequently present due to the convex chest slope. Alternatively, a modified Ravitch procedure that consists of costochondral resection and reconstruction has been used. Chest remodelling with external prostheses or braces that apply continuous pressure have limited success.

Poland's syndrome and tuberous breasts

See 'Congenital Breast Abnormalities'.

Further reading

Takeshi N. Long-term results of chest wall reconstruction with DualMesh. Interact Cardiovasc Thorac Surg 2010; 11:581–84.

Related topics of interest

- Burn reconstruction
- Congenital breast abnormalities
- Pressure sores
- Vacuum wound closure

Cleft lip

Cleft lip is a defect of the primary palate resulting from the abnormal fusion of the maxillary and medial frontonasal processes. The defect is more common on the left than on the right or bilaterally (6:3:1). Two thirds of cleft lip (CL) patients will also have cleft palate (CLP). Cleft lip, with or without an associated cleft palate (CL/P), is a different condition from the cleft palate only (CPO). The relative prevalances are CLP 50%, CL 20% and CPO 30%.

The number of patients in developed countries is decreasing due in part to a fall in the birth rate but also due to prenatal ultrasound diagnosis leading to a variable rate of abortions (low for isolated clefts but depends on cultural factors). CL/P can be diagnosed with routine ultrasound scanning at 13 weeks (limited by fetal position and maternal obesity), and earlier with transvaginal ultrasonography. The sensitivity is 20% when not looking for it specifically.

Although cleft patients carry a higher incidence of syndromic associations, the majority of cases are non-syndromic. Karyotyping is controversial due to its invasiveness and may be justified if there are structural abnormalities present or in bilateral clefts.

Parental counselling is paramount in the pre and postnatal period. Photographs are a helpful adjunct. It is important to clarify the aims of surgery and therapy and prepare them for the high likelihood of multiple operations with an end point that may be difficult to define and will evolve. The overall aim is to facilitate complete integration into society. Reassure parents that they are not to blame and inform them of the statistical risk of future children being affected. Introduce parents to the various members of the multidisciplinary cleft team.

- CL/P is more common in males.
- Racial variations in incidence are more marked than in CPO. The incidence of CL in Asians (2 in 1000) is twice the incidence in Caucasians (1 in 1000, compared to CPO 1 in 2500). It is uncommon in Afro-Caribbeans
- Familial risk (Caucasian) of CL/P in subsequent child

  - No family history = 0.1%
  - 1 parent or 1 sibling affected = 4%
  - 2 siblings affected = 10%
  - 1 parent and 1 sibling = 15%
  - 60% concordance with identical twins
  - Defects of greater severity may have a greater risk of recurring within a CL/P affected family
- CL/P may rarely (3%) occur as part of a syndrome: Patau (trisomy 13), Down (trisomy 21) and Van der Woude syndrome (AD—associated with lower lip pits due to accessory salivary glands, syndactyly and abnormal genitalia)
- Non-syndromic clefts are multifactorial with genetic predisposition

Apart from a cleft lip of variable degree (complete, incomplete or microform), there are other anatomical abnormalities:

- Abnormal muscle attachment to the nose: Muscles run parallel to the edge and inserts onto ala of the cleft side and columella of non-cleft side. The muscles between philtral midline and cleft are hypoplastic. This is in contrast to the non-cleft lip, where the deep parts of the orbicularis oris are sphincteric, whilst the superficial parts function mostly for facial expression and fine movements of speech (as a retractor). The pars marginalis contributes to the anterior projection of the vermilion border
- Complex nasal deformity: (see below)
- The alveolar cleft is at the canine position leading to an open nostril floor. It may be intact in incomplete clefts. The canine is likely to be deformed and malpositioned, whereas the other teeth are not usually malpositioned but may be deformed. There is outward rotation of the premaxillary segment and retroposition of lateral segment
  - The alveolar segments are classified according to gap width and degree of smaller segment collapse. This is relevant to treatment choice
  - Narrow non-collapsed segments do not need formal pre-surgical orthopaedics (PSO) or lip adhesion. A simple device or method to maintain segmental alignment may be all that is required

- – Other forms will generally benefit from PSO, although its use is controversial
- Shortened philtrum (50–75% of normal side) and vertical lip length: A Simonart band is a thin fibrous bridge over the upper lip cleft. A microform cleft (*forme fruste*) is the mildest form (but may be rather difficult to repair) and may manifest as a vermillion notch, a scar-like line/depression/band from lip to nostril floor or alar deformity

Treatment

Breast-feeding may still be possible with CL and feeding is not a major problem. Suckling is achieved via the milk letdown reflex and not by suction pressure.

Multidisciplinary approach

Results are surgeon dependent, but when performed meticulously, excellent results are possible despite widely varying protocols. Major controversies continue to be regarding many aspects of treatment: timing of lip surgery, use of pre-surgical orthopaedics, type of alveolar repair, and timing of primary and secondary rhinoplasties.

The important fundamental question of when the best time to operate remains elusive and is the subject of the on-going Scandcleft study. Studies are confounded by lack of consistent objective outcome assessments, variability of protocols and the long lag times involved. This is compounded by the multifaceted nature of the problem with interdependent effects. Early palate surgery may be better for speech development at the expense of facial growth.

There are many options with respect to the timing and type of surgery.

Timing

Reconstructing the orbicularis sphincter mechanism improves alveolar alignment. Delay permits gradual cleft widening that makes closure more difficult. It is thus preferable to perform lip repair sooner rather than later. However, this is tempered with the need to perform surgery safely. The traditional rule of 10 signifies this threshold: 10 weeks of age, 10 pounds in weight and a haemoglobin level of 10 g/dl. There is little firm evidence regarding optimal timing, but the overall trend has been for earlier surgery.

Successful scarless fetal cleft repair has been demonstrated in sheep models. There is no collagen scar if performed before the early third trimester but there is a lack of skin appendages at the repair site. This option remains experimental due to the unacceptable risk of inducing abortion for a non life-threatening problem. Furthermore, cleft treatment extends beyond any single operation and there is currently no evidence in-utero surgery decreases nor abolishes the need for other treatment. A thorough in-utero clinical assessment is impossible.

Neonatal surgery is generally defined as surgery within 48 hours. Whilst the surgery is technically more difficult, the main issue is fitness for surgery and airway concerns as neonates are obligate nasal breathers. Organising the surgery and coordinating appropriate staff at short notice whilst also excluding concomitant disease is a practical problem with the risk of missing undiagnosed anomalies. Whilst children with isolated clefts have no significant increase in mortality in 1st year, those who have associated abnormalities (35% of cases) do. The theoretical advantage of improved wound healing has not been borne out clinically. Neonatal surgery is not scarless. No significant overall advantage has been demonstrated to date.

Type of surgery

A conventional 2-stage repair is as follows:
- Repair of the lip and anterior palate at 3 months with a vomerine flap (primary nose correction, e.g. McComb, may also be performed). The previous view that early lip repair adversely affects nasal growth has not been proven but early repair of the bony alveolus and primary bone grafting is generally avoided as this will adversely affect subsequent growth of premaxilla and vomer. Primary gingivoperiosteoplasty however, is beneficial with no impairment of growth, with or without synchronous soft palate repair in wide clefts
- Repair of the hard and soft palate at 6–18 months (tendency for earlier repair between 6–9 months)

Delayed palatal repair is infrequent in modern practice. It aims to provide better midfacial growth at the expense of speech development due to prolonged palatal incompetence.

Surgical techniques

Chinese surgeons were among the first to treat CL by simply suturing the excised skin edges. Currently, there are many different techniques that use a variety of skin flaps to repair the upper lip. In general, the priority in all modern techniques is to reconstruct the continuity of the lip muscle after detachment from its abnormal insertions to maximise sphincteric function. This is more important than the skin or scar geometry.

The Millard and Tennison-Randall are the most popular techniques and good results can be obtained by either technique. A recent survey in Northern America (2008) showed that 84% of cleft surgeons perform variants of the Millard rotation advancement but over half use modifications, most commonly Noordhoff, Mohler, Onizuka/triangular flaps and some undescribed variants. Only 9% use a Tennison-Randall triangular repair technique. 86% of surgeons use the same technique all the time.

Although the primary pathology is tissue displacement instead of tissue deficiency, there are elements of both. In simple terms, the greater the vertical deficit, the more difficult the lip repair, whilst the greater the horizontal deficit, the more difficult the nasal repair.

- Millard rotation-advancement (**Figure 4**) is so-named because the cleft-side flap (A flap) is advanced into the defect after the non-cleft-side flap (R flap) is rotated downwards to lengthen the philtrum. This preserves the philtrum and Cupid's bow, and places tension in the alar base that may mould the alveolar process to an extent. However, it has a tendency to produce a constricted nostril. Small C flaps can be rotated to create the nasal sill or lengthen the columella. Back cuts are performed to the required degree. The M and L flaps of cleft vermilion are sutured together to close the nasal floor. Cosmesis can be very good as the scar is well hidden along the philtral border, except in the uppermost part. An important advantage of the Millard technique is intraoperative adjustment (cut-as-you-go). However, the learning curve is rather steep and is less effective for very wide clefts. An oblique scar that diverges from the line of the

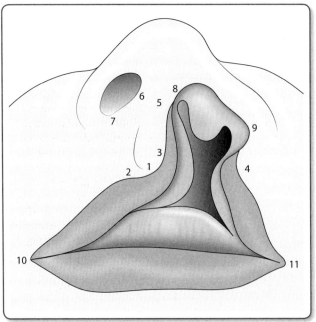

Figure 4 The cleft lip, with common pre-operative markings. 1,2 and 3 define the Cupid's bow and distances 1–2 equals 1–3. Similarly distance 2–10 equals 4–11. 5–9 defines the base of the nose.

philtrum as well as deficient lip length may result if applied to the latter

- Tennison–Randall repair, also known as the stencil method, is an easier technique to master for the inexperienced. It is a triangular flap technique where tissue from the lateral lip, in the form of a triangular flap, is used to augment the medial lip height that is deficient. It creates a pouting tubercle/attractive Z-plasty but at the expense of a scar crossing the lower philtrum (may be camouflaged by the male moustache), which itself may also be flattened. It is more useful in wide cleft repairs as it does not discard tissue and some reserve its use for this particular indication. It does have the side effect of lengthening of the lip, although sometimes excessively. The Tennison-Randall is quicker to perform and with less blood loss but does not permit intraoperative lip length adjustment
- Fisher repair (Toronto, Canada): This is the anatomical subunit approximation technique that is designed to keep the final scar almost entirely along the philtral column. The superior incision is curved along the medial footplate of the nose and no rotation advancement is achieved with this. The minor lengthening achieved with the Rose-Thompson effect (1 mm) is augmented with a Y-V flap above the white roll (originally described as the Chang Gung modification of the Millard repair) and of the vermillion (Noordhoff triangular vermillion flap). The argument for this over the Tennison-Randall is that the horizontal lip width is not sacrificed for vertical lip height. It leaves a triangle above the white roll that tensions the pout in the correct vector
- The majority of UK cleft surgeons use a variation of the Millard repair incorporating the best elements of the other techniques
- Elements used to achieve
  - Major increases in vertical height of lip: Millard rotation advancement +/– triangular white roll flap; Triangular white roll flap alone; Tennison-Randall triangular flaps. Options for location of

    Millard backcut: On lip between philtral columns; up onto columella (Mohler)
  - Minor increases in vertical height of lip: Rose-Thompson effect (angled lines gain length when approximated vertically)
  - Vertical height of vermillion: Noordhoff triangular vermillion flap (**Figure 4**)

Postoperative care

The aim is to protect the repairs:

- Avoid sleeping face down
- No bottle-feeding is allowed for 7–10 days. Syringes or special cups are usually used. Normal diet is usually possible by day 10
- Breast-feeding was traditionally discouraged on the grounds that it added extra strain, but evidence suggests that the problem is overestimated and the risks are outweighed by the benefits

Presurgical orthopaedics

Presurgical orthopaedics aims to narrow and improve alveolar alignment by passive (lip tape, adhesion) or dynamic/active appliances, e.g. the Latham device (appliance placed onto palatal segments with screws that need to be turned daily). These techniques aim to make use of the increased tissue malleability within the first 3 months attributed to high circulating levels of maternal oestrogens. Suggestions of growth detriment and increased dental caries risk have been largely disproved. PSO is time-consuming and costly (with need for appropriate resources and orthodontic support).

- McNeil first described modern PSO in 1950 but the overstated claims that it eliminated alveolar, palatal and orthodontic problems damaged the credibility of the technique, making it more controversial than it should have been
- PSO has limited benefits with orthodontic improvement and maxillary growth. The major advantage of PSO is restoration of the alveolar alignment that makes surgery easier. The lip repair is under less tension, healing is improved and poor scarring is reduced. Nasal alveolar moulding (NAM) with its nasal stent also permits

straightening of the columella from its oblique over the cleft position and brings the nasal cartilages into a more normal position, thereby reducing the extent of primary nasal surgery
- Some reserve the use of PSO for wide bilateral clefts only. NAM can expand the columella and often eliminates need for surgical columellar lengthening

Lip adhesion (suturing edges of cleft together converting it to an incomplete cleft, first described in 1961 as a prior step before bone grafting, and in 1964 by Millard before lip closure) is sometimes used as a substitute for PSO with similar aims but its use is also controversial. The adhesion is a straight-line repair that is 3 mm or more away from the incision lines for definitive surgery. The arguments against this are that the scar can still interfere with subsequent cleft repair and that the forces are less controlled. Some contend that lip taping (by reliable parents) may achieve similar results.

Bilateral clefts

The most prominent feature is the protruding premaxilla that will continue outward growth unfettered by connections to the secondary palate. The prolabium lacks muscle and is deficient of white roll and vermilion that is of different character with drier mucosa with a tendency to peel. The nasal lower lateral cartilages are pulled laterally and posteriorly with transversely orientated nostrils, whilst the domes part to leave a flat broad nose tip with a short columella and no sills.

These become increasingly difficult to treat with age (> 1/12) as the central segment pushes forwards and downwards. Even after repair, the prolabium will remain flat with a wide Cupid's bow. The dynamic height discrepancy (caused by a combination of differential growth rate of the segments, scar tethering and true height discrepancy) between the prolabium and lateral lip elements may lead to a whistling lip deformity. Techniques that remove the prolabium will result in severe deformities of nose and upper lip. There are many described repair techniques with numerous modifications as none are ideal. The principles of repair are:

- Symmetry with secure muscle repair across the midline under a raised prolabial skin flap
- Reconstruction of prolabium and median tubercle (usually from lateral lip, the prolabial vermilion is used for labial surface/sulcus)
- Reconstruct nasal tip and columella (usually from alar cartilage)

Skin only techniques

Older methods of repair focused on dealing with the skin problems particularly the short columella and broad nasal tip.

Two stage technique:

- First stage: Lip repair and banked forked flaps from lateral prolabial tissues into sill, sutured end on to the alar base to form a standing cone (lump of tissue that protrudes into the nostril). Prolabial vermilion is turned down as a flap for the inner lining
- Second stage: Columella lengthening is achieved by an inverted V columellar incision that joins the bases of the fork flaps, advanced in V-Y fashion to gain height
  - Banking of primary forked flaps is more suited to a wider prolabium. In narrower cases, the tension in the lip will stretch out the prolabium enough to harvest a secondary forked flap

Cartilage techniques

A criticism of the skin only techniques is that the anatomical derangements of the nose are not addressed and subsequent growth will lead to a bulbous tip, which may be difficult to correct. This led to a different set of techniques focused on the cartilages, with skin from the nasal tip used for the columella. There is perhaps even greater variation in bilateral cleft lip repair techniques compared to unilateral clefts. It is twice as difficult, and the results are half as good.

- McComb: Two stages. First stage: A gull-wing incision to expose, mobilise and suture the cartilages. The skin is redraped in a V-Y fashion to elongate the columella. Lip adhesion can be performed with a formal lip repair at a second stage

- Mulliken: Vertical tip incision for exposure of the cartilages supposedly maintains the blood supply to the prolabium better, but there is less columellar lengthening. This evolved into a technique with bilateral rim incisions for best access to the cartilages

Some have described the use of traction or tape, external bonnet contraptions, pin-retained retraction (Latham) and even external fixation to push back the premaxilla, avoiding surgery on this segment, if at all possible. Lip adhesion is avoided in bilateral clefts as it consumes tissue that is already in short supply. Surgical excision and premaxillary set back techniques are no longer used.

Secondary deformities

After the primary lip repair, further work is usually deferred until just before school age to optimise social interaction.
- Lip asymmetry: Discontinuities in muscle repair may cause grooving (repair muscle) or notching (lengthen with Z-plasty). The lip may be short (after Millard) or tight and long (after Tennison Randall)
- Nasal deformities: e.g. persistence of short columella or wide ala (see below)

Other surgeries to consider

- Pharyngoplasty for VPI at about 3 years in patients with CLP
- Bone grafting of the alveolus to encourage eruption of teeth. This is usually delayed until after 9 years of age to reduce adverse effects on maxillary growth
- Osteotomy, rhinoplasty when 17–20 years old

Nose in cleft lip

One of the biggest challenges in CL surgery is to optimise the nasal deformity, which can be complex. The stigmata of a cleft nose become more obvious in adolescence.
- Hypoplastic buckled ('M'-shaped) alar cartilage
  - The cartilage deformity is analogous to a half a rugby ball (cut lengthwise) and pulled apart at its two ends. The central convexity buckles forming a central concavity. The overall resultant shape is the "M". Twisting the lateral end inferiorly while maintaining the medial end in place simulates the inferior rotation of the lateral crus
  - No overlap with upper lateral cartilage
  - Angle between the crura is increased making alar base wide, with a flat alar facial angle and missing nasal sill
  - Rotated inferiorly: The medial crus lies in coronal plane and the lateral crus in sagittal plane
  - Alar base is rotated out in a flare and a skin curtain that is cartilage deficient distorts the rim
- Flattened nasal bones and underdeveloped maxilla leaving a deficient bony base
- Septum is bent with base dislocated to non-cleft side whilst the midseptum obstructs cleft side
- Deviation of nose to cleft side with the domes lower and bifid due to separation

The resultant nasal deformity is tempered by time. Although the pathology of each of the elements (skin, cartilage, mucosa, alar base position, etc.) is important, their relative position is equally so. This is akin to runners lining up to race on a circular track, whose starting positions have to be offset correctly so that all run the equal distance. Surgery on a single element, without restoring its correct relative position will result in the disparity being magnified with time. It is thus almost impossible to approximate normality without correcting deformity, replacing the deficiencies and realigning the skeletal base. Procedures that rely on suturing alone will show gradual recurrence. Ideally, maxillary surgery is performed first if there is a bony deficiency. Advancement is not recommended before the age of 14–15 years in females and 17–18 years for males.
- There is no consensus on the use of PSO
- 50% perform some form of primary nasal correction routinely but this does not seem to eliminate the need for future operations/nor diminish their magnitude
  - Asymmetry is the most common problem followed by nasal obstruction. In general, patients are usually more satisfied than doctors

- The late nose deformity is usually characterised by an asymmetric under-projected tip, short columella, long lateral crus, flat nostril and wide alar base. Treatment usually requires an open rhinoplasty with complete exposure and undermining of skin for redraping and cartilage grafts for support

  – Nasal stenosis is a very difficult problem to treat. Z-plasties, skin grafts, and Koken nostril retainers (Koken Co. Ltd., Japan) are options
  – Short columella: Use of lip skin such as forked flaps may be used. If severely lip deficient, an Abbé flap is an option

Further reading

Fisher D, Sommerlad B. Cleft lip, cleft palate and velopharangeal insufficiency. Plast Reconstr Surg 2011; 128:342e.

Related topic of interest

- Cleft palate

Cleft palate

Cleft palate only (CPO) is a separate disease entity from cleft lip, with or without a cleft palate (CL/P). It is less common (30%) with an incidence of 1 in 2000 with little evidence of racial variation. CPO is more common in females.

Embryology

The palatal shelves of the maxillary processes initially point vertically downwards. After the tongue descends, they normally rotate upwards, meet in midline and fuse. Any interference with this process may cause defects or clefts of the secondary palate. This is the hard palate located posterior to the incisive foramen. The underlying problem is theorised to be a lack of fusion (at 7–12 weeks) whereas in CL/P it is due to a lack of mesenchymal penetration after fusion of the processes (earlier at 4–6 weeks).

Pierre Robin Sequence (PRS)

A sequence is a single developmental deficit that results in a chain or cascade of secondary deficits. PRS may be a result of many syndromes. The leading theory is that the lead event appears to be an inability of head to come out of flexion, e.g. high intrauterine pressure or oligohydramnios (accounting for the potential catch-up growth), retrogenia (initiator) and glossoptosis (and relative macroglossia), causing airway obstruction. The hypoplastic mandible limits tongue descent that prevents fusion of the palatal shelves, causing the cleft palate. Other theories suggest neurological maturation problems.

- Wide U-shaped cleft palate
- A posterior and low hyoid contributing to airway compromise, whilst glossoptosis from a low tongue attachment tends to block the pharyngeal airway
- May also have cardiac, eye, ear and skeletal defects
- Chin grows over 3–18 months and usually catches up by age of 4–6 years to a normal profile, although the angle region may still be abnormal. The chin problem is primarily a retrognathia/genia rather than a growth problem. The term micrognathia applied here is inaccurate. Surgical airway improvement should thus only be used as a last resort in view of the high catch-up rate

PRS occurs in 1 in 8000 and is associated with up to 18 different syndromes.

- Stickler syndrome is a connective tissue disorder with AD inheritance and constitutes up to 30% of PRS patients, with associated features such as maxillary hypoplasia, hypotonia, joint hyperextensibility, mitral valve prolapse, pectus excavatum, eye problems (severe myopia, retinal detachment and progressive blindness) and sensorineural deafness
- Van der Woude syndrome: Lip pits
- Velocardiofacial syndrome is associated with a deletion on chromosome 22 (CATCH 22) that leads to thymic aplasia, vertically long face, narrow palpebral fissures, square nasal root, microcephaly (40–50%), learning/psychological disorders (seen in 10%), submucous clefts (SMCs) and cardiovascular anomalies such as VSD/TOF are common. Inheritance is AD and it is also called Shprintzen or Di George syndrome. VPI is common. The carotid arteries may be displaced medially putting them at risk with pharyngoplasty. Nasoendoscopy was recommended previously to observe pulsations of pharyngeal wall but MRA is more useful

Multifactorial environmental influences seem to be more important than genetic factors in CP: fetal alcohol syndrome, maternal smoking, anticonvulsant and retinoic acid therapy, and maternal diabetes have all been implicated. There is some evidence of folate deficiency being important, but studies on the effect of folate supplements are inconclusive.

- CPO is probably related to a single major gene (autosomal recessive) with minor genes contributing whilst CL/P is probably polygenic. However inheritance is weak overall. If one sibling or parent is affected, then a child has a 2% risk, with both being affected this rises to 15%

- Up to 50% of patients with CP occur in the context of a syndrome or in association with other abnormalities, e.g. Treacher–Collins syndrome, Velocardiofacial syndrome, Apert syndrome, Crouzon syndrome, Stickler syndrome and Pierre Robin sequence

Airway management

Airway management: Most airways problems spontaneously resolve within a year.

- Lie prone: Successful in 80%
- Nasopharyngeal airway: Adequate in an additional 18%. In general, a cut Portex endotracheal tube positioned just above the epiglottis that is replaced every fortnight for 1-3 months is used. Signs of improvement that include weight gain are expected after 7 days

Surgery may be needed if the patient requires prolonged nasal continuous positive airway pressure (NCPAP), desaturates while asleep or has increased end tidal CO_2 levels. Options include:

- Glossopexy: Routledge suture (1960) from the tongue to the inner surface of lip (tongue-lip adhesion)
- Tracheostomy (required in less than 1%): It may take up to 3 years to decannulate the tracheostomy. Tracheomalacia is common
- Mandibular advancement
- Distraction osteogenesis of mandible (Ilizarov technique - Tension stress causes bone proliferation). The major advantage of this is that the soft tissues, including nerves and vessels, are also stretched (distraction histogenesis), without which may contribute to relapse. It is safe to use in the young for many indications such as hemifacial microsomia and obviates need for a donor site, such as a rib. After a latency of 5–7 days (2 days in the younger) distraction can proceed at 1 mm a day (in one or both segments) until a slight class III occlusion is attained. This is followed by a period of consolidation (8 weeks for a child, 12 weeks for adults). Risks include infection, premature or fibrous union

Classification

Palatal clefts may be

- Complete or incomplete
- Unilateral or bilateral (depends on attachment to vomer on one or neither side respectively)
- Submucous cleft (SMC): This condition is characterised by Calnan's triad, comprising a uvula that is bifid to a variable degree, a palpable bony notch and a central pale blue line, the zona pellucida, indicating the separation of the palatal muscles. Twenty per cent of cases present with VPI, although not all cases require surgery. Thorough speech and language therapy assessment is thus paramount. Physical signs do not directly correlate to VPI severity. The indications for surgery are variable. Some centres operate on almost all SMCs at an early age, whereas others use the presence of bridging muscle on MRI to imply function and defer early surgery. Pharyngoplasty is the traditional treatment but a Furlow palatoplasty with intravelar veloplasty, or Veau-Wardill-Kilner with retroposition, are alternatives that attempt to restore both length and palatal function to a degree
  - The rate of bifid uvula occurrence (2%) is independent of race but is more common in males. It is not an accurate predictor of SMC palate and thus should not be regarded as a 'microform' CP

Methods of documenting clefts include:

- Kernahan's striped Y classification, modified by Millard and Jackson, is a useful diagrammatic representation
- LAHSAL is a modification of the striped Y: **L**ip, **A**lveolus, **H**ard palate, **S**oft palate, **A**lveolus, **L**ip
- The Veau classification is descriptive

Problems

Speech

The nose and oral cavity act as coupled resonators; one fixed and the other of variable volume. All sounds except m, n and ng require adequate velopharyngeal function. Hypernasality is the most common problem. Hyponasality is an obstructive issue, commonly iatrogenic, created by the presence of a large obstructing pharyngeal flap or pharyngoplasty. Facial grimacing may manifest as patients try to restrict airflow through constriction of nostrils and contraction of the facial musculature. It is important to remember that speech problems in cleft patients are multifactorial and include dental, occlusal, fistulae and hearing problems. Speech therapy may be adequate for some, but surgery may be indicated for others.

- Plosives (most consonants) require pressure build up and release. Ps and Bs require generation of maximal air pressure prior that is impossible in the presence of a cleft palate. This is due to nasal escape or emission. Plosives are substituted with glottal stops with cleft palates
- Fricatives are generated with a turbulent airstream produced by forcing air through a narrow channel. Approximating the lower lip against the upper teeth, such as for Fs, can create this. The narrow channel is created by curing the tongue lengthwise to direct air over the edge of the teeth for sibilants (a subset of fricatives) such as the Ss. Fricatives are substituted with pharyngeal fricatives in cleft palates
- One of the postoperative goals of speech and language therapy is to undo these maladaptive compensatory articulatory patterns

Feeding

Overall, babies with CP exhibit worse feeding than those with CL, but this is manageable in almost all cases. Although supplements are often needed, a trial of breastfeeding is always worthwhile. Frequent burping is advised due to the excessive aerophagy when feeding. The sucking reflex develops from the 34th week onwards and is underdeveloped in the premature (who are also more likely to have clefts). Particular attention is needed to oral hygiene after feeds especially in those not being breast-fed (babies have low saliva production). Optimising feeding as soon as possible after birth (whilst avoiding nasogastric tube feeding) is important to build up weight prior to surgery, and most usually catch up by 6 months post-surgery.

Those with syndromic CP tend to have more problems and are often below the fifth percentile for weight.

Bottle-feeding strategies

Certain modifications are useful in facilitating feeding such as the Haberman bottle.

- A one-way valve between the bottle and teat prevents the back flow into the bottle
- Bottle is soft and the teat has a large squeezable reservoir that allows the feeder to propel a small bolus into the baby's mouth, reducing infant effort and fatigue
- The teat opening is a slit that allows flow control by rotating the bottle. The air inlet grooves reduce the amount of aerophagy and promotes smooth, non-turbulent milk flow

Other issues

Other issues include:

- Otitis media (OM) with hearing loss. There is an abnormal levator veli palatini insertion and function. Earlier myringotomy may allow greater improvement in hearing but it is unclear whether cleft repair works by reducing OM or actually improves hearing
- Airway obstruction: Patients may have sleep apnoea or other airway abnormalities. CPAP may be required but adenoidectomy is to be avoided
- Dental problems: At risk from disordered dental occlusion and impaired midface growth

Management needs to be truly multidisciplinary. Its team members comprise the following and the composition changes as the child ages, as different considerations come to the forefront. Some roles may be amalgamated, depending on country and local setup.

- Primary surgeons
- Secondary surgeons
- Orthodontist
- Paediatric dentist
- Restorative dentist
- Specialist nurses
- Speech and language therapists
- Psychologist
- Paediatrician
- ENT Surgeon

- Multidisciplinary team coordinator
- Secretary
- Geneticist
- Audiologist
- Anaesthetist

The aim of surgery is to close the palate to produce optimal speech whilst minimising adverse effects on midface growth. However, the balance is determined by the timing of surgery as well as by the surgical technique. The differences in outcome between different techniques (in 2000, 201 cleft centres in Europe were using 194 different protocols) are less obvious. Papers in dental journals are biased towards facial growth as the preeminent outcome at the expense of speech, appearance, and social integration that are more difficult to evaluate. The CSAG study is often quoted as demonstrating poorer results in the UK compared to Europe, which led to the recommendation for centralisation of cleft services for centres falling below a minimum operative number of 30 clefts a year. This however is not due to low volumes being necessarily associated with poor outcomes, but instead because low volumes do not allow measurements of outcomes in a reasonable timeframe. Approximately 40 clefts per surgeon per year translate to an average of 15 unilateral CLP a year, which is the minimum number required for outcome measurement. Unilateral CLP is the operation that permits meaningful inter-operator comparison (other clefts are too variable).

Timing

There has been great variation in timing in the past, but the general trend is towards early two-stage surgery (for CLP). However, it is important to note that babies are obligate nasal breathers until approximately 6 months. As palatal surgery may compromise the nasal airway, it is deferred until after the 6-month mark.

- Repair of the lip and anterior palate at 3 months, with primary nose correction
- Repair of the hard and soft palate at 9 months (6–18 months) +/– myringotomy and grommet insertion (Assess with clinical examination, tympanometry and hearing tests. Distraction tests can

be performed from the age of 6 months onwards)

Surgical techniques
Repair of the hard palate

- Veau-Wardill-Kilner technique: Large triangular mucosal flaps based on the greater palatine arteries are raised and rotated medially to meet in the midline. The lateral donor sites are left to heal secondarily. New bone is then formed under the transposed periosteum. There are concerns that the extensive denudation of bone may inhibit maxillary growth. Fracture of the hamulus is no longer advocated. It is also known as the pushback but this lengthening effect on the soft palate alone is often insufficient to correct significant VPI as it does not realign the misaligned palatal musculature
- Von Langenbeck technique: Bipedicled flaps, based on the great palatine arteries, are raised with longitudinal incisions that are then sutured along the midline. The soft palate is not lengthened by this technique (possibly slightly shortened) but the postulation is that by avoiding the anterior palate, there is less disturbance of the maxillary growth centres and subsequent facial growth. Note however that the precise locations of the maxillary growth centres still remain elusive. The technique is simple and can close moderate sized defects but may be prone to develop anterior fistulae (where the suture line lies over the bony defect) and a shorter palate
- Bardach two-flap palatoplasty (first described in 1967) raises large posteriorly based flaps for closure of the hard palate defect and veloplasty without leaving large areas of denuded bone. Several series with long-term experience has been published and confirms that good results including speech (> 75%) are possible with a low fistula rate 2.4% (Murthy 2009)

There is little difference between these techniques with regards to speech outcomes and surgeon expertise at the technique may pay a more important role. Vomerine flaps can be used to supplement anterior closure.

Repair of the soft palate musculature

Veloplasty involves detaching abnormal muscle insertions at the back of the hard palate and reforming the aponeurotic sling. The posterior border of the cleft palatal bone tends to be oblique and muscle attachments (tensor veli palatini) too anterior. Dissecting them free allows retropositioning (drops posteriorly and inferiorly) which narrows the nasopharyngeal aperture. The effect of muscle reposition and soft palate lengthening does not directly correlate with speech improvement.

- Intravelar veloplasty (popularised by Sommerlad) involves radical muscle dissection under microscope magnification, realignment and repair in layers
- Furlow double opposing Z-plasties (opposing orientations on the nasal and oral layers) lengthens the soft palate. It allows incorporation of a veloplasty and when performed in this way, has been known as a Furlad repair in recognition of the namesake origins
- More recent variations utilise the buccal fat pad as a pedicled fascial flap to bridge soft tissue gaps and permit donor site reduction. Long-term results are not available

Postoperative monitoring

Airway monitoring is important, particularly in PRS patients. Obstruction may occur due to oedema, bleeding or secretions.

Complications

Routine preoperative nose and throat swabs for the detection b-haemolytic *Streptococci* are important to allow antibiotic treatment if present (and possibly delaying the operation) and decrease the complication rate. The rate is related to the severity/Veau classification.

- Fistula formation (5–30%) is becoming increasingly common with the trend for less aggressive undermining to avoid adverse effects on growth. It is more common with the pushback technique, as well as in single-layered wide cleft repairs. However, it is likely that the specific surgical technique is less important than the surgeon's experience. The intraoral view provides no indication of the 3-dimensional nature or course of the fistula
  - May cause nasal regurgitation with chronic inflammation of the nasal lining. Its effect on speech can be difficult to separate from VPI. Assess by examination (and probing) and enlisting an experienced speech therapist
  - There is no evidence that spontaneous closure will occur once the wound itself has healed. The usual treatment is to excise the fistula and achieve tension-free closure with large palatal flaps. Bone grafting may be required. Alternatives to bone include cartilage or acellular dermal matrices, while obturators (temporarily or permanently) may be used in selected patients
- Retarded maxillary growth is determined in part by the operations and their timing, although cleft palate patients may have inherent impairment of facial growth
- Airway obstruction is most common with pharyngoplasty, pushback, and combined procedures, particularly in patients with the Pierre-Robin sequence. Desaturation is most profound in first 30 minutes postoperatively. Significant obstruction is rare in the absence of excessive bleeding

Other treatments

Other treatments may be needed for the patient with cleft palate:

- Speech therapy at 3–4 years
- Myringotomy and grommets, usually at time of hard palate repair. Hearing tends to improve at 8 years as the midface grows and the Eustachian tube begins to drain with gravity
- Pharyngoplasty at 5 years, nasal correction if needed
- Alveolar bone graft at 9 (8–12) years or when the permanent teeth (canines)

erupt (or when roots are one quarter–one half erupted). Cancellous bone from the iliac crest or cranium is preferred to cortical bone. The latter tends to result in unpredictable take and tooth eruption. The aim is to optimise dental alignment and provide a stable base for further orthodontic work. Any fistulae can be closed at this time (vide supra)

- Six months of orthodontics may be required to get the alveolar segments into a position suitable for grafting. Postoperative orthodontic work can begin 3–4 years after bone grafting at the age of 12–13 years
- Primary bone grafts along with mucoperiosteal flaps were once popular in Germany but have largely been abandoned as they may hinder maxillary growth

- Midface advancement (Le Fort I) is the only viable treatment for midfacial retrusion and is best delayed until after the growth spurt. Mandibular setback may be required in combination to treat malocclusion. Larger degrees of midface retrusion are difficult to advance, as scarring is often the limiting factor
- Rhinoplasty
- Secondary lip, about 6 years or later (observe)
- Genetic counselling of patient: Related defects are found in 2% of CPO and 4% of CL/P overall

Bone grafts

- Osteoproduction is the production of new bone from surviving osteoblasts in the graft
- Osteoinduction is the stimulation of mesenchymal precursor cells in the recipient bed to form osteoclasts and osteoblasts
- Osteoconduction is the ingrowth of new bone into the graft bone or entry of osteoblasts from recipient tissues also known as creeping substitution

Osteoproduction is the predominant phenomenon in vascularised bone flaps. With non-vascularised grafts, only the surface cells survive and revascularisation takes months after vessel ingrowth. There is creeping substitution along with some osteoinduction with this. In general, take can be improved by ensuring good contact, retaining periosteum, rigid fixation, maximising the cancellous: cortical bone ratio and optimising vascularity.

- Cortical bone has high initial strength that decreases with resorption until regained by remodelling. It acts predominantly as a structural scaffold
- Cancellous bone by contrast, is initially weak but its strength gradually increases. Cancellous bone offers a more reliable take due to the larger surface area of contact. It can be used to stimulate healing, provide bulk or bridge small gaps but offers little structural support

Velopharyngeal incompetence

If the short palate is too short and immobile, its inability to completely close off the gap between the soft palate and posterior pharyngeal wall allows air to escape, resulting in hypernasal speech. Causes include structural (CP is most common, or following Le Fort I osteotomy maxillary advancement, or seen transiently after adenoidectomy) and neurological causes. VPI depends on both palate length and mobility. It is best assessed by:

- Speech therapists: Speech therapy may be sufficient for minor degrees of escape especially if not all phonemes are affected
- Videofluoroscopy allows real-time assessment of the problem with multiple views (especially lateral). Wall motion is graded 0–5 (5 being apposition of the sides)
- Nasoendoscopy: Allows direct visualisation of aperture and of movement of lateral and posterior wall, which is useful to guide the choice of operation

Operative repair

Repair is required in approximately one fifth of cases after cleft surgery. This rate is highly variable between populations and may reflect different cultural tolerances of speech defects and different language requirements.

Beware of anomalous (medially displaced) internal carotid arteries in syndromic patients (especially Shprintzen syndrome).

- Posterior wall augmentation with pharyngeal flaps. They may be superiorly or inferiorly based but here is little difference between the two. Inferior flaps may be marginally more effective but are difficult to inset into the friable adenoidal tissue and may cause more middle ear problems. The flaps are raised full-thickness off the vertebral fascia, sutured to the split soft palate and the lateral ports fashioned over catheters. The donor areas are left to heal by secondary intention
  - This provides a static repair. There is a central obturator effect with lateral channels and thus the width of channels (and flap) is determined by the amount of lateral wall movement. Estimating the flap width is the greatest problem with a risk of overcorrection (causing apnoea) and undercorrection
- Lateral wall procedures/sphincter pharyngoplasties are generally more effective particularly when the lateral wall movement is poor. The flaps are inset higher up on the posterior pharyngeal wall
  - Hynes: A pair of superiorly based flaps (salpingopharyngeus) are elevated and rotated up to meet medially where they are sutured one above the other
  - Orticochea: Posterior tonsillar flaps (palatopharyngeus) are elevated, transposed medially and interdigitated into a small inferiorly based posterior pharyngeal flap. The donor areas heal by secondary intention and the scar helps with closure of the gap. Jackson's modification is an end-to-end inset across the posterior pharyngeal wall, closing all wounds from tonsil to midline, leaving a solitary central hole. These provide a combination of static and dynamic repairs, although it may take more than 6 months for movement in the muscles to return. Criticisms include excessive narrowing of the nasopharyngeal isthmus
- Other choices
  - Soft palate lengthening by (redo) veloplasty, Furlow or V-Y advancement
  - Prosthesis (may displace or move due to mobility of the region) and speech therapy especially if movement is very poor overall. No repair is functional if the palate is totally paralysed
  - Back wall pyloroplasty: Horizontal incision sutured vertically
  - Autologous fat transfer

Bleeding and obstruction are the main complications. In the long term, these procedures may lead to snoring, sleep apnoea or frank airway obstruction. Revision is required in 10% of cases, especially in VCF syndrome patients.

Further reading

Reiter R, Brosch S, Wefel H, et al. The submucous cleft palate: diagnosis and therapy. Int J Pediatr Otorhinolaryngol 2011; 75:85–8.

Related topics of interest

- Cleft lip
- Craniosynostosis (CS)
- Hypoplastic facial conditions
- Tissue fillers

Cold injury and frostbite

Studies of cold injuries are complicated by the large number of variables such as the rate of cooling, minimum temperature reached, time sustained, and rate of thawing. In addition, responses are dependent on the cell types involved. The mechanism of tissue destruction in localised cold injury involves a mixture of direct and indirect injury.

- Direct injury is caused by ice formation that is first extracellular then intracellular. The relative proportions depend on the speed of freezing
- Indirect injury is caused by the thawing process where arterial vasoconstriction, vascular stasis, thrombosis and reperfusion injury occur, causing release of inflammatory mediators

Freezing

Most injuries related to cold weather exposure are due to slow freezing. Rapid freezing occurs with exposure to sub-zero degree cold, commonly solids such as dry ice, or cold volatile liquids such as propane, butane, helium, nitrous oxide or Freon.

Slow freezing

- Frostbite: Exposure in cold climates either due to insufficient precaution or associated with mental illness, drug or alcohol abuse. It often affects exposed regions such as the ears, nose and cheeks. The malnourished, infants and elderly are predisposed to this
- Hypothermia is a systemic response with effects such as hypertension and tachycardia that may progress to shock with reduced cardiac output and volume depletion from fluid sequestration. It is defined as a core body temperature (BT) of less than 35°C (mild 32–35°, moderate 28–32° and severe less than 28°C). Signs at initial presentation may be subtle

Rapid freezing

The primary causes tend to be either occupational or recreational. These mostly involve pressurised liquid gases with low boiling points that when in contact with skin, cause rapid evaporative cooling. Skin refrigerants such as ethyl chloride exploit this to produce topical anaesthesia. In some cases, the substance itself is very cold, such as liquid nitrogen.

Cryotherapy studies demonstrate that while many cells die from the freezing injury, the fibrocollagenous matrix and fibroblast are more resistant and thus preserved, potentially contributing to improved healing.

Staging

The early assessment of cold injuries can be difficult, except in obvious cases, with less than 50% clinical accuracy. They are thus generally treated more conservatively than thermal burn injuries.

Stages of frostbite are shown in **Table 14.**

Other symptoms

There is often a feeling of clumsiness or numbness, which is replaced by a severe

Table 14 Stages of frostbite	
Stage of frostbite	**Notes**
I: Frostnip	Superficial injury that looks slightly pale without blistering or peeling. There may be pins and needles. This injury is potentially reversible.
II: Superficial frostbite	Skin feels leathery and numb. Colour changes range from pale grey/white/yellow to slightly blue with blistering and peeling.
III: Deep frostbite	The skin has no feeling and is firm, swollen, cold to touch and variable in colour. There are usually fewer blisters, although they can form on rewarming with cyanotic/haemorrhagic fluid.

The severity or depth of injury can be classified according to the clinical appearance of the wound after rewarming (most injuries can appear similar initially). Complete necrosis is often referred to as stage IV or fourth degree.

throbbing pain after rewarming. This can persist for weeks, before changing to a mild tingling sensation. Sensory loss, increased cold sensitivity and hyperhidrosis can also develop and persist. Symptoms such as skin of normal colour that is indentable (indicating elasticity) may be predictive of a favourable outcome.

Treatment

The treatment of cold injuries is not without controversy. Rewarming injured parts may cause significant pain and local rewarming should only be started if there is no risk of refreezing.

Larger deeper injuries are better rewarmed rapidly in a water bath at 40–42°C for 15–30 min with analgesia. Studies have shown less tissue necrosis with this, compared to slow thawing. There are no specific medications or dressings that can change the course of cold injuries. Numerous adjuvants have been described but are of doubtful efficacy (dextran, heparin, warfarin, steroids, and vitamin C) or unproven benefit (HBOT, tPA, prostaglandin E1 analogues, nifedipine, pentoxifylline and superoxide dismutase). Dry heat (uneven effect and can cause thermal injury), rubbing and exercise is not recommended.

- Wound care with avoidance of pressure or friction, elevation and physiotherapy are the mainstays of treatment. Blisters should be left intact until the wound can be properly assessed
- Debridement is delayed until demarcation occurs, unless infection supersedes. Usage of studies such as radionuclide scans, thermography, laser Doppler and NMR have not proved superior to this. In particular, definitive tests in the first 3–5 days are not possible because of persistent vascular spasm and instability. Resultant tissue defects are reconstructed in a standard manner

Further reading

Imray C, Grieve A, Dhillon S, et al. Cold damage to the extremities: frostbites and non-freezing cold injures. Postgrad Med J 2009; 85:481–88.

Related topic of interest

- Acute burns

Compartment syndrome

Compartment syndrome is caused by increased pressure in a rigid soft tissue compartment to a degree that impairs vascular flow into it, causing ischaemia of its contents. This can be caused by a rise in intrinsic or extrinsic pressure or both. Intrinsic pressure is commonly secondary to intra-compartmental tissue swelling that worsens with progressive ischaemia. Extrinsic pressure is commonly secondary to reduced compliance of the tissues surrounding the compartment. Circumferential burns may have an extrinsic element from the eschar and an intrinsic element from tissue oedema.

It is most commonly post-traumatic. Neglect or failure to treat compartment syndrome results in ischaemic necrosis of the contents. Volkmann's contracture is an example of this.

Other less common causes include prolonged immobility with impairment of protective reflexes (lying on the forearm causes the pressure to rise from 6 mmHg to 180 mmHg), haematomas (fractures, venepuncture in the anticoagulated), fluid extravasation or muscle hypertrophy due to steroid abuse.

The basic mechanism is as follows:

- Intracompartmental pressure (CP, normal 0–8 mmHg) rises
- Venous pressure (VP) rises
- When CP/VP increases above capillary perfusion pressure, the capillaries collapse (30 mm Hg)
- Hypoxic injury causes release of mediators that increase capillary permeability, increasing tissue fluid and increase soft tissue swelling, elevating the CP further
- Compartmental effects: Tissues become ischaemic, leading to muscle necrosis
- Systemic effects: Necrotic tissue is now a source of breakdown products and inflammatory mediators. A significant risk of renal failure and mortality ensues

Diagnosis

Diagnosis is clinical with a high index of suspicion that is related to the mechanism and history. The hallmark is pain out of proportion to the signs, particularly with passive stretch. A sensation of burning or tightness precedes motor symptoms (sensory nerves affected before motor nerves).

- The compartment may feel swollen, tense or 'doughy' (compared to opposite side)
- The traditional five Ps of pain, paraesthesia, pallor, poikilothermia and pulselessness apply. The last three are notoriously unreliable and are at best, late signs

The diagnosis can be a problem in those with altered consciousness and in children. If in doubt, operate. Investigations that may be helpful include:

- Compartment pressure monitoring is performed by direct invasive measurement within the compartment. Commercial products such as the Stryker or home-made devices can be used, although the former is validated and more reliable
  - Absolute compartment pressure: A 30-mmHg threshold (some use 45 mmHg) is used. A low measured pressure does not exclude compartment syndrome and surgical decompression is indicated if clinical suspicion is high. The trend over time may be of greater diagnostic use than single values. Hypotensive patients will have lower thresholds
  - Pressure difference: Delta P = Diastolic blood pressure - CP, is used as a proxy for perfusion pressure. A value of 30 mmHg is usually taken as the threshold for intervention

Diastolic – CP

Treatment is surgical and comprises fasciotomy, under controlled conditions of an operating theatre with full asepsis and haemostasis. For the leg, it is common to use two incisions for release of the four compartments, as recommended in the BAPRAS/BOA Lower Limb Trauma Guidelines.

Two incision technique

Skin incisions are approximately 15 cm long and each compartment should be released independently with longitudinal incisions extending the full length of the compartment. Shorter incisions can be used in elective/chronic cases.

Anterolateral incision: The anterior and lateral compartments are approached through a single longitudinal incision placed in the middle third of a line between the tibia and fibula. This is located approximately over the anterior intermuscular septum, allowing access to both anterior and lateral compartments.

Posteromedial incision: The deep and superficial posterior compartments are approached through a longitudinal incision in distal part of leg, 2 cm posterior to posteromedial palpable edge of the tibia, thus anterior to the posterior tibial perforators. Dissection then proceeds in the subfascial plane, anterior to the posterior tibial margin (avoiding saphenous vein and nerve), where the fascia over the deep posterior compartment is released. The proximal part of the septum between the posterior compartments lies under the soleus muscle, and its origin from the proximal one third of the tibia may be mobilised for greater exposure to facilitate release of the fascia covering FDL and tibialis posterior.

Postoperatively it is important to anticipate reperfusion injury, acidosis, hyperkalaemia, myoglobinuria and renal failure. The wounds are left open. Skin grafting is rarely needed, if a full week is allowed for the oedema to settle. The two incisions described above retain the perforators, allowing flap options if required.

- Outcome depends very much on intervention. Near complete recovery can be expected with fasciotomy within 6 hours (before muscle necrosis)
- Elevation does not help. It decreases arterial pressure without significantly changing compartment pressure (i.e. decreased perfusion pressure)
- Fluid resuscitation is essential as hypotension accentuates CS but over-resuscitation (as may happen in burns) should be avoided
- Oxygen is useful. HBOT has some benefits as an adjunct and may protect against reperfusion injury

Further reading

Hammerberg EM, Whitesides, Seiler JG 3rd, et al. The reliability of measurement of tissue pressure in compartment syndrome. J Orthop Trauma 2012; 26:24–31.

Related topic of interest

- Acute burns
- Lower limb trauma and reconstruction

Patella head
fibula
medial edge of tibia
tibial tuberosity
. over Ant intermuscular septum
allows access to Ant & lateral
compartments
2cm
Ant tibial spine
lateral malleolus
medial malleolus.

Congenital breast abnormalities

Breast development

The breasts are ectodermal structures that develop in the 6th week, along the milk lines (primitive mammary ridges) that run from axilla to groin. Most of these ridges subsequently atrophy, except for the middle pectoral ridges at the fourth intercostal space. The areola develops in 5th month *in utero* whilst the nipple appears shortly after birth. Some breast enlargement may occur after birth due to circulating maternal hormones, but then involutes and remains quiescent until puberty (ducts and connective tissue). At thelarche, oestrogens stimulate duct and stromal growth while progesterone causes lobular growth. Breast development is generally completed by age 16–18.

Patients present after puberty and early if the deformity is significant. The complaint is deformity, asymmetry or both, and the complaint or its emphasis may change as the patient progresses through the teenage years. Timing of intervention is controversial during the period of breast development. The potential for remaining breast development must be balanced against its probability and contextualised to the individual's desires, social and psychological factors. The issue of age and informed consent may arise.

Poland syndrome

Described by Clarkson (1962) and attributed to the observations of Alfred Poland (1841), a medical student at the time, Poland syndrome is characterised by four essential features.

1. Unilateral hand hypoplasia
2. Syndactyly
3. Shortening of the index, long, and ring fingers (brachydactyly)
4. Absence of the sternocostal portion of the ipsilateral pectoralis major muscle (100%)

There may also be:

- Deficiency of NAC and breast (50%)
- Abnormal costal cartilage and ribs, sternal rotation and contralateral pectus and scoliosis
- Less commonly, the rotator cuff and latissimus dorsi muscles are affected

It is five times more common on the right side and three times more common in males. It occurs in 1:20–30,000 live births and most cases are sporadic. A popular causative (unsubstantiated) theory is one of diminished blood flow through the ipsilateral subclavian artery with variable degrees of differential flow reduction in its subsequent branches that account for the variety of manifestations. It remains a non-specific developmental field defect that occurs between the sixth and eighth weeks of fetal development.

Management

Postponing treatment until breast development is complete produces the best physical results. If valid psychological justifications warrant earlier surgery, the increased risk of revisional surgery must be accepted.

Customised implants alone usually suffice in males. In women, the restoration of the mound and anterior axillary fold is commonly achieved through a combination of an expander implant-based reconstruction with a pedicled LD flap. Particular attention is given to reconstructing the anterior axillary fold by repositioning the tendon appropriately (Hester). The muscle edge is sutured to the IMF and the regions of the sternal and clavicular heads, with careful inset along infraclavicular region to avoid a depression (which can be difficult to treat).

- If the ipsilateral LD is absent or underdeveloped, a free contralateral LD flap may be used. Preoperative angiography is not universally used, but hypoplastic or aberrant thoracodorsal vessels have been described albeit rarely
- The rationale for chest wall reconstruction is that an ideal breast reconstruction requires an ideal foundation for it. It remains controversial and its adoption is not universal. Options include resection and rotation of a chest wall segment, usage of mesh-reinforced MMA, customised implants and stacked acellular dermal matrices

Tuberous breast

This common breast deformity is under recognised and its presentation is bimodal. Patients classically present in during or shortly after the period of breast development. However, an increasing proportion present later in life for breast augmentation, albeit with a milder form. It is characterised by:

- Deficiency of skin envelope especially base, usually asymmetric
- Deficiency of parenchyma especially inferiorly
- NAC deformity with herniation of tissue into areola
- A raised IMF and a short (craniocaudal) breast footprint

As the severity increases, the normal conical breast shape deforms to a cylindrical or tubular form. It has been described as such as a tubular breast or a Snoopy dog deformity. It is important to note that the hypoplasia does not necessarily affect the remaining breast tissue. There is a subset of breast reduction patients who present with large tubular breasts.

Von Heimburg classification (1996)

- Type I (hypoplasia of the lower medial quadrant)
- Type II (hypoplasia of the lower medial and lateral quadrants with sufficient skin in the subareolar region)
- Type III (hypoplasia of the lower medial and lateral quadrants with deficiency of skin in the subareolar region)
- Type IV (severe breast constriction with minimal breast base)

Components of treatment

The essential features of a tuberous breast are constriction of the breast tissue, which may lead to herniation through areolar ring and management needs to be aimed at these issues.

- Reduce and correct NAC
  - Periareolar skin excision to reduce areolar size. Excess tissue is de-epithelialised
- Lower the IMF and increase lower pole skin height
  - Anatomical expander/implants are particularly useful to achieve differential lower pole expansion and preserve the increased caudocranial height of the footprint
- Expand breast base width
  - Redistribute parenchyma
    - Lower pole width is increased with multiple vertical parenchymal splits of the lower pole to allow redraping
- Increase volume of breast +/– mastopexy
  - Fill the volume void, commonly with an implant
- Newer alternatives
  - Primary lipomodelling with extensive Rigotomies to release lower pole tethering
  - Becker adjustable expander-implants that allow serial adjustment to match the normal rate of breast development
  - Gradual substitution of expander with serial lipomodelling once breast development is complete

A periareolar Benelli type incision is commonly used. With a mild medial defect (type I) Wise type incisions can also be used and lateral tissue can be shifted in after undermining. With type II/III tuberous breasts, variations of periareolar mastopexy with augmentation are commonly used. More severe problems are best dealt with using two-stage operations with the implant/expander placement as a first stage and implant exchange/port removal with areolar surgery as a second stage. As the deformity increases in severity, the increasingly short IMF to nipple distance and the constricted breast base makes reconstruction, including placing an implant more difficult.

Inadequate expansion or inadequate release of the transverse lower pole restriction will result in a double-bubble deformity, where a transverse indentation occurs at the level of the native IMF, resulting in a bulge superior and inferior to it. (Note that here we refer to an American double-bubble deformity, as commonly referred to in the US literature. In the UK, a double-bubble deformity is associated with inferior glandular prolapse over a superior submuscular implant.)

Further reading

Mandrekas AD, Zambacos GJ. Aesthetic reconstruction of the tuberous breast deformity: a 10 year experience. Aesthet Surg J 2010; 30:680-92.

Related topics of interest

- Breast reconstruction
- Congenital upper limb anomalies

Congenital upper limb anomalies

Development

The arm buds appear at the third week. At the 5th-6th week, the cartilaginous versions of the bones of the arm, forearm and hand bones appear. Apoptosis of the webs at the seventh to eighth week leads to finger separation. Thereafter, changes are minor and mostly of size and proportion. Control of growth in the three dimensions is simplified as follows:

- The apical ectodermal ridge (AER) directs proximo-distal development. The progress zone theory is the most popular but like all other theories to date, does not fully account for all processes involved. FGF is a major signalling factor here
- The dorsal ectoderm controls dorso-volar development primarily through Wnt-7a in the presence of Lmx-1. Engrailed-1 is specified on the volar surface to permit palmar development
- The zone of polarising activity (ZPA) is a block of mesoderm at the posterior base of the limb bud that controls radio-ulnar (pre-axial-post-axial) differentiation through Sonic hedgehog (Shh). The ulnar three digits are controlled by the temporal gradient of Shh and the index specified by a long-range diffusible form of Shh. ZPA duplication results in ulnar dimelia (mirror hand). The thumb is not dependent on Shh and thus radial dimelia is not possible through this mechanism

The postnatal hand starts to develop fine pinch at 10 months, but handedness is not established until 3–4 years. Proper hand eye coordination requires 4–5 years to develop.

Classification of congenital upper limb anomalies

The Swanson classification (1976) is commonly used, but is of little practical value and does not fully encompass all congenital upper limb anomalies. Conditions may belong in more than one category.

An alternative classification, such as one proposed by Tonkin (APSICON 2011), is based on the fact that formation and differentiation are parallel phenomena and are categorised into malformations, deformations and dysplasias. However, the Swanson remains the most widespread.

- Failure of formation
  - Transverse: Amputations are named after the level of termination, which is most commonly below the elbow. There is of little or no role for reconstruction
  - Longitudinal: Named after the absent or deficient bones, with radial problems being more common. Phocomelia (associated with thalidomide use) is the condition of shortened limbs, as though the hands are attached to the trunk. This is due to absence of a segment, which can be complete (hand to shoulder), proximal (forearm to shoulder) or distal (hand to arm)
- Failure of differentiation (separation)
  - Syndactyly, camptodactyly (usually PIPJ), clinodactyly (bent in a radio-ulnar direction), symphalangism (sym–fused longitudinally, syn–fused side to side), synostosis, contracture (arthrogryposis–flexion contracture of multiple joints associated with hypoplastic muscles and stiff joints), carpal coalitions (such as between lunate and triquetrum)
- Duplication: In the radio-ulnar axis (polydactyly, ulnar dimelia) or proximodistal direction (triphalangeal thumb)
- Overgrowth: Macrodactyly, most commonly affecting the index
- Undergrowth: Hypoplastic thumb, Poland syndrome
- Constriction band syndrome: Proximal portions often normal, with autoamputated distal portions or hypoplasia with a definite band in between
- Generalised skeletal deformities: Dystrophic dwarfism, Madelung disease, Marfan syndrome, achondroplasia

The overall incidence of congenital hand anomalies is 1 in 600 (with 1 in 10 being functionally or cosmetically significant). By comparison the overall congenital anomaly rate is 1 in 15. The cause is unknown in more than 50% of cases and of the remainder, 60% have multiple gene disorders, 20% with a single gene disorder, 10% chromosomal and 10% environmentally influenced. Genetic counselling and assessment to exclude other anomalies is paramount. These commonly include Apert syndrome, VATER/VACTERL, Holt-Oram syndrome, thrombocytopaenia absent radius (TAR) and Fanconi anaemia.

- Most anomalies are simple (sporadic or AD inheritance and not associated with involvement of any other system)
- Defects associated with craniofacial anomalies are generally AD (e.g. Apert and Pfeiffer syndromes)
- Multisystem syndromal anomalies can be AR or AD, such as Fanconi anaemia and Holt-Oram respectively

Sequences (localised insult, usually vascular, that causes a secondary pattern of rather specific, predictable and multiple anomalies, e.g. VATER) are distinguished from associations (non-random association of abnormalities that are not part of a distinct syndrome). Sequences usually occur sporadically.

General principles of treatment

The diagnosis of a congenital limb anomaly primarily impacts the parents. There is frequently a mixture of anger and guilt and many parents have unrealistic expectations. Counselling focuses on the likely outcomes, including the need for multiple staged operations with possible failure rate. Scars on hands and donor regions are necessary, as is potential sacrifice of normal parts for reconstruction. Parents often find it difficult to accept pollicisation (loss of index) or toe-to-hand transfer. Children become aware of differences from normality much later on and parts that are always visible to them (hands > face) rank higher in priority.

In the management of congenital hand deformities, maximising function is the priority (sensation is prerequisite) with cosmesis a close second. The patient's mental capacity, demands and general condition modifies this somewhat. For example, creating a tripod, instead of separating all digits, may satisfactorily treat an Apert mitten hand as the child is unlikely to be able to utilise it fully. Although Flatt makes the point that 90% of activities of daily living can be done with one hand, the aim is usually to maximise the function of both.

The aim of corrective surgery is to orientate the hand in space and provide adequate prehension (fine grip and power) that requires:

- Thumb, web-space and opposable digits of adequate length (preferably two or more for finer grip)
- Sensate parts and a stable ulna or radius
- Proximal joints are important. Whether the elbow is fixed or flexible has a tremendous impact

Not all deformities are amenable to treatment. Sometimes surgery improves appearance with little impact on function (cleft hand), and whilst a radially dysplastic hand is an obvious deformity, its correction may worsen function, particularly if the elbow is stuff (patient can no longer feed self). When normalisation of the hand cannot be achieved, the order of priorities is:

- Thumb to two-finger tripod pinch: Can still give good fine pinch function
- A precise thumb to single finger pinch is the basic aim in digit aplasia. Finger grip with power requires length and IPJ movement
- Crude thumb-finger pinch, where the fingers cannot touch but capable of limited opposition, can be enough to hold objects of certain size
- Key pinch (thumb to side of finger) requires less precision and sensation but is strong and useful. Key pinch is the aim when the fingers lack movement and the thumb has limited mobility, especially abduction and opposition
- At the most basic level, a sensate palm paddle with a mobile wrist or thoraco-

humeral pinch for a short arm is the minimum

Timing

The age at which surgery is needed is variable, being dependent on the severity/urgency of the condition. Timing has little impact on future growth except in constriction bands and complex/border syndactyly. Nevertheless, early treatment is advocated in most cases to maximise growth, avoid the formation of fixed deformities and exploits both tissue and cortical plasticity. Other factors to consider include:

- Immunity: Before 5th week (passive immunity still present) or after 5 months (maturation of immune system)
- Psychological: Children do not recall surgery before the age of 2
- Technical: Delay to allow structural growth to a sufficient size for easy surgery, or until an age when post-operative compliance can be achieved are common

Due to the rapid growth rate, X-rays (if required) should be performed pre-operatively instead of at presentation.

- Neonatal: If the procedure is simple (ligation of extra digit) or urgent (constriction band/ring with distal compromise)
- First year of life (healthy child, 6 months to 1 year)
  - Syndactyly: Especially digits of unequal length, border digits, complex syndactyly and acrosyndactyly
  - Deep constriction rings
- After 1st year: includes most other anomalies such as
  - Non-complex syndactyly and polydactyly is generally treated in the 2nd or 3rd year or prior to school age. Earlier surgery may be justified for other reasons, such as skin grafts that can be taken from the instep before child walks (10 months)
  - Trigger finger: These may resolve with age and complications such as flexion contracture are rare. However should the latter occur, they are more difficult to treat after 5 years of age (may need osteotomies)

- Waiting can be justified when there is
  - Relearning of alternate hand patterns, e.g. radial deficiency with fixed elbow extension
  - Camptodactyly, windblown hand, extensor tendon drift can often be treated with splint/stretching first

Syndactyly

This is the most common congenital hand deformity occurring in 1 in 2000 live births and is more common in Afro-Caribbeans. There is a positive family history in up to one third (AD with variable penetrance). The condition occurs due to lack of differentiation/separation and usually involves the third web (3, 4, 2, 1 in order of decreasing frequency). The first web is involved in only 1% of cases. Half are bilateral and symmetrical. Males are affected twice as frequently.

- Apert syndrome: Multiple and bilateral complex syndactyly with symphalangism of PIPJ, synostosis of fourth and fifth metacarpal (MC) bases and short radially deviated thumbs (delta phalanx). The hand is usually treated in stages (see below)
- Poland syndrome: A hypoplastic forearm with brachysyndactyly and symphalangism
- Radial deficiency

The condition can be described as:

- Incomplete vs. complete: The latter describes fusion along the entire length
- Simple vs. complex: The latter is defined as having fused bones
- Complicated: Other abnormalities present.
  - Symphalangism is the fusion of phalanges (proximo-distal) due to failure of segmentation and usually involves the MP and PP with absent or poorly developed PIPJ (undifferentiated capsule, ligament, cartilage or ankylosis). Creases are absent over the fused joint. The fingers tend to be shorter (especially MP) and narrower. Isolated symphalangism is often left alone or treated with arthroplasty/ arthrodesis when the patient is older. Earlier surgery is indicated when

there is also syndactyly, although the outcome of surgery is generally poor

- Acrosyndactyly: Usually sporadic. There is bony fusion but only at the tips, with fenestrations between the digits proximally (their configuration and extent sub classifies the condition). It represents refusion, and is often associated with constriction bands
- Acrocephalosyndactyly is a more complicated form of syndactyly, usually occurring in tandem with symphalangism. Is is found with craniofacial anomalies and is usually inherited in an AD manner. The best-known types are those of the Apert and Pfeiffer syndromes. In the former, the hand deformities are classically described as mitten, spade and rosebud types, with the fusion pattern resembling the namesake. With the Apert mitten hand, the little finger that is near normal is released first while the first web is deepened with grafts to increase span and provide tripod pinch (**Figure 5**)

Principles of treatment

Border digits (1/2 or 4/5), complex syndactyly and acrosyndactyly are usually treated earlier to maximise growth and minimise deformity progression.

- Broad webs are preferred. The new web should be positioned approximately halfway between MC head and PIPJ. Note that the second and third web-spaces are more distal than the fourth. The dorsal flap should be two thirds of the distance from MC head to PIPJ, with matching triangular flaps along the digits (Cronin) at 45° angles and crossing midline of digits. The palmar base is an inverted T with the vertical limb joining the Z and the horizontal limb tilted between the bases of the digits (**Figure 5**)
- For shared nails, these should be trimmed down (including the germinal bed), whilst the lateral defects in complete syndactyly are closed with hyponychial pulp flaps
- As complexity increases, the bifurcation of the common digital vessels arises more distally and the position/presence of arteries on other side becomes more unpredictable. Test the circulation with

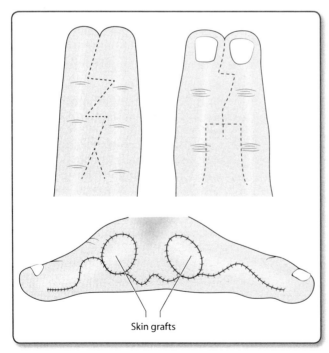

Figure 5 A common technique for syndactyly release. The need for skin grafts depends on the 'looseness' of the skin envelope; these should be placed near but not within the web.

Skin grafts

a finger Allen's test before any vessel division

- FTSGs give better results than SSG. Skin grafts in webs should be avoided to reduce formation of web contractures and should be preferentially placed on the side of the digits where any impact of contracture is minimal. There is a 22% geometrical deficiency of the skin circumference with syndactyly. Skin is almost always needed except in looser syndactyly or lesser degrees of incomplete syndactyly where flaps alone may suffice. Groin skin tends to hyperpigment and a better colour match may be obtained with hypothenar or instep grafts, but is limited in quantity
- A delay of 6 months is advised between surgery on adjacent digits to maximise viability and soft tissue pliability. Bilateral limb surgery should be restricted to patients younger than 18 months, otherwise compliance and postoperative disability is an issue

Postoperatively, conforming dressings (boxing gloves work well in children) are used to reduce movement that may lead to graft loss, dehiscence, and fusion of surfaces. The hand is protected for 2–3 weeks. Play therapy is used subsequently to encourage motion. Complications include lateral contracture/curvature whilst web-space creep occurs in 2–24% of cases. The revision rate is 10%.

Camptodactyly and clinodactyly

Camptodactyly: Flexion deformity of PIPJ (most commonly little finger) that is bimodal in distribution (infants and adolescent girls). It worsens during the growth spurt. Almost two thirds of cases are bilateral. The causes are bone or soft-tissue related. Soft tissue causes include abnormal lumbrical or FDS insertions that may be perpetuated by skin shortage. It is rarely a functional problem. Splintage may be occasionally successful (in children). Surgery is only indicated if it undergoes rapid progression or if the angulation is greater than 60° and impacts function. Surgery is often only partially effective.

X-rays features suggesting poor results include remodelling or indentation of the end of the proximal phalanx and a narrowed joint space. Severe deformities may be untreatable and osteotomy or arthrodesis may be considered.

Clinodactyly is lateral deviation of a digit. Radial deviation of little finger is most common and is due to abnormal middle phalangeal development (trapezoidal or triangular in shape; severe forms have a delta phalanx). It may be AD, often bilateral. No treatment is required unless there is functional impairment. Wedge osteotomies can be used to straighten and lengthen digits simultaneously if required.

Undergrowth

Short digits are due to transverse arrest of development (where proximal structures may be hypoplastic) or due to amputation from constriction (proximal structures are usually normal). The most common type of undergrowth deformity is symbrachydactyly, which is usually unilateral.

- Symbrachydactyly: Short fused fingers caused by longitudinal deficiency of digits and limbs, related to absent mesoderm. Digits may harbour ectodermal remnants. The four types based on clinical findings are
  1. Short finger
  2. Cleft hand type
  3. Monodactylic
  4. Peromelic type
- Brachydactyly: Digital shortening that is usually radial

Treatment

- Web spacing deepening, usually with Z-plasty
- Vascularised toe-transfer
- Bone grafting: Interposition or end-on with bone from iliac crest or toe phalanx (preferable, as the cortex/periosteal envelope promotes less resorption and greater growth potential). There are conflicting results from end-on toe grafts regarding the degree of epiphyseal growth. Distraction may be needed if the digit is of insufficient length

- Distraction osteogenesis can potentially provide sensate tissue with a nail plate with growth potential (average 85%), although the result is usually a stiff digit

Brachydactyly (symbrachydactyly without the fusion)

Bell classification

A. Shortened MP
B. Shortened/absent MP and DP, deformed thumbs and halluces
C. Deformities of MP and PP of the middle and ring fingers (hypersegmentation), ulnar deviation of index finger
D. Short broad DP of thumbs and halluces
E. Metacarpal shortening

Overgrowth

Macrodactyly is a congenital localised enlargement of the bones and soft tissues of toes/fingers (most commonly index finger) that is usually unilateral. True macrodactyly should be distinguished from other causes of a big finger/toe such as exostosis, vascular malformations and others (see below). As such, a common classification is:

I. Lipofibromatous haematoma, usually median or ulnar
II. Neurofibromatosis
III. Polyostotic fibrous dysplasia
IV. Hemihypertrophy (Klippel-Trenaunay, Proteus syndrome)

It can be
- Static: Proportions fixed from birth onwards
- Progressive: Usually related to area supplied by digital nerves (nerve territory orientated macrodactyly)

Operations include debulking (long term follow-up suggests that resection of nerve is not useful), epiphyseal destruction (epiphysiodesis)/stapling and osteotomies. However, the digits tend to have poorly developed tendons and vasculature, giving rise to a large but poorly vascularised and stiff digit. Amputation may be the best functional option in selected cases.

Constriction ring syndrome

The incidence is 1 in 15,000 with rings of variable severity oriented perpendicular the long axis of the limb. The middle finger is most commonly affected and most patients (80%) have other hand deformities. Clinical examination should focus on the extent of wrist motion, the presence of tendons, metacarpals and the soft tissue envelope. Paterson classification:

I. Simple constriction rings (incomplete or complete) that are treated with excision of entire groove including walls and closure with multiple Z-plasties
II. Deformity of distal part with or without lymphoedema
III. Fusion of distal part (acrosyndactyly): Early release within the first year is advocated
IV. Intrauterine autoamputations: These are ideal for free tissue transfer

This is one of the few conditions that can affect the fingers but leave functional thumbs. Hand function is potentially better preserved as the proximal structures are unaffected. Toe transfers may be thus be good options to provide pincer grasp. The growth of transferred toe is 90% of the normal toe whereas 10% will have premature closure of the epiphysis.

Thumb anomalies

Trigger thumb: The thumb rarely triggers, and the most common presentation is fixed IPJ flexion (locked) that is often unnoticed for months after birth. Notta's node is a palpable thickening of the FPL tendon at the MCPJ level that is bilateral in 25% of cases. It is reactive in nature and may spontaneously resolve (30% in 1st year). Splintage is the first line treatment. If this fails (50% of cases), cautious release the A1 pulley before age of 3 years is performed to avoid persistent deformities. Steroids are unhelpful.

Congenital clasped thumb manifests as a thumb held adducted against palm with flexed MCPJs. It is often bilateral and affects males more often. Splintage may help in mild cases but surgery may be required to correct contractures. Joint fusion after skeletal maturity is reserved for contractures that fail to release.

Thumb duplication occurs in 0.8 per 10 000 live births. It is a preaxial/radial duplication that is more common than its postaxial counterpart in Asians and Blacks. Most isolated cases are unilateral and sporadic except for the triphalangeal thumb (AD inheritance, associated with Holt-Oram syndrome). By comparison, postaxial duplication occurs in 1 in 300 Blacks, which is ten times more common than it is in Caucasians.

Wassel classification

Odd numbers bifid, even numbers duplicated. Progresses from distal to proximal.
- I and II: Bifid and duplicated DP respectively
- III and IV: Bifid and duplicated PP respectively
- V and VI: Bifid and duplicated MC respectively
- VII: Duplication with triphalangia (20%). This is distinct from isolated triphalangia

The most common is type IV (40%). The thumb is often hypoplastic and angulated (due to a variety of reasons such as shared tendons, conjoint tendons, abnormal/improperly attached muscles, unstable collaterals and altered/abnormal bone shapes). The muscles supplied by the ulnar nerve typically insert on the ulnar thumb whereas those supplied by the median nerve tend to insert onto the radial thumb. The nail is often ridged, and it is usually preferable to split the nail making it smaller.

The general strategy is to augment the proper thumb with tissues of the accessory digit. Postoperatively, instability of MCPJ and smaller thumb size may result with late Z-deformity (ulnar deviation at MCPJ, radial deviation at IPJ) if the collateral ligaments are not reconstructed or migrated appropriately.
- Part sharing is frequently used, where parts of the larger digit (larger than 80% normal side, usually ulnar) are kept and reconstruction of radial collateral ligament (RCL) and reattachment of the intrinsics to the MP joint is performed. The alternative

for symmetrical distal duplications seen in Wassel types I and II is central excision of equivalent portions and fusion of the remaining halves (Bilhaut Cloquet technique). Tendons are centralised and temporary arthrodesis with K-wires maintained for 6–8 weeks. Stiffness and deformity may be due to damage to joint, growth plate and nail bed
- For types III and IV, the most common option is total ablation of one thumb, usually the radial. This preserves the more important ulnar collateral ligament and ulnar sensation. RCL reconstruction is required. Type IV duplications should be treated early to prevent displacement of the normal components by the accessory part due to asymmetrical growth
- Type V and VI thumbs can be treated with muscle rebalancing, web space widening and osteotomies. The radial thumb may be more mobile mobility and can be preserved along with the ulnar with an on-top plasty
- VII: Fusion of DIPJ or on-top plasty

Hypoplastic thumb: The thumb is the commonest digit involved in the undergrowth syndromes. A hypoplastic thumb is often associated with other upper limb anomalies such as the radius with Fanconi's and Holt-Oram, but the majority are non-syndromic.

The Blauth classification (modified by Buck and Gramcko) is a useful guide to treatment.
I. Minor hypoplasia of the thumb with functional muscle. Smaller but otherwise normal. No treatment is required
II. Minor underdevelopment of skeletal elements with adduction contracture, MCPJ ulnar collateral ligament laxity and thenar muscle hypoplasia. Repair and correct tendons and ligaments, release web and adductor. Opponensplasty may be required (commonest is Huber transfer: ADM tendon to APB)
III. Marked skeletal hypoplasia especially first MC and atrophy/instability of the first ray, intrinsic muscle aplasia and rudimentary extrinsic tendons. There are two subtypes A and B (carpometacarpal joint (CMCJ) functional or deficient respectively). The former is reconstructible and the

latter should be treated by ablation and pollicisation

IV. Floating thumb (*pouce flottant*): Thin soft tissue bridge and rudimentary phalanges. Treat with amputation

V. Total thumb absence

In simple terms, thumbs that are II and IIIA are reconstructed while III B or more severe should be treated by index pollicisation. Surgery is best performed before age of 3 years as the new thumb is more easily integrated into hand function. Reasonable results are possible in the absence of additional radius abnormalities. Distraction lengthening is rarely used because of the absence of thumb joint motion while toe transfers are potentially problematic as proximal structures are absent/rudimentary.

Deficiencies

Radial dysplasia/deficiency occurs in 1 in 100,000 and more common in males. It may be related to environmental causes (thalidomide). Some occur as part of a syndrome:

- Holt-Oram with cardiovascular anomalies
- VATER with gut anomalies
- TAR, Fanconi with haematological anomalies, e.g. blood dyscrasia, these cases tend to be bilateral

The term 'radial club hand' has been replaced with 'deficiency' or 'dysplasia' to avoid the negative connotations. Most are unilateral and on the right. The ulna is never normal and is short and curved. Wedge osteotomy of ulna or Ilizarov distraction straightening may be needed to correct ulnar bowing of more than 35°. The whole arm/forearm is generally shorter, with radial deviation due to forearm muscles that normally arise from medial epicondyle having abnormal insertions. In addition, there may be stiffness and flexion contractures of joints that include the elbow and digits. Syndromic cases tend to be more severe.

- There is a range of additional abnormalities of the radial vessels (e.g. absent radial artery) and nerves (median nerve also displaced), and other parts including the humerus, forearm, radial carpus and thumbs (absent in one third)

- Many cope very well without treatment, but bilateral deformity with stiff elbows makes independent living near impossible. Early comprehensive correction is warranted. Relapse is common

Bayne classification

I. Hypoplastic radius. Distal epiphyseal growth is delayed/deficient but present. A short distal radius results

II. Hypoplastic radius. Both ends are defective resulting in a miniature radius

III. Partial absence, usually distal, with fibrous *anlage*. This is the most common

IV. Total absence

Treatment should begin within the 1st year, before the formation of significant fibrotic contractures and to allow ulna remodelling (distally wider). The principle is to centralise the wrist in stages aiming to be complete by 2 years of age.

- Stretching preoperatively with serial splintage, passive stretch by parents or frame-based distraction. In the latter, partial centralisation is achieved simultaneously, delaying formal centralisation until complete

- Surgery aims to place wrist on the distal ulna (centralise with a pin through third ray or radialise through second MC), which requires transposition of redundant ulnar skin to the radial side in form of Z-plasty or bilobed flap, release of fibrotic soft tissue, transferring radially deviating vectors to the ulnar side and tensioning the extensor mechanism appropriately. Subsequent pollicisation of index improves grasp (at a later date)

- Prolonged splintage: Maintenance of position postoperatively with K wires and plaster splints for 6–8 weeks, with continued splintage until 6 years old and a night splint until the bones mature

- Pollicisation not before 6 months post-centralisation

Contraindications to surgery include:

- Mild deformities
- Older patients who have adjusted well
- Life threatening conditions coexisting in the patient
- Proximal joint fixed, e.g. elbow

Ulnar deficiency is an uncommon deformity where the forearm tends to be stable at the wrist (the carpus remains articulated) but unstable at elbow.

I. Deficient ulna, minimal deformity
II. Partial absence with fibrous *anlage*, radial bowing and displaced distal epiphysis. This is most common
III. Total absence with *anlage*
IV. Humeroradial synostosis

Central deficiencies are usually bilateral and may involve the feet as well (**Table 15**).

Treatment of typical central deficiencies includes release of first web syndactyly and transposition of index finger to the base of middle MC (Snow-Littler procedure).

Table 15 Comparison between atypical and typical forms of central deficiency

Typical cleft hand	Atypical (after Barsky) or cleft-hand type symbrachydactyly
Autosomal dominant	Sporadic
Several limbs involved, often bilateral	Unilateral, foot involvement rare
Syndactyly common especially border digits	Syndactyly rare
V cleft with absence of central MCs	U cleft with central three rays absent
Narrowed first web, hypoplasia of radial rays	Hypoplasia of ulnar rays
Hypertrophic skeleton adjacent to cleft	Hypoplastic/atrophic skeleton adjacent to cleft

Further reading

Kajikawa A, Ueda K, Katsuragi Y, et al. Aesthetic repair for syndactyly of the toes using a plantar rectangular flap. Plast Recontr Surg 2010; 126:156–62.

Related topics of interest

Craniosynostosis

There are five ossification centres in the cranial vault with six main suture lines. This arrangement allows over-riding of the bones during childbirth. The anterior fontanelle is larger and closes at 2 years of age, while the posterior fontanelle closes earlier at 2 months. CS is the premature fusion of the sutures and occurs in 1 per 2000 live births. Premature fusion can occur at any of the sutures or in combination, leading to distinctive abnormalities of skull shape as growth perpendicular to the suture line is predictably retarded (Virchow's principle). Compensatory growth occurs in the direction parallel to the fused sutures.

There is a male predominance (4:1) in sagittal synostosis, while females predominate (3:2) in unilateral coronal synostosis. Gender differences are less obvious in other synostoses. The common forms of are metopic, sagittal and coronal. Positional plagiocephaly is the commonest cause of skull deformity and is non-synostotic, but must be distinguished from synostotic plagiocephaly.

The causes of CS include genetic disorders, gestational toxicity or a sporadic occurrence. The dura mater underlying sutures may be important in the timing of closure through osteoinductive growth factors. The primary event in CS is unclear, the pathogenesis complex and multifactorial. The various sutures that can be involved in craniosynostosis are shown in **Table 16**. A common classification is:

- Primary CS: Due to a suture problem **(Table 16)**
- Secondary CS: Due to another a non-suture factor such as failure of brain development, endocrine disorders (e.g. hypothyroidism, hypoparathyroidism and vitamin D deficiency or haematological disorders with marrow hyperplasia). This type of CS is more common and less likely to be associated with raised ICP

Other descriptions include:

- Simple vs. complex: Simple CS affects one suture and is usually sporadic. Complex CS affects two or more sutures

- Syndromic vs. non-syndromic: Syndromic CS is associated with other abnormalities (more than 100 different syndromes have been described). It is usually complex and more likely to be inherited but 50% are new mutations. Coronal synostosis is likely to be syndromic. Non-syndromic CS is usually sporadic and not inherited

Physical examination may demonstrate recognisable patterns. The commonest craniosynostotic syndromes are Crouzon, Apert and Pfeiffer, which are associated with mutations of the fibroblast growth factor receptors (FGFR).

Investigations

- Plain radiographs
- CT including 3D reconstruction
- MRI: Particularly for posterior fossa/cranial base

Raised intracranial pressure

The brain is 25% of adult size at birth, triples in size in the 1st year, and bony restriction of this expansion may lead to raised ICP. With a single suture synostosis, ICP is raised (defined as > 15–20 mmHg under unstressed conditions) in 13%; with multiple sutures/syndromic, it is raised in 42% (Marchac) particularly in patients with Crouzon's (66%) and less so in Apert's (43%). The cause of raised ICP is not always clear but may be related to venous hypertension. The signs of raised ICP are irritability, vomiting, bulging fontanelles, papilloedema (pathognomonic feature) and optic atrophy. Ophthalmic review is appropriate in complex/syndromic cases.

Radiological features include the loss of the usual lucency of suture interdigitations with increased sclerosis. CT is useful in detecting fusion (there may be heaping up of bone at the suture line) and demonstrating any coexisting abnormalities. With persistently raised ICP, the bones may have a 'copper-beaten' or 'thumb-printed' appearance.

Hydrocephalus is relatively uncommon, although it is more common in syndromic cases (~10%) and is usually of the communicating type. CT may be used to assess ventricle size but this does not directly correlate to the presence of hydrocephalus or raised ICP (Apert patients tend to have ventriculomegaly without hydrocephalus). Progressive changes on serial scans may be a better indicator. Decreased cranial volume per se is inadequate justification for surgery.

Mental retardation

The risk of mental retardation is increased in craniosynostotic patients and may be related to a raised ICP, hydrocephalus, prematurity and primary brain abnormalities. Whilst an association between cranial capacity, ICP and mental retardation may seem logical, it is not always the case.

Although most surgeons advocate early treatment especially with multiple suture involvement, the effect of surgery (particularly on mental retardation) in patients with a single synostosis is unclear. Some suggest that moderately severe retardation in those with single suture synostosis is more likely to be due to a primary brain problem than the synostosis, with some studies showing no effect from early surgical correction, indicating that some brain impairment had taken in place *in utero*. Furthermore, some studies have shown that while surgery improves the deformities, it does not affect mental development (IQ scores), although Marchac maintains that surgery can be helpful, particularly in younger patients.

Neuropsychiatric abnormalities ranging from mild behavioural disturbance to mental retardation may exist. The abnormal head shape can cause severe embarrassment, worsening the slow learning. Some studies showed increased self-esteem with surgery but with little effect on social interaction. Normalisation of measurements did not equate with increased perceived attractiveness.

Crouzon syndrome

This is the commonest of the craniosynostoses, occurring in 1 in 25,000. The four essential components are exorbitism, proptosis, midface hypoplasia and paradoxical retrogenia. Although most cases are sporadic (with the risk of another affected child being born to healthy parents being less than 1%), some exhibit AD inheritance with widely variable penetrance. It is associated with FGFR2 mutations on chromosome 10 and is characterised by:

- Skull abnormality – Most commonly a flattened skull (turribrachycephaly) due to bicoronal synostosis (tall forehead), but other sutures can be involved. The fusion is not immediate and takes 1–2 years to complete. Hydrocephalus may also coexist, contributing further to the raised ICP
- Nystagmus and strabismus are associated features, along with shallow orbits and maxillary hypoplasia that cause exorbitism (the most consistent feature, bulging eyes with risk of exposure or trauma) and hypotelorism
- Severe midfacial hypoplasia, beaked nose and a class III dental occlusion (relative prognathia, the mandible is shorter than normal) with a concave profile are common, although the severity varies widely

Problems include:

- Vision may be affected by the raised ICP, exorbitism, nystagmus and strabismus
- Airway problems may be more acute just after birth as neonates are obligate nasal breathers and forcing the neonate to mouth breathe expends more energy

These features are also found in Apert syndrome, although craniofacial development is different and distinct. The overall craniofacial features are more severe in Apert syndrome but the degree of exorbitism/proptosis may be more severe in Crouzon syndrome. The other main differences include:

- Hands are normal in Crouzon syndrome
- Mental retardation is uncommon in Crouzon (5%). There may be a conductive hearing loss
- Non-cranial anomalies affecting the bone and cartilage of the spine and elbow may be present with Crouzon

Treatment

- Anterior vault and upper orbit reshaped and advanced at 1 year. Revision may be necessary within 5 years if ICP is raised (15%)
- Le Fort III/Monoblock/facial bipartition (FBP) at age 5–7 or later (see below)
- Mandible is treated using a Le Fort, genioplasty or subsagittal split when skeletal maturity is reached (14–16 years in females, 16–18 years in males)

Apert syndrome

Apert is another acrocephalosyndactyly syndrome (Type I, Crouzon is Type II). Most cases are sporadic (possibly related to increasing paternal age), but some are inherited in an AD manner. There are similarities to Crouzon syndrome, but is generally more severe/complex (except for midface) and more uniform in presentation. The features include:

- Abnormal head shape - Tendency towards turribrachycephaly with a long forehead and anteriorly displaced vertex.
- Complex syndactyly commonly involving the second to fourth digits with a common nail. It is common to release thumb and marginal webs before the central webs
  - Class 1: Spade hand: The thumb is joined with simple syndactyly, the middle three digits are syndactylised with a flat palm, and the fourth web space is a simple, incomplete syndactyly. Thumb clinodactyly is common and may also be broad
  - Class 2: Mitten hand: The thumb is joined with simple syndactyly, the middle three fingertips are fused, forming a concave palm, and the fourth web space is a simple, complete syndactyly
  - Class 3: Rosebud hand: Complex syndactyly of the thumb and middle three digits with a single conjoined nail. The fourth web space is a simple, complete syndactyly
- Cleft palate is found in 20%. Conductive deafness is also present in a similar number. The abnormally long soft palate/ uvula causes unusual speech
- Small nose with down-turned tip, antimongoloid slant, proptosis and hypertelorism. Midfacial and mandibular hypoplasia is present but the latter less so than the maxilla. Airway problems can arise due to the narrowed nasopharynx, retrodisplaced maxilla and long soft palate
- Acne/hyperhidrosis: Affects forearms and thick sebaceous skin is present especially over the nose
- Polycystic kidneys
- Raised ICP in 40% of cases. Mental retardation can occur in the absence of a raised ICP due to hydrocephalus or other primary brain abnormalities such as agenesis of the corpus callosum

The treatment schedule is similar to Crouzon but with an increased need for revision due to increased ICP. The emphasis in Apert is usually early surgery to prevent further dysmorphia due to the abnormal cranial base, while surgery in Crouzon is generally to treat/prevent raised ICP. Early surgery (for fronto-orbital regions) generally does not improve midface growth.

Position moulding

Positional moulding describes the misshaped head that results from prolonged pressure in a particular direction without premature suture fusion. Approximately 98% of posterior plagiocephaly is due to moulding. Causes include:

- Sleeping position: Tendency to nurse babies supine to reduce sudden infant death (SID)
- Prematurity: Softer skull and *in utero* compression
- Intrauterine compression, e.g. from the pelvis or a twin
- Abnormal vision leading to preferred head position
- Torticollis: This is found in 1 per 300 live births and in 30% of breech deliveries. Lumps may be felt in the lower third of the sternomastoid especially in the first few weeks of life, although these usually resolve without need for surgery. It is due to a shortened muscle on the same

Table 16 Features of craniosynostosis involving various sutures

Suture involved	Deformity	Notes
Plagiocephaly (Greek for oblique or crooked)	Coronal (anterior) or lambdoid (posterior, less common). In coronal CS, there is a single frontoparietal bone plate that defines the deformity.	Most cases are 'positional' whereas 'true' plagiocephaly is due to CS and may be associated with oligohydramnios or other causes of uterine constraint. Harlequin orbits (shallow with an elevated upper outer corner on AP X-ray) are a feature of anterior plagiocephaly and may cause severe proptosis with ulceration and blindness though most cases have few functional problems. May need formal reconstruction at 1 year (bifrontal craniotomy with supraorbital advancement) and a bilateral approach is often preferred to ensure symmetry.
Posterior plagiocephaly	Lambdoid synostosis is the rarest type and tends to be progressive.	There is flattening of the occiput with displacement of the ear, posteroinferiorly on the ipsilateral side with deformation of the cranial base. The foramen magnum is deviated to the affected side. Treatment consists of a craniotomy with radial cuts, barrel staves and dural plication.
Trigonocephaly (triangular) 10% of isolated, nonsyndromic cases. There is a wide variation in shape. Some have primary frontal lobe underdevelopment.	**Metopic** (usually fuses at 2 years) with palpable ridge. Skull is narrow in transverse dimension with mild hypotelorism. Keel shaped with bitemporal narrowing and compensatory parietal growth.	Less than 10% are syndromic but these are more likely to be associated with mental retardation (up to 1/3 compared to 4%). Cosmetic results are generally good. Simple ridges can be burred away. In some, it may resolve with time with no functional impairment, but treatment, if needed, requires suture release with bifrontal craniotomy, advancement of supraorbital bar, barrel staves osteotomy to modify volume if needed at age of 1.
Scaphocephaly (narrow and long, like an upturned boat)	**Sagittal.** It may not involve the whole suture.	**Commonest isolated CS** (>50%, usually sporadic) and midface is usually normal. Males are affected 3–4 times more frequently. Optimal management is still debated. Some favour early simple suture release (strip craniectomy) but most advocate formal release and reconstruction to shorten the AP and widen the transverse diameter. This is achieved through a bifrontal craniotomy, reshaping with radial osteotomies and barrel staves in the parietal region.
Brachycephaly (short)	**Bilateral coronal synostosis.** Compensatory anterosuperior bulging with open metopic suture.	**Commonly syndromic** and results in a short skull with compensatory growth superiorly. If untreated, a tower-like appearance results, with bulging of the upper frontal area with an anterior vertex, known as turribrachycephaly (more common in Apert's). Orbits are often shallow. Treatment is instituted at 1 year, where frontal and occipital craniotomies facilitate reshaping. A central handlebar that includes the sagittal suture line is shifted posteriorly to move the vertex. Supraorbital advancement and volume modification is achieved with barrel staving.
Kleeblattschädel (clover leaf head)	Often due to synostosis of multiple sutures except the sagittal/metopic and squamosal.	There is severe exophthalmos and nasal atresia and marked hydrocephalus. It is often associated with limb abnormalities.

side (scarring or ischaemic changes) that leads to inclination and tension in the neck and facial deviation. Early treatment with physiotherapy or headband/helmets gives better results. Muscle release is rarely needed. The typical skull changes are an ipsilateral cranio-orbital flattening with contralateral occipital flattening (positional plagiocephaly) that often resolves with conservative measures. Cases that persist beyond 12–18 months may require surgical treatment. Adult torticollis may be associated with spasm and possibly psychological disturbance.

A positionally plagiocephalic head adopts a parallelogram shape (although forehead deformities tend to be minor). This is in contrast to a synostotic head that adopts a trapezoidal shape instead (only one pair of parallel sides due to retarded growth along one side of the skull).

Other features of positional plagiocephaly:

- Frontal bossing ipsilateral to the flattening instead of contralateral
- Ear is more anterior on flattened side instead of being more posterior and low set

In positional plagiocephaly, the skull shape starts off being normal at birth before becoming increasingly flat from 2–8 months. It subsequently improves as the baby becomes more active and sits up, and resolves by 12–18 months. Treatment is rarely required. Playing in the prone position (tummy time) and sleeping with the head on alternate sides is to be encouraged. Moulding helmets can be used but are uncommon.

Treatment of craniosynostosis

It is important to differentiate between positional moulding that rarely requires surgery, from true synostoses. Those with multiple suture involvement may be part of a recognised syndrome and should be referred to geneticists. In general, whilst the surgery can be protracted and multistaged, the priorities are rather simple:

- Correct breathing problems: This may be as simple as a tonsillectomy, but may require a formal skeletal advancement/ distraction. Temporary tracheostomy may be necessary
- Protect the brain: Elevated ICP should be relieved quickly as there is a risk of chronic herniation of the cerebellar tonsils
- Protect the eyes: Exorbitism may to lead to corneal exposure
- Optimise feeding: Adequate nutrition and good dental hygiene is important

Sorting out these basic priorities will allow the patient to be in optimal shape for subsequent treatment that aims to improve head shape. The controversial issues are the optimal timing for surgery and risk-benefit ratios.

Timing

Good comparative studies do not exist and thus the optimal timing remains unknown. Advocates for early surgery argue that benefits to brain development are maximised and moulding is still possible. Furthermore, the magnitude of subsequent corrective surgery may be reduced. Advocates for delayed surgery cite lower revision rates and thus lower complication rates. This approach may be less appropriate in syndromic cases with raised ICP, even though there is little strong evidence to show that surgery has any influence on mental retardation. Most surgeons agree that operating when the patient is below 1 year of age is best, but many avoid the 3–6 month period when the haematopoietic capacity is lowest. Early craniofacial advancement surgery may improve self-esteem particularly before school, at the expense of an increased requirement for secondary surgery.

- Less than 1 year: Bone is malleable, easily reshaped (cut with scissors and moulded with greenstick fractures) and defects ossify spontaneously
- 1–3 years: Bone is more brittle and less likely to bend but can be selectively weakened with channels. The capacity to ossify defects is reduced
- Older than 3 years: Direct reshaping and fixation in the adult position/shape. Malleability and reossification of defects is minimal

Type of surgery

Surgery can be simple or comprehensive, open or endoscopic. The method and requirement for fixation is also controversial. Stabilisation may impair growth and screws may internalise.

- Early suture release
  - Craniectomy or cranial vault reconstruction at 3 months if the ICP is high or before 6 months for syndromic patients. Reoperation rates are higher for surgery before 9 months. Early strip suture excision may allow spontaneous normalisation of the skull shape but is insufficient for all but the isolated sagittal CS. Further surgery is likely for

all other types of CS
- Fronto-orbital advancement of the supraorbital rim (1.5–2.5 cm) should be performed within a year to protect globe in severe exorbitism. This should be delayed in its absence, as the recurrence rate is higher if performed before the age of 5. It can be combined with vault reshaping
- Reassess midface at 5–7 years of age when features are roughly 85% of adult size. Treatment at this or a later stage (some wait for eruption of permanent dentition at 12 years) can be regarded as permanent. Any maxillary/midface deficiency at this stage is treated with midfacial advancement
  - Le Fort III (subcranial approach) to correct lower skeletal and generalised midfacial deficiency/retrusion. The effect is limited to 1 cm, although it can be followed by distraction
  - Monobloc (Le Fort III segment along with fronto-orbital advancement, Ortiz-Monasterio) for recessed supraorbital ridges and shallow orbits. The communication between cranial and nasal cavities increases the risk of infective complications and separate procedures are usually preferred
  - Facial bipartition is particularly useful for orbital hypertelorism in Apert patients with flat, wide faces. The facial skeleton is divided vertically in the midline and segments reunited after removal of the central portion
  - Distraction osteogenesis
- The mandible may outgrow the maxilla and require orthognathic surgery in the form of a Le Fort I osteotomy or sliding genioplasty. Fine adjustments may be needed in later life, particularly in the superior forehead position for overall balance, and the supraorbital ridge

Postoperative

Deaths are rare (1–2%) but are most commonly due to uncontrolled bleeding and infection. The most common complication is incomplete correction, and is most frequent in those with unilateral/asymmetric deformities.
- Blood loss is the major intraoperative and postoperative concern and the small blood volume of patients makes any blood loss proportionately more significant. Major bleeding can come from the sinuses (with risk of air embolism) and bleeding from the bone edges may be significant
- Postoperative fever is not uncommon and is usually due to degradation of clots, prolonged use of lines and transfusion reactions, rather than SSI per se. Antibiotics are often used but the risk of meningitis is low, except in the presence of prolonged CSF leaks that should be repaired (intraoperative check with Valsalva 40 mmHg). Leaks found later on can often be treated with head elevation and drainage/decompression before considering surgical exploration

Further reading

Czerwinski M, Kolar JC, Fearon JA, et al. Complex craniosynostosis. Plast Reconstr Surg 2011; 128:955–61.

Related topic of interest

- Cleft palate

Ear reconstruction

Ear reconstruction is commonly required with
- Congenital malformation such as microtia (children)
- Acquired loss post-traumatic or post-extirpation for cancer (adults)

The ear develops from six hillocks (appearing at 5 weeks of development), three from the second arch and three from the first arch. The latter contributes only to the tragus and crus of the helix.

Microtia

This condition occurs in 1 per 7000 Caucasians and is slightly more common in Asians.
- Twice as common on the right (right: left: bilateral = 6:3:1)
- Males are affected three times more frequently

The cause is unknown and is multifactorial. There have been reported associations with maternal rubella and thalidomide exposure. There is low concordance in twins. One-third have other associated abnormalities and 10% of these are part of defined syndromes such as Treacher-Collins, hemifacial microsomia or Goldenhar syndrome. Some regard microtia as a 'microform' of hemifacial microsomia with shared features such as asymmetry (right more common) and an association with facial nerve palsy that is more common in males.
- There is an increased risk of cholesteatoma in those with ear canal atresia
- The hairline is often low on the abnormal side
- Auricular dystopia is an ear (either normal or microtic) that is displaced secondary to deformity of the facial skeleton and is a common feature of hemifacial microsomia. The remnant is often a bit anterior and inferior to the proposed/optimal position for reconstruction and the halfway point is usually used as a compromise. The presence of a formed external auditory canal limits positional adjustment and complicates the surgery. The facial nerve is at greater risk

Classification

There is a wide spectrum of deformity. The presentation varies from a rudimentary skin appendage to a smaller version of an otherwise normal ear. The widely-used classifications overlap to a degree.

The lobular type of microtia is a sausage-shaped mass consisting mostly of the lobule remnant, which is relatively normal but displaced. This is analogous to the classic type described by Brent. The external ear canal is often absent.

Conchal microtia is more ear-like in appearance and the ear canal is variably present. This is a less common variant and more likely to be displaced. It is analogous to the atypical type.

Microtia can also be graded:

- Grade 1: Small but normal, with or without an intact ear canal
- Grade 2: Small but missing some features; equivalent to the 'atypical' or 'conchal' variants
- Grade 3: Ear with a malformed rudimentary lobule and a mass of disorganised cartilage with fibrous tissue; the 'classic' or 'lobular' form
- Grade 4: Anotia

The two main options for these patients with respect to the external ear are reconstruction or using a prosthetic ear. Local preferences are a strong determining factor in the choice of technique. Autologous reconstruction is the treatment of choice in countries including the USA, UK, Japan and France, while prosthetics is preferred in Sweden (home of the Brånemark prosthesis).

Reconstruction

To reconstruct an ear, cartilage or its equivalent is used to recreate a framework, which is then covered by skin/soft tissue. There is a choice of materials available for the framework.
- Silicone scaffolds are prone to extrusion even if covered by temporoparietal (TP) flaps (Cronin) and have largely

been abandoned. Results with porous polyethylene (MEDPOR) covered by TP flaps are more encouraging (Reinisch). Patients must be counselled of the risk of late exposure

- Autologous material
  - Costal cartilage remains the most popular choice
  - Tissue expansion for gaining skin is generally not useful

The results depends more on the quality of the overlying skin than the intricacy of the carving as the details tend to be blunted. The skin is often thick and in short supply, but yet has to drape freely over the framework. The primary goal is to have the framework in an appropriate size and orientation.

Timing of surgery

Although there are many different techniques, the fundamentals are similar. Many surgeons have contributed to the evolution of modern ear reconstruction; they include Tanzer (1940s, credited with the modern four-stage technique which evolved from six stages), Brent (1980s, three-stage sometimes four), Nagata (1990s), and Firmin (2000s). The latter two described two-staged techniques with modifications to allow early lobule placement and used a cartilage wedge for elevation.

At the age of 5–6 years, the normal ear is >85% of adult size and can be considered to be fully developed (though not fully grown, as it continues to widen and its relationship to scalp changes) and can be used as a reference (if bilateral, can use siblings or parents). The other delay is waiting for the costal cartilages to be sufficiently large for an adequately sized construct (chest circumference >60 cm). On average, reconstruction occurs between the ages of 8–10. Costal cartilage becomes increasingly calcified with age, making it brittle and difficult to carve.

The trend seems to be towards adopting a Nagata approach or similar, though criticisms include the large amount of cartilage needed, potential vascular compromise in lobule movement and the scars from TP harvest. Those that cannot accept these risks tend to prefer a Brent type approach, which also tends to leave a more natural lobule (less tissue is used to line the concha and tragus).

Preoperative preparations

Careful planning is crucial. Undeveloped X-ray film is used to make a template from the other ear; taking care to match the angle and position. The template should be slightly smaller by a few millimetres to allow for thickness of soft tissue. The following description approximates to the technique described by Brent.

- First stage: A costal cartilage framework is constructed and placed into position
  - The contralateral sixth to eighth costal cartilages are made into a framework with an exaggerated rim and a pronounced antihelix. A segment of cartilage for framework elevation can be banked in the lateral part of the donor wound
  - Through an anterior incision, residual cartilage remnants are removed and a pocket that is 1 cm wider than the framework is dissected out. Mattress quilting sutures are used to improve definition of the ear contours, with or without bolsters. Suction drains, conforming dressings and an ear bandages may be used while minimising pressure on the ear
- Second stage: This is undertaken after 4–6 months to allow reestablishment of the blood supply and settling of oedema. The scaffold is elevated from the side of the head through an incision 5 mm superior and posterior to the framework. This exposes a bare postauricular sulcus that may be covered with fascia (temporoparietal or postauricular) and a skin graft over a bolster. There may be reconstruction of the lobule and tragus at this point (Brent) or with the first stage, depending on the exact technique (Table 17)
- Third stage: Definitive reconstruction of the tragus and lobule. Costal cartilage is used for tragus (or a composite graft) and cartilage excavated to reconstruct the conchal depression

Nagata's two-stage technique involves transfer of the lobule in the first stage, along with reconstruction of the tragus and posterior wall of the concha. The more extensive dissection translates to a greater risk of skin necrosis while the greater demands for cartilage may lead to a more obvious donor site deformity. Work suggests that with hyaline cartilage can regenerate in the presence of intact perichondrium. Preserving the perichondral sleeve during harvest and refilling the defect with diced cartilage remnants not only preserve contour, but permit further harvest from the same site in future (Nagata).

Postoperative care

Patients are advised to avoid sleeping on the reconstructed ear for at least a month. Contact sports are to be avoided for 4–5 weeks to protect the new ear as well as the donor site. Specific complications include

- Infection: Rare but prophylactic antibiotics are routinely used
- Loss of skin graft with exposure of cartilage (generally due to the pocket being too tight or postoperative compression from dressings/bolsters). Small areas can be dressed whilst larger areas should be covered with skin or fascial flaps
- Pneumothorax from costal cartilage harvest is rare and should be detected intraoperatively if it occurs

Hearing restoration surgery

Hearing restoration surgery can be performed by ENT surgeons in between stages, if necessary (bilateral microtia). Surgery before external ear reconstruction is avoided to reduce tissue scarring that may compromise the vascularity of skin flaps.

Patients with microtia are 10 times more likely to have problems at school, which may be related to several factors including hearing difficulties, behavioural and psychological

Table 17 Comparison between Nagata and Brent/Tanzer techniques of autologous cartilage ear reconstruction		
	Nagata technique	**Tanzer/Brent technique**
Timing	Age 10–12 years for better carving.	Age 6 years for better psychological result.
Ribs used	Ipsilateral (6)789, leaving posterior perichondrium. Wired together in two layers to make three planes: 78 as main base, 9 as helix, concha, antihelix/antitragus and helix lobule level. 6th rib cartilage is banked in the costal margin.	678 of contralateral side: 6–7 base, 8 rim.
Lobule reconstruction	First stage with subcutaneous pedicle.	
Elevation framework	Additional cartilage wedge covered with temporoparietal fascial flap (TPFF) and thin split skin graft (SSG).	
Postoperative	Suction drains and bolsters secured with sutures kept for 2 weeks.	Suction drains, Vaseline packing. Remove stitches after 1 week.
Next stage	Elevate framework 6 months later, taking skin with a 3 mm margin. Retrieve banked cartilage for elevation of 12 mm. Cover with TPFF and full-thickness skin graft (FTSG)	SSG causes more contraction.
Criticisms	Greater donor site deformity. Skin flap necrosis. Extrusion of wires. Thick framework. Routine TPFF use may burn unnecessary bridges. TPFF is otherwise the salvage option for cover.	Multistage operation. Tragus and conchal shapes often unsatisfactory.

problems related to self-consciousness and low self-esteem. Most have hearing at a bone conduction level that is traditionally improved with a BAHA (bone anchored hearing aid). BAHAs have a skin-protruding anchor that docks with the hearing aid. More recently, the Vibrant Soundbridge middle ear implant system has proved to be a superior device that tackles both conductive and mixed hearing loss without a skin-protrusion. The external audio processor attaches to the buried implant through a magnet, affording better cosmesis and superior sound quality in the high frequencies.

Ear prosthesis

The Brånemark (1995) technique uses an externalised osteointegrated titanium bone anchor to host the ear prosthesis. After implantation, the titanium anchor forms an interface with bone and is capable of supporting stresses. The skin over the anchors may need to be thinned to reduce movement against the implant and thus irritation. The common reasons for preferring prostheses to autologous reconstruction are

- Failed autologous reconstruction: Previous scarring hindering surgery. Patient reluctance for numerous staged surgeries and donor sites
- Hypoplastic soft tissue/skeleton: Insufficient tissue. Ear reconstruction is rarely the highest priority in these patients. Augmentation of facial skeleton may be required either with bone grafts or distraction osteogenesis
- Low hairline: This would leave a hairy upper pole but this can be treated using standard hair removal techniques although the skin remains thicker. It is actually the lower pole and overall positioning that is much more important for cosmesis
- Acquired defects, especially with an intact tragus that can disguise the anterior margin of the prosthesis
- Scarring, skin/soft tissue loss and irradiation

However, for prostheses:

- Meticulous hygiene is required. There is a surface layer of titanium oxide that may reduce the infection risk
- The anterior margin is difficult to disguise (unless the tragus is intact) and the patient has a constant reminder of a false ear
- The materials degrade and the prostheses need to be changed every 2–5 years. The average overall cost is higher than for autologous reconstruction. Ear prostheses are generally more successful than orbital or nose prostheses (midline structures that are obvious and reflects light differently)

Avulsed ear

Options include:

- Throw away the ear and opt for delayed reconstruction if it is crushed/ traumatised, no vessels are available on examination under anaesthesia (EUA) or if patient is unfit for a long operation. Revascularisation often requires vein grafts and often uses the superior temporal artery/temporoparietal fascia that would otherwise be useful for future reconstruction (burns bridges)
- Composite graft techniques have been tried but are unreliable for an entire ear. Skeletonisation/filleting the cartilage out and banking/covering immediately with skin or fascia in the retroauricular region (or in forearm to be raised later as a composite flap) is often unsatisfactory. The cartilage invariably loses strength distorts/flattens and is prone to infection. Furthermore, the retroauricular skin that would otherwise be used for delayed reconstruction is sacrificed for an unsatisfactory result
- Baudet's technique: The medial skin is removed and the cartilage fenestrated to increased contact between avulsed ear (lateral skin) and recipient bed. A tie over dressing is used and if successful, grafting of the sulcus is performed 2 months later. This supposedly causes less flattening than with pocket placement

Further reading

Breugem CC, Stewart KJ, Kon M. International trends in the treatment of microtia. J Craniofac Surg 2011; 22:1367–79.

Related topics of interest

- Craniosynostosis
- Facial anatomy
- Hypoplastic facial conditions
- Hair removal

Electrical burns

Electricity can cause both thermal and non-thermal injury.
- Thermal: The skin resistance to the flow of electrical current generates heat (Joule effect), resulting in charring at the contact points (also called the entry and exit points). Bones are heated the most due to their high resistance (nerves have lowest resistance). As they lie deep, the heat will not dissipate easily (this simplified picture has been challenged). Heat generation is also related to cross-sectional area or current density and thus is greatest in the extremities. Vascular damage causes vessel thrombosis
  - Clothing may ignite causing a flame burn. It is important to clarify the exact mechanism of injury as thermal burns may masquerade as 'electrical burns' due to a flash/explosion or other things catching fire
- Non-thermal: Massive depolarisation damages excitable tissues such as
  - Cardiac conduction system: Resulting in cardiac arrest due to VF or other arrhythmias
  - Central nervous tissue: May cause loss of consciousness or brain damage
- Associated injuries:
  - Be on the alert for fractures/spinal injuries

Classification

Electrical burns are classified according to the magnitude of the voltage involved.

Low voltage (<1000 V) Low <1000 v

This is the most common type of electrical injury and occurs mostly in the home. Tetany can occur, resulting in patients being unable to let go of the source. The strong muscular contractions may also cause fractures or dislocations, but extensive muscle damage is uncommon. The cutaneous injury at entry and exit points may appear similar to thermal burns. With alternating current, the exit points will also be entry points.

High voltage (> 1000 V) > 1000V

Higher voltages cause deep and extensive muscle injury (with deceptively little damage of the overlying skin). The resultant rhabdomyolysis and myoglobinuria may lead to blockage of the renal tubules and renal failure. Muscle damage may be indicated by
- Hyperkalaemia and acidosis
- Raised creatinine and creatine kinase (CK)
- Raised plasma and urinary myoglobin

It is important to be watch for CS. Clinical assessment is less reliable than in other situations, as the nerve symptoms from direct electrical damage may be indistinguishable from CS. Compartment pressure monitoring may be useful in this situation. Tissue damage without significant temperature change occurs by electroporation. The current disrupts the lipid membrane forming pores that increase passive permeability. MRI may demonstrate muscle necrosis while radionuclide scanning may be oversensitive.

The patient may be thrown with force, causing fractures or dislocations. Arcing (high voltage ionised air particles can arc a distance of 2–3 cm for every 10,000 V, up to 3 metres) may cause very high temperatures (2–20,000°C) resulting in full-thickness burns. Exit wounds tend to be larger than entry wounds.

Alternating current (AC) is more dangerous than direct current (DC). A risk of ventricular fibrillation exists at exposure to AC at 40-200 Hz. Arrhythmias, especially ectopics, right bundle branch block and supraventricular tachycardia are found in a third of high voltage injuries. The risk of VF actually decreases with very high currents. The passage of current from hand-to-hand (across the heart) is associated with much higher mortality compared with hand-to-foot passage.

RBBB
SVT
1/3rd

Ultra high voltage (lightning)

Lightning is a current arc between the clouds and the ground. The voltage is very high (20 million volts) but very brief. Injuries from a direct strike have a typically high mortality but injuries can also be from side flashes.

Side flashes are due current discharge either through the ground or air, from an adjacent structure that suffered a direct strike.

Most of the current travels superficially with little deep organ damage. Very brief secondary local currents may occur that cause non-thermal electrical damage. Shock to the cardiac and central nervous systems may be transient or permanent depending on severity of injury. Skin changes may be seen in more severe cases but entry and exit points can be deceptively small. Contact burns may occur from metallic accessories or jewellery. Flame burns may occur if the clothing ignites.

Management

Remove the patient safely from the cause. A third of lightning strikes are fatal but many die due to lack of first aid from safety concerns. The current discharges quickly and it is safe to help immediately. The greatest risk comes from a repeated lightning strike.

- Airway: The cervical spine may be damaged by intense contractions or a fall
- Breathing: Electrical effects on the medulla may cause respiratory arrest
- Circulation: Gross cardiac damage is relatively rare but electrical injury may cause cardiac arrest or arrhythmias. Prolonged cardiopulmonary resuscitation may be required in such patients

The secondary survey is a head-to-toe inspection. In particular, check for:

- Cutaneous burns and entry/exit wounds: Lichtenberg figures are arborescent skin patterns that are pathognomonic of lightning strike and generally disappear within 24 hours. Nerve dysfunction, such as brief loss of consciousness, weakness or paraesthesia is common. The latter can be

partly due to transient extremity ischaemia from local vasoconstriction
- Fractures and injuries of the eye and ear may result. Perforation of the tympanic membrane is one of the most common reported complications

An ECG is required on admission with electrical injuries. Continuous monitoring (telemetry) for 24 hours is advisable in those who have suffered a cardiac arrest or had trans-cardiac current applied (vide supra). The literature suggests that patients with low voltage injuries and a normal admission ECG do not require ECG monitoring.

Resuscitation should be aimed at both the thermal and electrical components. Crystalloid resuscitation should be titrated according to the urine output rather than the burn surface area, which may be deceptively small. Muscle necrosis will increase fluid requirements. A urinary output of 1–1.5 ml/kg/h is reasonable without creating oedema. Myoglobinuria may require aggressive resuscitation, forced alkaline diuresis (solubilises free haemoglobin and myoglobin) or dialysis. Mannitol may be considered. Hyperkalaemia is likely with muscle necrosis and may be exacerbated by the potassium content of Ringers Lactate.

Debridement of non-viable skin and muscle according to standard principles is warranted. Muscle necrosis after an electrical burn is recognised to be non-progressive. There is no consensus regarding the timing of surgery. The chronic sequelae include

- Cataracts: The onset may be delayed by 6–12 months. The mechanism is unknown
- Neurological problems: Epilepsy, peripheral nerve demyelination and spinal cord problems
- Post-traumatic stress disorder

Further reading

Collinge C, Kuper M. Comparison of three methods for measuring intracompartmental pressure in injured limbs of trauma patients. J Orthop Trauma 2010; 24:364–68.

Related topics of interest

- Acute burns
- Compartment syndrome

Eyelid reconstruction

Anatomy

The skin of the upper eyelid is the thinnest in the body. Eccrine glands are found throughout whereas the apocrine (Moll) glands are limited to the margin. The sebaceous glands of Zeiss are associated with the eyelashes.

- Tears are produced by basic secretors (from small glands and the palpebral part of the lacrimal) that lubricate and from the pre-corneal film during sleep. Reflex secretors (from the main orbital lacrimal gland) respond to sudden changes in environment or emotion. The Schirmer test is designed to measure and distinguish between the two
- The marginal artery runs close to inferior lid margin, but is further away from upper lid margin (3–3.5 mm)
- The superior tarsal fold lies 8–11 mm above the margin in Caucasians (shorter in Asians 6.5–8 mm), while the lower fold tends to form a divergent oblique line between 5 mm medially to 7 mm laterally. The tarsal plates are sheets of connective tissue (not cartilage) that contain the Meibomian glands and are 2 mm thick. They are wider at the lid margins and almost triangular in cross-section at this point. The plates are continuous with fibrous strands that converge to form the medial and lateral canthal tendons

Muscles: 90% of eye opening comes from upper eyelid retraction.

- Orbicularis oculi comprises three parts. The orbital part over bony margin for forced eye closure, the pretarsal for blinking, tear distribution, lacrimal sac emptying, and the preseptal for blinking. The preseptal and pretarsal portions are components of the palpebral part over the eyelids
- Levator palpebrae superioris (LPS): This arises from the lesser wing of the sphenoid, just anterior to the optic foramen and passes over Whitnall's ligament, which acts as a fulcrum. It inserts via the anterior aponeurosis (10–15 mm) into the superior tarsal plate. It is innervated by the third cranial nerve and provides 10–15 mm of upper lid movement
- Muller's muscle is a smooth muscle under sympathetic control that provides 2–3 mm excursion. When paralysed, it will cause partial ptosis (such as in Horner syndrome). The lower lid has a small muscle analogous to Muller's muscle that lies just posterior to the capsulopalpebral fascia (CPF). The CPF originates from inferior rectus muscle and splits anteriorly to surround the inferior oblique. The suspensory ligament of Lockwood marks the refusion point of the two fascial layers

The eyelids consisting of lamellae
- Anterior lamella: Skin and orbicularis oculi
- Posterior lamella: Tarsal plate and conjunctiva

Eyelid defects arise mostly from trauma or cancer surgery. The most common tumour affecting the eyelids is BCC, which mostly affects the lower lid. Only 10% of malignant tumours of the eyelids are found on the upper lid. SCC is less common (2%) but tends to be more aggressive. Sebaceous cell carcinoma is the third most common tumour here.

Reconstruction
Partial thickness defects

- Skin: FTSG (particularly contralateral lid, postauricular) is preferred. Healing by secondary intention is possible for small areas of concavities such as the medial canthus
  - Local flaps are preferred. The Tripier (bipedicled upper eyelid skin and muscle flap performed in two stages, pedicle is divided after 10 days), hemi-Tripier, Fricke (laterally-based on upper brow skin) and rotational cheek flaps are good matches. Other sources of skin such as the glabellar and nasolabial fold (NLF) do not provide as good a match. Local flaps can be combined with mucosal grafts for small full thickness defects

- Conjunctival defects can be closed by advancement in many cases. Small defects on the undersurface of lids that do not involve the fornices, usually heal without deformity by secondary intention. Grafts are prone to contraction. Buccal mucosa contracts by 50% when thinned, nasal mucosa contracts by 20% while skin grafts irritate the cornea. Conformers should be used if grafts are placed into fornices
- The upper lid does not (usually) require reconstruction of rigid support. Lower lid defects require formal reconstruction of tarsal support (especially for defects >30%), which can be performed with
  - Nasal septum (strong stable cartilage that can be shaped by scoring)
  - Palatal mucosa (metaplasia after months, pliable with less shrinkage)
  - Conchal cartilage (useful if skin also required but less reliable take)
  - Tarsoconjunctival flaps or composite grafts from the other lid
  - Alloplastic material such as acellular dermal matrices of high rigidity (Enduragen) or chondroplast (irradiated bovine cartilage)

Full thickness defects

If there is full thickness loss, the two lamellae can be replaced separately with different combinations, such as vascularised skin-muscle flaps covering tarsoconjunctival graft.

Flaps are more commonly used to reconstruct full thickness eyelid defects as they have more reliable vascularity, will tend to contract less (though they may be more bulky).

Lower lid defects

Direct closure

Full thickness lesions should be excised as a shield or pentagon shape (whereas partial thickness should be closed in a fusiform manner) and closed in layers. The conjunctiva should reasonably apposed by closure of the adjacent layers, sufficient to not require separate closure itself.

It is conventional to classify defects according to their relative size (**Table 18**) and there are many options available (**Table 19**). The treatment algorithm is as follows – after excision as a wedge, a stitch through the margins is placed and used to test closure.

- If it is too tight then a lateral canthotomy/cantholysis allows additional 5 mm of advancement
- If still too tight, undermine the cheek laterally (Tenzel, see below) with or without a superior back-cut (with an inferior cut to make a Z-plasty)

If still insufficient beyond this point, closure will require a formal cheek flap (arched upwards to the brow level, with or without the SMAS layer and anchored to reduce tissue ptosis) with a mucosal graft (often septal).

Table 18 Classification of eyelid defects (percentage size relative to eyelid)		
	Younger patient/tight skin	Older patient/lax skin
Small	25–35%	35–45%
Moderate	35–45%	45–55%
Larger	55–total	65–total

Table 19 Options for upper and lower eyelid reconstruction		
	Upper eyelid	Lower eyelid
Small	Direct closure and cantholysis	Direct closure and cantholysis
Moderate	Tenzel flap Cutler-Beard flap Tarsoconjunctival flap (sliding) + SSG	Tenzel flap
Large	Cutler-Beard + ear cartilage	Hughes flap and FTSG Mustarde flap with nasal cartilage graft

Tenzel flap

A Tenzel flap is a semi-circular musculocutaneous flap of periorbital tissue undermined inferiorly and laterally up to the level of the brow, used in conjunction with a lateral cantholysis. The pre-existing lateral canthus is thus advanced along the inferior lid margin. The reconstructed lid margin will not bear lashes nor tarsal plate.

Hughes flap

It is a common two-staged method of lower lid repair. The major disadvantage is use of an undamaged upper lid for reconstruction. It essentially combines sharing of the upper lid posterior lamellae (that is pulled downwards) and covered with a sliding advancement musculocutaneous flap of the lower lid tissue (alternatively a FTSG can be used if the muscle layer can be mobilised sufficiently). The lower border of the upper lid flap should be at least 4 mm superior to the lid margin to preserve a rim of tarsal plate. The flap is divided 4–6 weeks later.

Cheek flaps (Mustarde)

The cheek advancement flap popularised by Mustarde, is combined with septal cartilage if support is needed (>30% loss). Mustarde argues against using the upper lid, pointing out that lower lid deficiencies are usually well-tolerated as long as the upper lid is functional but deficiencies of upper lid may lead to ulceration/impairment. The flap is raised in the subcutaneous plane in a 'cut as you go' fashion and is anchored to the orbital margin and at lateral canthus just above canthal ligament for support. Late ectropion still remains the most common complication. There is a risk of apical flap loss but reliability may be improved by including the SMAS layer in the flap.
Modifications:

- Callahan recommends a highly arched flap to recruit temporal skin.
- McGregor combines a lateral Z-plasty for defects up to 60%. The lateral incision is extended with an inferior back-cut with corresponding superior cut to form a Z-plasty to tackle the dog-ear.

Upper lid defects

Cutler-Beard

This is a lid sharing procedure that reconstructs the upper lid using the lower lid. A full thickness lower lid flap of 15 mm height is raised with its upper edge 5 mm below the lower lid margin and 2 mm wider than measured defect. This is passed under the remaining bridge of lower lid margin tissue and advanced into upper lid defect. It does not replace the tarsus of the upper lid and therefore there is less theoretical support. A flap modification allows the incorporation of a sandwich cartilage graft by splitting the flap into skin-muscle and conjunctival layers. The second stage is performed 6–8 weeks later, where the flap is divided 2 mm below the desired upper lid margin. This latter manoeuvre recreates some desired eversion.

Lid switch (lower to upper) Heuston

This can be raised either laterally or medially and is essentially an Abbé flap of the eyelids. It replaces like with like but sacrifices an undamaged lid (which is left three quarters of its original size). When raised laterally, the arc of rotation is smoother and the second operation is easier but the flap has less reliable vascularity. The medially based flap is more difficult to rotate and inset but is preferred if a cheek advancement is planned to close the lower lid defect (with nasal septal chondromucosal graft).
There are a variety of alternative techniques:

- A sliding tarsoconjunctival flap from remaining tarsus can be advanced to the lid margin and covered with FTSG. Shallow marginal defects may be repaired by advancing remaining tarsus (if >3 mm remains).
- A reverse Hughes flap, a lower lid flap up to upper lid defect, covered with skin and divided 5–8 weeks later.
- Tripier flaps of skin and orbicularis muscle can be combined with buccal mucosa for lining. These flaps are classically bipedicled but can be reliably unipedicled if the pupillary sagittal line is not crossed. A Fricke flap is another option.

- A variety of islanded flaps have been described in the literature. Supratrochlear (two-staged), nasojugal, paramedian forehead and flaps based on the anterior branch of superficial temporal artery are viable options

Orbital reconstruction

- Evisceration: Removal of contents of globe *preserving sclera*, extraocular muscle attachments and Tenon's capsule
- Enucleation: Removal of the globe, preserving Tenon's capsule
- Exenteration: Removal of the entire contents of orbit

Congenital orbital defects

The commonest congenital problem is microphthalmos. There is hypoplasia of the bony orbit and the lack of a continuous expansile stimulus. The eye is usually non-functional and requires removal. The reconstructive aim is to match the contralateral aesthetic. The cardinal manoeuvres that facilitate this are

- The rim base should be made higher to provide a bony shelf
- The cavity should be shallower to avoid an excessive posterior space. An excessive space necessitates a larger and thus heavier implant that will fatigue and stretch the lower eyelid

Options for the bony orbit reconstruction include

- Expanders: These are associated with high complication rates
- Implants (regularly changed every 6 months) are usually preferred. The implants can be made of silicone, MEDPOR (porosity and tissue integration can removal difficult) or hydroxyapatite. They are wrapped in fascia lata, temporalis fascia or pericranium
- Autologous cranial bone grafts from peri-occipital area can be used to supplement or correct volume deficiencies. Osteotomies may be necessary but risks making the orbit too large

Soft tissue options include

- Cavity filling with muscle, bone or dermofat grafts
- Conjunctival sac: Grafts are often needed to create deep fornices, with a choice of buccal mucosa or skin (debris tends to collect, but there is greater availability)
- Eyelids: The lower lid can usually reconstructed from hemi-Tripier flaps, while the upper lid can be reconstructed with an FTSG in a cosmetic subunit from the brow to lid

Post-tumour resection

The effect of surgical resection may be compounded by the effects of RT. The effects are ischaemic, fibrotic effects and growth-related (younger patients).

- Bony orbit: Reconstruct, supplement volume and build up inferior rim with cranial bone as onlay grafts (with the expectation of greater resorption in irradiated fields). Avoid using alloplastic materials or placing osteotomies in irradiated tissues
- Volume/content replacement: The lining needs to be soft, conforming and well vascularised. Choices include the temporalis flap or free flaps
- Lid reconstruction may need to be staged. The FTSG-grafted temporalis muscle flap is then split, and then the dissected pocket lined with grafts. The eyelashes can be reconstructed with brow grafts or hair transplantation

As oncological surveillance is often a concern, a SSG lining with an osteointegrated (OI) implant may be preferred. This 'glass' eye is made from glass or acrylic with 'soft tissue parts'. The attachments for OI implants are placed on the inner aspect of the orbital rim; usually 4–5 of them to provide some redundancy should any fail.

Post-traumatic

Approximately 15–20% of patients with orbital fractures develop enophthalmos. This is most frequently due to increased bony volume following inadequate reduction. Changes in volume of as little as 5% can affect globe positioning. Other less common causes of enophthalmos include atrophy of fat or muscles.

- Acute fracture: Reduce, usually no need for bone grafting
- Mild/moderate enophthalmos: Bone grafting through small incision
- Severe enophthalmos: Reposition zygoma, bone graft and detach masseter muscle

Further reading

Ehmke M, Schwipper V. Surgical reconstruction of eyelids. Arch Facial Plast Surg 2011; 27:276–83.

Related topics of interest

- Nasal reconstruction
- Orbital fractures
- Zygomatic fractures

Extensor tendon injuries

The excursion of the extensor tendons tends to be shorter and adhesions cause less joint limitation (compared to flexors). In most cases, a small loss of active extension tends not to interfere with hand function. The repair of extensor tendon injuries of the hand is often delegated to junior surgeons. Inappropriate management can still lead to significant loss of flexion and extension from adhesions and inaccuracy in length restoration.

Anatomy

The extensor digitorum communis (EDC) arises from the common extensor origin on the lateral epicondyle (LE) of the humerus and acts to extend MCPJs. The individual tendons pass under the extensor retinaculum into the dorsum of the hand to split over the PP and the tendon to the little finger is absent in almost half of the patients. The central slip inserts into the base of the MP, and the terminal extensor tendon (formed by the convergence of the lateral slips and the lateral bands from the intrinsics) inserts into the base of the DP. The wide hood-like extensor aponeurosis that covers the dorsal aspect and sides of the PP is formed by an aponeurosis from the tendons of the intrinsics (lumbricals and interossei) that run dorsally towards the EDC.

The extrinsic tendon ends as the central slip inserts onto the MP. The intrinsics form the lateral bands that unite over the MP to insert into the DP. There is thus a dual extensor system where tendon divisions retract very little and can often be treated by immobilisation/splintage (in extension). However, it also means that there is little tolerance for length errors. Due to the complexity of arrangement, complete extensor failure in this region may not be reconstructible.

- The insertions of the intrinsic muscles pass volar to the axis of MCPJ and dorsal to the IPJ (due to indirect action via the lateral bands) and thus will flex MCPJ while extending the IPJs

- The orientation of the retinacular ligaments of Landsmeer (that run from the volar PP to the dorsal DP) is volar to the PIPJ while being dorsal to the DIPJ. This is important for joint synchronisation between these two joints. It has transverse (retinacular ligament) fibres and oblique (retinacular ligament) fibres (previously known as Landsmeer ligament). This terminology is important in reference to the historical literature

In general, injuries in odd-numbered zones are more difficult to treat because they overlie joints (zones 1, 3 and 5) or involve multiple tendons (zone 7).

Management
Common injuries

Common injuries include:

- Open trauma: Lacerations and fight/ punch injuries
- Closed injuries: May occur with forceful flexion of the extended joint or through crush injuries
  - Attrition is most commonly due to rheumatoid arthritis particularly at the wrist level (due to a combination of ischaemia, synovitis and friction), starting from the little finger and progressing radially. Wrist fractures, especially the ones that are minimally displaced, can lead to tendon attrition. This is theorised to be due to the intact retinaculum that holds the tendons close to the roughened bone

Passive and active movements at each joint should be systematically tested. Loss of tendon continuity will result in extensor lag, with reduced active extension of the MCPJs against resistance. However, the juncturae tendinae may disguise injuries and limit retraction of tendon ends. The single digit extensors, such as the EIP and EDM, lie ulnar to the EDC tendons to the respective fingers. Testing requires flexion of the middle and ring fingers to eliminate the contributory action of the EDC.

- Partial lacerations proximal to the MCPJ may not need to be repaired, as there are many inter-tendinous connections. They can be splinted in wrist hyperextension and some degree of MCPJ flexion
- Tendons should be repaired early, except in infected (such as fight bites) injuries that should instead undergo delayed closure to allow resolution. Independent tendons, such as the EPL, should be repaired early as they shorten more quickly
- Exposure: The dorsum can be incised in the straight midline. There are a variety of methods for repairing extensor tendons. The strength of repair is to the number of sutures crossing the repair, but it is important to avoid bunching and excessive shortening that will instead compromise function
  - Continuous horizontal mattresses or 'figure of eight' sutures are easy, quick and produce minimal shortening when done correctly
  - Modified Bunnell or Kessler sutures are stronger and commonly used in thicker tendons
  - The MGH (Massachusetts General Hospital) repair (four strands) with crossing running suture is more resistant to gaping and is recommended for zone 6 (between MCPJ and extensor retinaculum), where early mobilisation may be preferential
  - Some surgeons prefer absorbable sutures (PDS) to Prolene as the risk of extrusion is lower in the presence of the thin dorsal skin

Specific injuries

DIPJ, Zone 1

As this lies distal to the central slip insertion, the division of the conjoint tendon at this level will result in reduced extension at the DIPJ and a mallet finger deformity. This may lead to a secondary swan-neck deformity at the PIPJ due to tendon imbalance and volar plate laxity. Significant functional impairment with pain and stiffness may result if left untreated.

- Open injury (Type II mallet): Primary tendon repair should be carried out if possible. The ribbon-like tendon may be difficult to suture. Postoperative splintage for 6 weeks with 2 weeks of night splintage is needed. Some prefer pin fixation of the DIPJ to maintain slight hyperextension
- Closed injury (Type I mallet): This can occur following minor blows to the tip of the finger forcing it into flexion. Presentation may be delayed. A mallet splint can be used to maintain hyperextension (to allow tendon healing as the ends do not retract significantly) for 6 weeks followed by 2 weeks of night splinting, with active extension afterwards. It will take several months for full movement to recover. This is adequate for the vast majority but this regime requires high patient compliance. The patient must understand that splintage needs to be continuous, without any interruption
  - If there is a small fracture, K-wires can be used for fixation for 6 weeks, followed by splintage for 2 weeks after its removal. There is a small risk of osteomyelitis
  - A large or rotated fracture fragment requires accurate reduction and fixation, but ORIF can be difficult and is associated with a rather high rate of complications such as joint stiffness or avascular necrosis of the fragment. Alternatives include extension block K-wiring (Ishiguro technique) or using miniature external fixators
- Type III injuries involve the loss of tendon and soft tissue that require coverage
- Type IV injuries are avulsion fractures. Splintage is used unless the fragment is subluxed, in which case internal fixation is required

Persistent mallet deformity can be treated by
- Further splintage (though less successful, but still worth trying for up to several months afterwards)
- Resection of a more proximal tendon segment
- Arthrodesis of DIPJ. The angle of fusion depends on the digit and the functional needs of the patient

Though open reduction aims to restore articular surfaces and reduce the risk of osteoarthritis, it is generally used only if closed reduction (with a longitudinal K-wire) is not possible.

Zone 2 injuries can be repaired and splinted in the same way if active extension is intact. Otherwise, repair is advised. This applies to zone 4 digit injuries and zone 2 injuries of the thumb.

PIPJ, Zone 3

Check for full active joint extension. A small amount of local anaesthetic may be needed to facilitate this. With tendon injuries, a 15–20° extensor loss with the wrist and MCPJ flexed is present. There is also weakness in extending the flexed PIPJ. The central slip test can be used (but not well validated): Flex the PIPJ over the edge of a table or on a large book with the MCPJ straight.

- Actively extend the MP at the PIPJ: If the central slip is transected, any extension is via lateral bands and causes hyperextension of DIPJ with weak/absent PIPJ movement
- Flex at PIPJ: If the central slip is intact then the DIPJ will be floppy and cannot resist flexion as the lateral bands are only able to extend PIPJ. If resistance is felt, then the lateral bands have subluxed and are directing force across DIPJ

Injuries in this region may lead to a boutonnière deformity due to the MP head buttonholing through the disrupted central slip. There is an immediate imbalance of forces but little extension loss may be evident in the acute situation. This is due to the lateral bands still being able to produce PIPJ extension by virtue of their dorsal position. The deformity starts more than 2 weeks later as the transverse retinacular ligament (TRL) stretches and the lateral bands move progressively more anterior to the axis of the PIPJ, eventually becoming flexors of the PIPJ and hyperextensors of the DIPJ. Splinting may be able to correct early imbalance before the deformities become fixed and difficult to correct.

- Open injury: Lacerations over the PIPJ mean a central slip rupture until proven

otherwise. The tendon is repaired with the PIPJ in full extension and then preferably splinted with K-wire. This leaves the DIPJ free to flex, drawing the lateral bands and central slip dorsally taking pressure off the repair
- Closed injury: Selected injuries can be treated by splintage or K-wire. The latter is the most reliable method for immobilisation, but may still require additional supportive external splinting. It is particularly appropriate in the uncooperative. Involvement of a large bony fragment or significant extensor lag especially at the PIPJ requires open treatment

MCPJ, Zone 5

This is commonly a fight injury involving the middle and ring fingers. The tooth lacerates the tendon and contaminates the joint (which is directly underneath and can be difficult to separate from the tendon). There is often a delay in presentation due to intoxication at the time of injury but is potentially serious and may require amputation if neglected.

- Broad-spectrum intravenous antibiotics
- X-ray to exclude tooth fragment or other foreign body
- Primary tendon repair can be considered if there is no evidence of clinical infection. Otherwise, delayed repair is advisable (consider a continuous irrigation system)

The fingers should be splinted in comfortable full extension for 3 weeks with the IPJs free and with greater extension in the middle and ring fingers.

Rehabilitation

Due to narrower tendon cross-sectional area (and the stronger antagonistic flexors), it takes about 12 weeks for extensor tendons to recover to full strength. However, the extensor system is more tolerant of immobilisation. Adhesions tend to remodel well and there is less movement block as the neighbouring tissues are relatively mobile. The exact program of rehabilitation depends on the level of injury (the level of the MCPJ is a common dividing line) as well as the preferences of the surgeon. Most regimes involve protective mobilisation.

- Injuries distal to MCPJ: (mallet, boutonnière) The DIPJ and PIPJ are immobilised in extension for 6 weeks
- Injuries at or proximal to MCPJ: Maintain MCPJ extension for 2–4 weeks, then splint in a position that allows active flexion and passive extension. The PIPJ/DIPJ should be left free to move

Wrist stabilisation is also important. The excursion across the wrist is 5–6 cm and hyperextension will relax the repair and allows for some MCPJ flexion. Uninjured fingers should be immobilised in greater flexion to take tension off the repair by advancing the common muscle tendon unit. Light (clerical) work is allowed at 6 weeks, medium work at 8 weeks and heavy work at 10 weeks. The patient can drive at 6 weeks, with contact sports delayed until after 12 weeks. There is a worse outcome with distal injuries (zones 1–4, beyond the MCPJ), and those with infection and associated bony/soft tissue injuries.

Complications

- The most common complication is adhesion, causing stiffness with loss of extension and loss of flexion. The latter may also be due to extensor tendon shortening and is often the biggest problem. Extrinsic and intrinsic tendon tightness often follows crush injuries
  - Overall 80% of motion is restored on average
- Tendon rupture
- Dorsal skin necrosis from inappropriate splintage
- Infection

Further reading

Sameem M, Wood T, Ignacy T, et al. A systematic review of rehabilitation protocols after surgical repair of the extensor tendons in zones V-VIII of the hand. J Hand Ther 2011; 24:365–72.

Related topics of interest

- Flexor tendon injuries

Facial anatomy

Embryology

During the fourth week, the fish-like head forms a series of ridges that resemble gills that are termed branchial arches. Each arch bears the three germ layers (ectoderm, mesoderm and endoderm) supplemented by neural crest cells. Despite their ectodermal origin, the neural crest cells are pluripotent, they migrate in the mesodermal layer and subsequently differentiate into their terminal cell type. They contribute to muscle (though most muscle arises from the initial mesodermal core), nerve, connective tissue, endocrine tissue, as well as pigmented cells. The first three arches are most well developed; the fourth less developed; the fifth absent; while the sixth cannot seen externally although its components remain.

The face is mostly formed by the paired maxillary and mandibular prominences (from the first arch) and the frontonasal prominence that forms ventral to the forebrain. As they fuse, the mesoderm migrates widely, even though there may still be surface grooves.

Eye

The eyes lie at the junction of the upper and middle thirds of the face. The distance between the eyes is roughly equivalent to the width of one eye (actually slightly wider) or the root of the nose (actually slightly narrower). The curvatures of the upper and lower eyelids differ. The margin of the upper lid lies along the circumference of a smaller circle (two thirds the radius) than the lower lid. The highest point of the upper eyelid lies one third the way from the medial canthus, while the lowest point of the lower lid lies one third the way from the lateral canthus. These points correspond to the medial and lateral corneal limbi respectively (**Figure 6**). There is a slight upward tilt (positive canthal tilt) with the lateral canthus being higher than the medial.

- Ptosis: This is drooping of the eyelid when looking straight ahead. Normally the upper lid covers 2–3 mm of the cornea/upper limbus, while the lower eyelid just touches the lower limbus, with no scleral show (sclera intervening between the limbus and the lower lid, although a tiny amount of scleral show can be an attractive feature)
- Lid retraction: This is the process or condition that causes scleral show, which may be related to ageing, thyroid disease or post-operative tissue contracture of the lid following blepharoplasty
- Supratarsal fold: The typical Caucasian fold is higher (one third to one quarter of the lid to brow distance centrally) than the Asian. The latter also tends to converge with the lid margin medially and may continue inferiorly as an epicanthal fold. This feature tends to increase in prominence with the flatness of the nose, and may give an impression of pseudotelecanthus
- Grooves on or near the lower lid: The nasojugal groove is a deep groove located at junction of eyelid and cheek skin, where it may be related to a muscular gap. In some cases, the base of the depression is the bony infraorbital rim, when it is often referred to as a tear trough deformity. Malar bags and festoons may not be true skin redundancies and thus any skin excision should be approached with extreme caution

Assessment of the brow/forehead should be a part of the work-up of a patient contemplating a blepharoplasty.

- Ideal brow position: The medial brow is level with a vertical line joining the alar base and medial canthus. It terminates laterally at its intersection with an oblique line that runs from the alar base to lateral canthus. The brow lies at the supraorbital rim in men, but is located several mm higher in women

Lip

The upper lip is formed by fusion of the medial nasal prominences (philtrum) and the maxillary prominences. Failure of fusion leads to a cleft lip.

- Failure of the mandibular and maxillary prominences to fuse at the commissure causes macrostomia (Tessier 7 cleft)
- Failure of the mandibular clefts to fuse in the midline leads to a Tessier 30 cleft
- Failure of fusion of the medial nasal prominences leads to a rare median cleft lip (Tessier 0)

The vermilion is the red portion of the lip that owes its colour to the lack of a keratinised layer and a rich superficial vascular plexus. It has no sweat or sebaceous glands (the name describes the orange red pigment mercuric sulphide that was originally made from Cinnabar). It contains the deep part of the orbicularis oris that inserts into the modiolus (from the Latin for socket or hub) and has a sphincteric function. The superficial part of the muscle is more peripheral, plays a role in facial animation and inserts into philtral columns. The vermilion border (**Figure 7**) represents the junction of skin and mucosa whereas the white roll is a subtle prominence adjacent to the vermilion border that reflects light (hence white). It is best to avoid cutting across the vermilion border where possible,

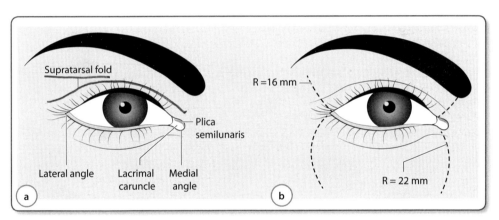

Figure 6 (a) Anatomical features of the eye. (b) The upper and lower eyelid margins follow different circles.

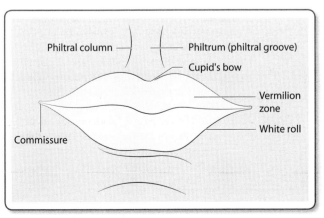

Figure 7 Anatomical features of the lips.

and when unavoidable, incisions should be made perpendicular to its border. Precise alignment of the edge of the lip is vital as even a minor misalignment (1 mm) can be noticeable. The other important landmark to preserve is the junction between the dry vermilion and wet vermilion, also known as the wet-dry border.

The skin above the upper lip has slight concavity, whilst the upper lip itself has a central vermilion tubercle with lateral fullness separated by depressions. The lower lip border shows a complementary shape with paramedian fullness. Volume is concentrated in the centre.

Ear

The external ear is formed from the three hillocks of His, around the future EAM that is derived from the dorsal end of the 1st groove. It starts in the cervical region and migrates upward to its final position. Congenital anomalies such as microtia tend to thus be inferiorly displaced.

On average, the coronal axis of the ear is 10–20° from the vertical, which is roughly the incline of the dorsum of the nose (the ear is usually more vertical). The width is approximately 55% of the height (typically 5–6 cm). The ear protrudes from the skull by about 21–25°. An angle > 35° manifests as a prominent ear deformity. The superior attachment of the external ear lies just above the upper eyelid, with the apex of the ear at the eyebrow, approximately one ear height from lateral end of the eyebrow.

Note that there are multiple planes in the ear that need to be recreated in ear reconstruction. The helix is the folded-over rim of the pinna that starts behind the tragus as the crus/ root. The antihelix is the Y-shaped fold in the upper half of the ear that delimits the scapha, fossa triangularis and concha from superior to inferior. The extension of the helical root divides the concha into cymba and cavum (**Figure 8**).

Multiple sensory nerves that overlap in territory and vary greatly supply the sensation of the ear.

- Great auricular nerve (GAN): Inferiorly and on both sides
- Auriculotemporal nerve: Superolaterally
- Lesser occipital nerve (LON): Superomedially
- Auricular branch of Vagus nerve (Arnold's nerve or Alderman's nerve): EAM and a small part of the posterior pinna

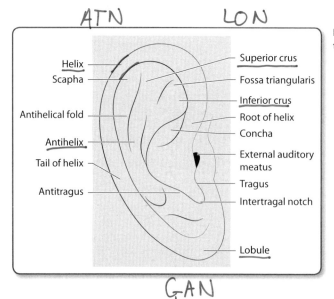

Figure 8 Anatomical features of the external ear.

Nose

The nasal placodes form at the lateral inferior portions of the frontonasal prominence and deepen to form the nasal pits with the medial and lateral nasal prominences either side. These normally fuse with the maxillary prominence.

- Lateral nasal prominences form the ala
- Medial nasal prominences fuse to form the philtrum, nasal tip, premaxilla and nasal septum (Figure 9)

Nasal subunits and zones

According to Burget, there are nine nasal cosmetic subunits: dorsum, sidewalls (2), tip, alar (2), soft triangles (2) and columella (meaning 'little column' in Latin). As a rough rule of thumb, if a defect involves more than half the size of a subunit, better cosmetic results may be obtained by replacing the entire subunit. The skin of the external nose can also be split into zones:

I. Dorsum: Dorsal nasal skin is thin, smooth and mobile. It can be satisfactorily reconstructed with preauricular FTSG or local flaps
II. Tip: The tip has thick sebaceous skin and dense adherent tissue. It is often too thick and stiff for use as local flaps and FTSG/SSGs offer a poor match (Menick advocates FTSGs from forehead for a

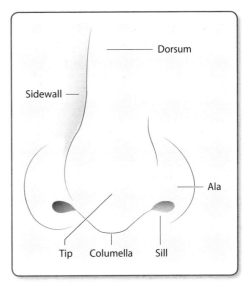

Figure 9 Anatomical features of the external nose.

better match). It is common to reconstruct with nasal skin, nasolabial or forehead flaps
III. Ala: Alar skin is similar to zone II

The underlying cartilages are important in maintaining the shape of the nose. It is important to note the surface anatomy of the lower lateral cartilages. There is no native cartilage in alar rim but cartilaginous support is usually required when reconstructing it.

Further reading

Thornton JF, Griffin JR, Constantine FC. Nasal reconstruction: an overview and nuances. Semin Plast Surg 2008; 257–68.

Related topics of interest

- Blepharoplasty
- Cleft lip
- Ear reconstruction
- Eyelid reconstruction
- Lip reconstruction
- Nasal reconstruction
- Rhinoplasty

Facial reanimation

Facial expression is a function of both voluntary and involuntary action of the facial muscles that are supplied by the facial nerve. The post-parotid portion of the nerve lies deep to the SMAS layer, except over the zygomatic arch and when it reaches the midface. It innervates the muscles from their deep surfaces with the exceptions of mentalis, buccinator and levator anguli oris. The facial nerve has somatic (motor and sensory) and visceral (motor and sensory) components at its origin. However, the extracranial portion (post-stylomastoid foramen) is purely motor and carries approximately 7000 nerve fibres. The important considerations with restoration of facial nerve function are

- Duration of paralysis: This determines end-organ availability. After a prolonged period of denervation, the muscle motor end plates atrophy, making nerve restoration futile
- The cause and level of palsy: This determines the availability of proximal and distal nerve stumps for anastomosis
- Clinical level testing: These include tests for stapedial reflex, taste, salivation and lacrimation (see below)

Causes of facial paralysis

The most common causes in adults are Bell's palsy, trauma and Ramsay-Hunt syndrome. The paralytic side bears a lesser degree of age-related wrinkling and may have ptosis.

- Acquired palsy:
  - The commonest cause is Bell's palsy (75%) with a typical prodrome. Most cases tend to recover well. Good prognostic factors an intact stapedial reflex, normal tearing, and age < 60
  - Iatrogenic, such as following parotid or acoustic neuroma surgery. Incomplete paralysis is a good prognostic indicator
  - Trauma
- Congenital palsy:
  - Moebius syndrome (1888): Multiple idiopathic cranial nerve palsies (especially abducens and facial nerves),

which may be bilateral but usually asymmetrical. The nerve palsy causes secondary changes in the facial bones. There are pectoral and limb anomalies such as clubfoot in one third of cases. There is a 10% rate of mild mental retardation
  - Goldenhar's syndrome (or Goldenhaar, after Dr Maurice Goldenha(a)r, 1924-2001, a Belgian physician): These patients have significant disability and deformity due to hemifacial microsomia and facial nerve palsy. It is often associated with dermoids and vertebral anomalies

Level of paralysis

- Forehead sparing indicates an upper motor neuron lesion
- Bell's phenomenon: Upward movement of eye along with incomplete closure when eye is closed with effort. It suggests a lower motor neuron lesion but can also be present in normal patients (normal defence mechanism)
- Schirmer's test in selected patients: Filter paper at lateral 1/3 for 5 min: 15–30 mm wetting is normal, 5–10 mm indicates hyposecretion, whilst < 5 mm implies a risk of dry eye after surgery. The significance and accuracy of this test is controversial
- Stapedial nerve and hyperacusis: This can be assessed with an audiogram
- Chorda tympani: Taste test on anterior two-thirds of tongue, although it is rather subjective
- Individual branches: Temporal (brow elevation), zygomatic (forced eye closure), buccal (pucker lips), mandibular (bare lower teeth)

Severity

The severity of facial paralysis can be difficult to measure objectively but it is common to use the House-Brackmann Scale of facial nerve weakness:

I. Normal symmetrical function in all areas
II. Mild dysfunction at rest that is noticeable only on close inspection. Complete eye closure with minimal effort. Slight smile asymmetry
III. Moderate dysfunction at rest but not disfiguring. Complete eye closure with maximal effort. Asymmetric smile and mass movement with maximal effort. This is the best-expected result with reanimation
IV. Moderately severe dysfunction with obvious disfiguring weakness, spasm and mass movement. Incomplete eye closure
V. Severe dysfunction with barely perceptible motion. Spasm usually absent
VI. Total paralysis

The success of reanimation decreases with the age of the patient and the duration of paralysis. It is vital to convey realistic outcomes to the patient, as complete normality post-repair is impossible. It is unrealistic to expect a result better than House-Brackmann III. There are functional and aesthetic aspects to consider including eye function and oral function (speaking and eating without drooling), smiling and the loss of soft tissue bulk particularly in the malar regions with prolonged facial paralysis. Thus, an alternative simpler classification scheme is:

- Symmetry at rest: Normal, moderate or little/none
- Eyelid closure: Complete, partial or poor
- Mouth movement: Voluntary, mild or little/none

Eye problems in facial nerve palsy

Evaluate sensation, tearing and Bell's phenomenon (vide supra).
Supportive management: Lubrication should be provided in the form of drops, ointments (cause blurring) or more viscous cellulose mixtures. At night, the standard patch and tape is inadequate and an occlusive guard with moisture is recommended.
Surgical options include:

- Tarsorrhaphy is generally not a permanent solution. A temporary tarsorrhaphy can be fashioned using 5–0 Prolene horizontal

mattress sutures tied over bolsters for up to 4 weeks (eye drops required). A longer lasting result may be possible by shaving the lid margins and splitting the tarsal groove before suturing
- Canthal/eyelid repair: After a full thickness canthotomy of 15 mm and lysis of the inferior limb of lateral canthal tendon, the redundant tissue is trimmed and the tarsus resuspended from the inner aspect of the lateral orbital rim (above normal tendon). The skin-muscle flap is suspended from the zygomatic periosteum. Alternatives to canthopexy include wedge resection or a temporalis sling
- Eyelid gold weights work reasonably well and are reversible (they may alter astigmatism). The effect can be previewed by sticking the weights (1 g) on the skin. The weight is sutured loosely into a pretarsal pocket to avoid warping the tarsus. It is common to aim for a lid position 2–3 mm below limbus with passive eye closure when sitting. Some have reported on the use of platinum with its higher density and thus smaller size, whilst others have used linked weights with a better degree of conformity to the curve of the globe
- The palpebral spring is made from stainless steel and looks somewhat like a safety pin. They aim to improve blink closure but have an increased risk of complications
- Soft tissue repositioning: A direct brow incision lift is often useful to correct an overhanging brow, taking care not to compromise eye closure. Endoscopic methods are less useful
- Slings: These are made of silicone, polytetrafluoroethylene (PTFE), fascia lata, acellular dermal matrix or other materials

Procedures can be divided into two categories:

- Dynamic: Movement, particularly a symmetrical smile, is the basic aim
  - Nerve restoration (particularly zygomatic and buccal divisions) while the muscles still have potential function
  - Muscle transfer when the facial musculature is no longer functional such as after prolonged denervation

- Static: This aims to produce a more acceptable face at rest, rather than additional movement. These procedures are best regarded as being adjunctive, since dynamic reconstruction is always preferred. Some procedures have a specific protective role (see 'Eye Problems')
  - Facelifts can be performed with slings (e.g. zygomatic arch periosteum to the corner of the mouth, or other slings to the brow or forehead) that may have functional effects. A lifted brow may improve vision and reapposition of the sagging cheek against the teeth improves feeding, speech, and may help nasal valve dysfunction
  - Botulinum toxin injection can reduce synkinesia, hypertonia and improve symmetry

Techniques can also be combined. A nerve graft to repair the zygomatic branches to the eye can be performed in combination with a masseteric transfer for the angle of the mouth.

Dynamic facial reanimation

Nerve restoration

Nerve repair can be classified according to timing (**Table 20**).

When both proximal and distal nerve stumps are available, such as after trauma or during parotid surgery,

- Direct repair of nerve at the time of damage has the best chance of success but there will still be a degree of weakness and synkinesia (see above). Immediate repair has the advantage of having the anatomy while still at its best and free of scar. The distal branches will still respond to nerve stimulation and the muscles are not atrophied yet. Thereafter, the

ends will be more difficult to find. Match fascicles if possible and use epineural 8–0 sutures (there is no evidence to suggest that other methods are any better) to approximate the ends without tension. An additional 20% of shrinkage is expected and may compromise a tight repair. Use grafts if necessary. A repair that is position-dependant to reduce tension is suboptimal. If the nerve has been severed at or in the temporal bone, then bony dissection to expose the nerve with rerouting for extra length is possible (consult ENT colleagues). The nerve typically regenerates at 1 mm per day and may take up to a month to cross an anastomosis

- Nerve grafting is also best performed early (within 6 months), when success rates approach 95%. If the facial nerve trunk is involved, synkinesia (mass muscular action) is likely to result due to the loss of individualised innervation of specific muscles. Tone returns first. The best results are obtained in the middle of the face with return of movement to forehead and lower lip being less common
  - The sural nerve (up to 35 cm available, but mostly sensory and has a high connective tissue content) or nerves of the cervical plexus such as the GAN (10 cm) are common donors for grafting. A graft that is 20% longer than the gap is needed. Epineural repair is preferable to fascicular repair
  - Nerve conduits (veins or PGA sheaths) that allow nerve regeneration across small gaps (< 3 cm) may have a role for sensory nerves (less critical) but not facial nerve repair
- Neurotisation is the direct implantation of a nerve into muscle that may be used if the distal stump is not available. Better results are seen if done early (within 6 months). Significant delay or congenital facial nerve palsy patients are poor candidates for this as results are poor in these groups. It may be regarded as a salvage procedure

If only the distal stump is available, direct grafting is not possible. A donor nerve such as the contralateral facial nerve is used instead.

Table 20 Classification of timing of nerve repair	
Class	Time lapsed since injury
Early	< 3 weeks
Delayed	< 2 years
Late	> 2 years

Cross-facial nerve grafting

- Cross-facial nerve grafting (CFNG, Scaramella): The repair has reasonably good resting tone and restoration of symmetrical voluntary movements is possible. Typically, a sural nerve graft is sutured to the contralateral facial nerve and the affected ipsilateral nerve stump. The surgery may be done in one or two stages, with the latter being more common (9–12 months between stages). There are many differing wiring patterns and opinions. Scaramella prefers to connect up the main trunks with a single graft while Anderl uses four grafts to connect the smaller distal branches
- In most cases, success is limited by the weak action produced (half of the donor is used and only half will cross) and there is less success with temporal and mandibular branches. The best results are achieved if the procedure is done very early (3 months, with noticeably worse results after 6 months) in young patients. However disadvantages include
  - Donor defect: Iatrogenic damage to contralateral face and facial nerve
  - The nerve has to cross two suture lines and takes 6–9 months to cross the face
  - Long overall denervation time for the muscle. This can be minimised with a babysitting procedure with a partial hypoglossal nerve crossover (Fisch)

Nerve crossovers

Hypoglossal nerve crossover has been used to treat facial nerve palsy following acoustic neuroma surgery for many decades. The patient moves their face by pushing the tongue against incisors. The glossopharyngeal (IX), spinal accessory (XI), ansa hypoglossi and phrenic nerves are less commonly used alternatives.

- The anastomosis can be made end-to-end or end-to-side. It involves only one suture line (though some use interpositional free nerve grafts) but at the expense of a possibly significant donor defect. Using the hypoglossal nerve will lead to moderate tongue atrophy in >50% of the patients, and severe atrophy in up to one quarter. There may be difficulty with speech articulation and handling of the food bolus during chewing/swallowing but most patients do not have complaints. Although the results can be unpredictable, 80% have good results with intensive physiotherapy and training. Satisfaction is highest in those whose palsy is secondary to cancer resection
- There is a tendency for uncoordinated mass movements or synkinesis and hypertonia. As such, crossovers are generally reserved for those patients not suitable for CFNG. These are frequently older patients in whom surgery is contemplated after a lengthy delay. It can also be used as a temporary babysitting procedure to maintain muscle innervation (and thus reduce atrophy) while awaiting a CFNG. In these cases, usually only 30–40% of the nerve is used so that the donor deficit is less pronounced

Muscle restoration

When facial palsy has been prolonged, restoring the nerve alone will be pointless as the end organ will no longer be functional due to degeneration (motor end plate and muscle atrophy). It typically takes 1–3 years for this to occur. Under such circumstances, functional muscle will need to be transferred. An EMG is useful to assess the integrity of the end organ/muscle.

One cannot hope to reconstruct all the facial muscles. The basic aim is to at least reproduce the action of the zygomaticus major (Manktelow), which can produce an almost normal smile (albeit without the lateral and depressor function of the buccinator). The major drawback with both free and local muscle transfer is that the size of the motor units in donor muscle is often ten times larger than the average facial muscle, making the resultant movement(s) much coarser. Even with the best results, there will still be a visible bulky mass that will get bulkier with contraction.

Local donor muscle

The aim is to overcorrect as some degree of stretching is expected. As these muscles (temporalis and masseter) are innervated by the trigeminal nerve, emotional smiling is unlikely without extensive retraining.

- The masseter is a common choice and can be combined with the temporalis. It is usually split into three slips, pivoted on the zygomatic arch, and inset into the dermal layer around the oral commissure and NLF with non-absorbable sutures. Harvest of the entire muscle is preferred to partial harvest, which increases the risk of damage to the motor nerve. The intermingling of the masseter fibres with the local muscles allows a degree of neurotisation (at least in theory) and thus the best results are found in denervation of short duration. Loss of the normal function of the muscle may cause difficulties with mastication. The vector of contraction is more lateral than superior, compared with the temporalis. The best choice will be determined in part by the vector of the patient's normal smile
- Temporalis can be turned over and slips transposed to the eye and mouth area. Additional fascial grafts may be needed due to the short muscle length or the zygomatic arch can be resected to improve the reach (and to reduce bulkiness). The depression at the donor defect can be rather obvious and some advocate taking only the middle third of the muscle. The donor defect can be filled by either prosthesis or fat transfer

Local muscle transfers are generally not very successful for treating the eye and a gold weight often remains the best option.

Free muscle

Patients with Moebius syndrome usually require free muscle transfer and nerve grafting to gain useful facial movement. The results are never normal and may take 2 years to achieve peak effect. A smile may be learnt but spontaneous smiles are rare.

- Pectoralis minor is a popular choice for children although patients need to be well motivated and young. A multi-directional functional result is possible, but the muscle has a short variable and sometimes complex pedicle, making the learning curve rather steep
- Gracilis is unidirectional and has a long and consistent pedicle with a nerve supply from the anterior division of the obturator

nerve. However, the muscle is rather thick and often needs debulking unless only a portion (usually anterior) is harvested. Intramuscular dissection can be used to create separately innervated strips to use for the eye
- Less common choices are the (partial) latissimus dorsi, serratus anterior (lower four slips), RA (predictable anatomy but bulky) and platysma (thin, has been used for reconstruction around the eye). The results with extensor digitorum brevis have been poor, most probably related to its small size and its use has largely been abandoned
- Single stage procedure: the muscle is transferred and the motor nerve sutured to a (contralateral) facial nerve branch
  - Only a single suture line is present, with no donor defect from the nerve graft
  - The donor muscle suffers from prolonged denervation and duration of paralysis is a prime consideration for this. The resting tone recovers by 4–5 months and movement by 7–8 months
- Two-stage procedure: This is preferred by most, particularly if the paralysis has been of long duration
  - A reversed sural nerve graft is used as a CNFG. It is anastomosed to the buccal branch and its end banked in the ipsilateral tragus
  - After demonstrable regeneration (usually after 6–9 months) using an advancing Tinel's sign (or histologically), free muscle is transferred with its nerve anastomosed to the CFNG stump. This reduces the amount of atrophy and fibrosis in the muscle

An early EMG can be used to investigate patients with an uncertain recovery after 1 year. A suggested treatment plan may be:
- Hypoglossal crossover to babysit and maintain muscle tone while allowing more time for reinnervation
- CFNG if muscle is working
- CFNG and free muscle otherwise
- Local muscle options for medically unfit or if patients decline further extensive surgery
- Static repair as adjunctive surgery

Further reading

Biglioli F, Frigerio A, Colombo V, et al. Masseteric-facial nerve anastomosis for early facial reanimation. J Craniomaxillofac Surg 2012; 40:149–55.

Related topics of interest

- Botulinum toxin
- Hypoplastic facial conditions

Finger fractures and dislocations

The AO general principles of fracture management are:

1. • Restoration of articular surface congruity
2. • Rigid fracture fixation
3. • Early mobilisation

Fracture management warrants consideration of the battle between the diametrically opposed forces of healing and motion. Immobility facilitates fracture healing at the expense of stiffness. Early mobilisation prevents stiffness from setting in, at the expense of suboptimal fracture healing. However, while the strength rigid fixation (ORIF with plates and/or screws) permits early mobilisation, the surgical injury of open reduction generates adhesions that produce stiffness. Conversely, non-rigid fixation (K-wiring) generates fewer adhesions and thus stiffness, but requires prolonged splint immobilisation that encourages stiffness. The choice between ORIF and non-rigid K-wire fixation is not clear and depends on the circumstance and aim.

With joint dislocations, a stable reduction of the concurrent fracture or dislocation may be sufficient to allow apposition of the torn ligament ends to heal. Transarticular K-wires are frequently used to maintain stability during the healing period. The common exceptions to this are:

• Volar dislocation of the PIPJ (central slip rupture)
• Dorsal dislocation of the PIPJ (volar plate rupture with limited flexion post-reduction as the torn end of volar plate interposed within the joint cavity)
• Complete ulnar collateral ligament (UCL) tear of the thumb MCPJ (interposition of the adductor pollicis tendon between the torn ends of the UCL, i.e. Stener lesion)

Conversely, fractures may be reduced and held in reduction by ligamentous traction (ligamentotaxis). A common example of this is the use of a Suzuki frame to maintain reduction of a volar lip fracture of the middle phalangeal base.

When considering surgery for fractures, it is important to realise that surgical injury compounds the traumatic injury and increases the risk of adhesions and scarring. This risk is greatest with open treatment and is least with closed reduction and percutaneous K-wires (which, although not absolutely rigid, it is sufficient for most fractures). Consequently, ORIF is only indicated for some metacarpal fractures and a few phalangeal fractures which would be problematic to treat otherwise.

• Rotational deformities are not well-tolerated; they may not be that apparent on radiography and is most obvious on clinical examination
• Comminution is almost always more serious than X-rays suggest
• Primary soft tissue repair of soft tissue injuries is the priority as secondary bony repair is almost always possible

In general, a fracture that is minimally displaced and stable after closed reduction can be treated by simple immobilisation in a plaster if:

• There is no rotational error,
• Other errors of alignment are less than 10°, and
• Less than 3–4 mm of shortening

Dislocations

Joint injury is suggested by local tenderness and pain that is aggravated by stressing; local blocks may help with the diagnosis.

PIPJ

PIPJ dislocations are the most common hand dislocations (second to fifth digits) and may be classified according to:

• I. Hyperextension injury with avulsion of volar plate from MP and a minor longitudinal split in the collateral ligaments. The articular surfaces remain intact
• II. Full dislocation with volar plate avulsion
• III. Force has sheared away a portion of the volar base of MP leading to a fracture dislocation

Dorsal dislocations (forced hyperextension, often sports related) are most common and mostly simple. Fracture dislocations are stable except in a minority where >40% of MP volar articular surface is avulsed – most of the collateral ligaments remain with the fragment thus ligamentous support of the MP is lost and dorsal dislocation tends to recur. These will need fixation and possibly open treatment if closed techniques (pin for 2–3 weeks) fail.

- Lateral dislocations are less common, often reduce spontaneously and can be treated with buddy taping
- Volar dislocations are rare (blow to partially flexed finger) and often involve extensor tendon central slip disruption that can lead to boutonnières if left untreated

Most dorsal dislocations and fracture dislocations are treated non-operatively. They can usually be reduced using regional wrist blocks, flexing wrist and MCPJ to decrease tone in the flexor tendons. After a closed reduction, the joint should be checked for:

- Stability (patient should be able to actively move up to last 15° of extension without dislocating again) and
- Radiologically (failure to reduce implies trapped ligament or volar plate and is thus an indication for open reduction)

PIPJ dislocations types I and II are usually stable after reduction, and along with stable type III dislocations, can be treated with dynamic splinting for 3–6 weeks. K-wire fixation is needed only if there is recurrent dislocation. Unstable type III injuries may be treated with open reduction and K-wire fixation, dynamic skeletal traction and volar plate arthroplasty (the plate can be used to resurface joint irregularities).

DIPJ
Open injuries are relatively more common

MCPJ
- Dorsal dislocations are most common and simple injuries can be treated as per PIPJ. Complex injuries may need an open approach (usually dorsal) for reduction but are usually stable afterwards
- Lateral dislocations are due to forced adduction/abduction and often missed; partial tears can be treated with splintage whilst gross injuries may need repair

Carpometacarpal (CMC) joint
These are intra-articular and are generally unstable, requiring fixation.

Thumb MCPJ
These injuries are more common than finger dislocation, especially, ulnar collateral injuries.
- Acute injuries are due to sudden force; adductor pollicis may become interpositioned between ruptured ends (Stener lesion) and require surgical repair
- Chronic injuries are usually due to stretching, i.e. gamekeeper's thumb

Phalangeal fractures

- Distal phalanx: tuft fractures from crush injuries are common and if not displaced will heal satisfactorily with splinting. Nail-bed injuries should be actively excluded by direct inspection and repaired, and is preferred over delayed correction
- Middle phalanx
  - Distal fractures should be reduced accurately (closed) and pinned.
  - Middle fractures are usually unstable due to the FDS insertion, and should be treated by closed reduction (fluoroscopy), pinning, and splinting
  - Proximal fractures may involve the volar plate. Minimally displaced fractures can be treated with early mobilisation whilst intra-articular fractures are often complex, comminuted and more serious. Treatment by traction may be the only option and full recovery is not to be expected. Bone fragments may need to be removed leading to shortening that will then require volar plate advancement
- Proximal phalangeal fractures are typically tilted apex volar due to proximal displacement from flexion forces of intrinsics at MCPJ and extension of distal fragment via central slip of extensor tendons
  - Neck fractures are unstable and should be reduced and pinned where possible

– Base/proximal fractures are often comminuted as strong forces are involved; the MCPJ may also be injured

Metacarpal fractures

The ligaments and muscles around the metacarpals may limit the distortion somewhat but shortening, angulation and rotation can still occur. Angulation of >15° will lead to noticeable knuckle depression and protrusion of the head into the palm, whilst greater angulation leads to a claw type of deformity. Treatment priorities include correction of rotational errors, limit shortening to 3 mm and angulation to 15° (20° in fourth/fifth digits which are more mobile).

- Shaft fractures can be treated with pinning after closed reduction. Rotational deformities are often unstable and need fixation with screws/plates is usually preferred to pins
- Neck fractures are most common, and are often angulated and comminuted

In thumb metacarpal fractures, angulation is better tolerated (up to 30°) and non-articular fractures can often be treated by closed traction/manipulation. Intra-articular fractures include:

- Bennett's fracture: the small fragment stays attached to the carpus whilst the shaft subluxes away. The shaft should be reduced back onto the fragment and fixed with a K-wire through the index metacarpal or trapezium, and not the small fragments
- Rolando: comminuted fracture that usually requires open treatment

Postoperative

The hand should be immobilised with a splint in the 'position of function' but there is a tendency for hand fractures to be immobilised for too long. The aim is to wait until sufficient callus is deposited to allow minimal stress to be placed on the fracture that will then accelerate the rate of healing, and 3–4 weeks are sufficient for most hand fractures. This is determined clinically instead of radiologically (which lags behind actual healing). Active mobilisation is allowed afterwards. Failure to pay attention to this and adherence to a strict 'timings' reduces the risk of non-union but at the cost of many stiff and impaired hands.

Further reading

Wilkinson A. Towards evidence-based emergency medicine: best BETs from the Manchester Royal Infirmary. Bet 2: finger fracture. Emerg Med J 2011; 28:441–43.

Related topics of interest

- Extensor tendon injuries
- Flexor tendon injuries

Fingertip injuries

Anatomy

The fingertip is arbitrarily defined as the part distal to the DIPJ. The pulps consist of highly innervated skin with thick epidermis and rugae that are connected to the periosteum by fibrous septae. The nail provides support that is both protective and an integral part of pinching. It grows at an average rate of 0.5 mm per week and complete regrowth takes 2–4 months.

Injuries

Approximately 80–95% of distal phalangeal fractures will have nailbed lacerations. Subungual haematomas are common, typically painful and differentiation from melanoma is important.

- Large haematomas (> 25% of area of nail): Remove nail to allow inspection and repair if necessary (60% of patients with a haematoma that covers > 50% of nail will have a nailbed laceration). Use fine absorbable sutures prevent long term ridging and then replace the nail plate to splint the nail folds and eponychium. Defects of the nailbed can be grafted with skin/dermis or nail-bed from a toe
- Small haematomas can be drained via a hole made in the overlying nail plate

Fingertip amputations

The objectives of treatment are to close the wound while preserving function (sensation and length) and an aesthetically pleasing appearance. The length/level and orientation (transverse/oblique, palmar/dorsal/lateral) of the amputation are important considerations. Numerous classifications exist but a descriptive method is frequently most useful. As a rough rule of thumb, distal injuries that retain more than half of the supported (with bone) nailbed will allow straight nail growth. Conversely, those with less than half are associated with a higher risk of hook nail deformities.

Allen classification
I.   Skin distal to nailbed
II. Nailbed to bone
III. Bone involved
IV. Proximal to nailbed

Treatment
Treatment options include:

- Composite graft using the tip/tip skin works better in children and if reattached before the sixth hour
- Secondary healing is an excellent method for treating areas less than 1.5 cm^2, especially in children and the elderly. The wound is covered with a semi-occlusive dressing and allowed to heal over several weeks. Innervated pulp skin is pulled over the defect as it contracts. This method requires either pre-coverage or trimming back of exposed bone. The latter is unsuitable for the thumb. There may be delayed healing, granulomas, stump tenderness and nail deformities, particularly with larger and more dorsal defects. Cold intolerance may occur, but no worse than with other methods
- Skin grafts allow immediate one-stage coverage and may also be used as a temporary measure. With the latter, contraction is desired and thus a thin SSG is used. If planned to be permanent, a FTSG is more durable and contracts less
  - Ridged skin from the instep or hypothenar eminence provides an excellent texture match. One way to harvest a hypothenar graft is to shave the first layer with Goulian knife but leave it attached, and then shave a second layer for use whilst the first layer is replaced as a dressing for donor site. Half report a good result compared to 90% with conservative therapy
  - Skin grafts are insensate
- Local skin flaps can be homodigital, heterodigital or local. They permit restoration of both skin loss and soft tissue padding such as pulp. Loss of more than one third of the pulp usually requires a flap. There are many techniques but to be truly useful they must safely provide reliable sensate tissue with minimal donor

deformities. Flaps will not necessarily improve outcome or speed up recovery. Flaps may be most useful for secondary tip revisions or primary coverage of exposed bone when length preservation is prime

- Transverse defect - Kutler flap, Segmüller   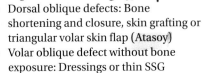 _side V-Y_
- Dorsal oblique defects: Bone shortening and closure, skin grafting or triangular volar skin flap (Atasoy)
- Volar oblique defect without bone exposure: Dressings or thin SSG

 Atasoy

Heterodigital

Cross-finger flaps (Cronin) use a random dorsal skin flap from the adjacent digit MP that can be based on any of the borders but most commonly laterally. It is a relatively simple technique but is two-staged and the donor needs a graft. Joints are immobilised in 30–40° of flexion for 10–14 days, after which the flap is divided. Physiotherapy may be required for stiffness afterwards. The thin tissue is not an ideal pulp replacement. The volar aspect of the middle finger may be used to cover the thumb tip. The average two-point discrimination is 9 mm with recovery maximal after 1 year (better in the young). Inclusion of a sensory nerve does not improve this significantly. Many variations exist, such as the reverse cross-finger flap that is a fascial flap. It is performed first by raising a skin-only flap, based further away from the side to cover. The definitive fascial flap underneath is then raised over the paratenon and based at the opposite end (on the side to cover) and turned-over. The skin-only flap is replaced and the fascial flap covered with a thin SSG.

Neurovascular island flaps are most useful for thumb pulp reconstruction using innervated skin from ulnar pulp of the middle finger (also median nerve). The transfer requires the pedicle be dissected well back and sacrifices the digital artery to the adjacent finger. The first dorsal metacarpal artery flap is an alternative based on similar principles.

Homodigital

Homodigital flaps do not damage a normal finger and involve less immobilisation but tissues used must be outside of zone of injury otherwise flap failure is more likely.

- Volar V-Y advancement flap: This is suitable for dorsal oblique/transverse amputations less than 1 cm in proximo-distal length. The flap is elevated in plane above flexor sheath on both pedicles with blunt but meticulous dissection (Atasoy-Kleinert). Excessive flap tension will lead to unsatisfactory results such as vascular compromise, sensory loss or hook nail/parrot beak deformity that can be difficult to correct. A distal axial K-wire may be used to hold the flap in place temporarily
- Lateral advancement flaps (Kutler flap, Segmüller) are useful for oblique pulp amputations and can be raised bilaterally for transverse amputations in a V-Y pattern. The original Kutler flap incised skin only with gentle traction to slowly transect fibrous bands under magnification. Greater mobility is possible (10–14 mm) if the flaps are taken down to periosteum as neurovascular flaps (Segmüller). The extended Segmüller flap extends the proximal V to the PIPJ and provides even greater mobility (Evans)
- Moberg volar neurovascular flaps are generally reserved for thumb tip reconstruction
- Reverse flow homodigital island flaps from the lateral aspect over the PP are based on a digital artery with retrograde flow from the contralateral artery (Lai). The soft tissue around the pedicle is maintained for venous drainage. A digital Allen's test is essential. These are particularly useful for pulp reconstruction of the fingers. The dorsal branch of the digital nerve on the donor side can be incorporated in the flap and anastomosed to one of the post-trifurcation branches in the damaged pulp for improved sensation

Other choices

- Regional skin flaps such as the classical thenar flap can lead to PIPJ contracture and thus reserved for use in children. It is only suitable for the index and middle fingers, as the others will not reach comfortably
- Free toe pulp is popular in some centres for fingertip amputation, especially the thumb. It provides nail, pulp, length and

sensation. The functional results depend on the return of skin sensation and joint mobility (less important in the thumb as it still achieve good function as a stiff post to oppose to). It allows earlier mobilisation compared to the cross-finger or thenar flap

- Distant flaps such as the groin flap or superficial epigastric artery flap (contralateral side involves less discomfort related to immobilisation). Reverse flow radial or ulnar artery flaps
- Free flaps such as the lateral arm flap are thin and have a good layer of fascia. Similarly, the temporoparietal fascial flap is useful in secondary tendon reconstruction

Amputations

There may be culturally dependent negative connotations and stigmata associated with amputations. However, there is a tendency to overestimate the physical impairment and the patient's psychological response usually bears little relation to the physical loss. Similarly patients are often quite sceptical about the need for bone shortening and may take some convincing. Cases must be judged individually. When dealing with multiply injured digits, the worst damaged digits may be used to salvage the least damaged, instead of amputation. While there are well-described levels for elective amputation, for traumatic amputation, the basic rule is to maintain as much length as possible provided there is good soft tissue cover, even if it requires the use of flaps.

For bone loss of over 50% of the DP or severe damage to nail matrix, amputation offers a one-stage procedure allowing early mobilisation and desensitisation (which is particularly important in older, stiffer hands or where occupational considerations are accounted for).

- The protruding bone is trimmed to the level of the remaining nailbed allowing tension free closure with a volar skin flap. Over-debridement of bone may cause hook nail. If there is < 5 mm of sterile matrix, nail adherence tends to be poor and the nailbed should be ablated

- Flexor and extensor tendon insertions on base of the DP should be left intact; otherwise the phalanx should be disarticulated
- Nerve ends should be handled carefully to avoid neuroma. Traction can be used to allow transection as proximally as possible. Diathermy, clips and buried ends have been used in attempts to reduce neuroma incidence
- When amputating through a joint, the condyles should be smoothened down with rongeurs. The need for cartilage removal is no longer absolute as the risk of chondritis is much reduced in modern practice

Thumb fingertip injuries

- Moberg flap can be used for defects < 2 cm or < 50% of the volar skin of the DP. With bilateral mid-axial incisions, a volar flap is dissected proximally off the periosteum and tendon sheath to the level of the MCPJ crease and then advanced with the IPJ flexed moderately (with a risk of joint contracture). It is most suited for the thumb with its dual circulation as the flap takes both digital bundles, and is less suited for other digits. There is a risk of tendon devascularisation. Modifications to this flap are in the closure of the donor defect
- Sensory flaps from other fingers such as Littler's neurosensory flap are used infrequently in the adult due to lack of cortical plasticity for sensory re-education (the flap still feels like the donor finger in its new location). The pedicle from ulnar side of the middle finger and tunnelled subcutaneously across the palm. Flap transfer usually requires division of the radial digital artery of the ring finger that then becomes solely dependent on ulnar digital artery. Venous congestion is not uncommon
- The Foucher flap is a neurovascular flap from the dorsum of the PP of index finger based on the first dorsal metacarpal artery. It is only suitable if the paratenon on the recipient is preserved. The donor area needs to be grafted

- Free tissue: Great toe pulp, wraparound or total (glabrous)

Replantation

Life before limb

The history should include general health, comorbidities and willingness of the patient to comply with rehabilitation and tolerate an average of 6–7 months off work. The aim is to improve the function of the hand/limb by replantation compared to simple closure/amputation with or without prosthesis. Consent and preoperative counselling should include:

- Unrealistic expectations of results and the time and effort involved in the recovery and rehabilitation, as well as the need for revision
- Possible need for vein, nerve and skin grafts or flaps, with the possibility of eventual amputation if it fails
- Replanted parts may have poor movement may be due to tendon adhesions, stiff joints, muscle contractures and reduced sensation (average final two-point discrimination is 11 mm)
- Late complications such as chronic regional pain syndrome (CRPS) and cold intolerance

Assessment of the injury

- Sharp amputations do better than avulsions or crush injuries. The signs of avulsion include the red streak sign along the lateral aspect of the digit and coiled or spring-like vessels. These coiled arteries tend to break off proximally, have long segments of intimal damage and grafts are often needed after trimming appropriately
- Ischaemic time for digits: Cold 24 hours, warm 8–12 hours. Proximal amputations with muscle are the most time sensitive and should not exceed 2–4 hours. The part should be wrapped in saline gauze and placed in a plastic bag on ice for transport. The digit should not be placed directly on ice

Indications

Replantation is indicated for multiple digits (replants can be performed by structure (faster) or by digits) or in children. The wisdom of single digit replants in adults is open to debate:

- Proximal to PIPJ: Even with good viability, there is a high risk of functionally impairing stiffness due to adhesions in Zone II. Patients may eventually request amputation for this hindrance. A replanted index is often ignored, as the original functions of the index are taken over by the middle finger automatically
- Good motion and sensory return are achievable for replants at the MP level, distal to the FDS insertion
- DP replants have a good outcome if they survive
- The thumb is almost always replanted as it contributes 40% of hand function according to most analyses. The larger vessels and nerves mean that the surgical results are generally better
- Other specific considerations: young women, cosmetic or specific occupational needs

Contraindications

- Absolute: Multiple level injuries or serious associated injuries or illness
- Relative: Single digit, avulsion, prolonged ischaemic time, old age (poor recovery expected), massive contamination, self-inflicted injuries

Surgical sequence

- The exploration of the amputated part can be performed under magnification whilst the patient is being anaesthetised. Expose vessels and nerves in part and tag them with fine sutures. Trace them back to segments that appear normal
- Stabilise the bones first. Shortening may be required and should be anticipated, particularly for more proximal injuries
- If there are many structures to repair, consider vascular shunting first
- Repair extensor tendons first, then muscles, then flexor tendons. The A2 and A4 pulleys should be kept intact or repaired
- Coapt nerves, using grafts if needed
- Anastomose two veins per artery and two arteries per digit, if possible. When ischaemia has been prolonged

(> 2 hours), arteries can be repaired first to reduce reperfusion injury. Prophylactic fasciotomies should be performed for more proximal replants involving muscle
- Vein grafts can be harvested from the arm, foot or leg
- With DP replants, veins may not always be available in which case venous

bleeding can be encouraged by leeches, nailbed bleeding. Veins are larger on the volar surface beyond the DIPJ or thumb IPJ
- Cover with soft tissue. Avoid tight skin closure as it may lead to venous compression

Further reading

Shi D, Qi J, Li D, et al. Fingertip replantation at or beyond the nail base in children. Microsurgery 2010; 30:380–85.

Related topics of interest

- Leeches and maggots
- Microsurgery and tissue transfer

Flexor tendon injuries

Tendons are tough fibrous structures made of dense collagen bundles that connect muscles to bones, enveloped by endotenon and a loose layer of paratenon.

- Flexor digitorum profundus (FDP): It has a common belly, although the index finger may have a separate belly. The tendons insert into the base of the DP. It is the more superficial tendon distal to the web spaces and is thus usually the first tendon to be cut in the finger
- Flexor digitorum superficialis (FDS): It has four bellies, one for each finger. The tendons lie superficial to the FDP until the level of the proximal digital flexor crease, where it decussates around the FDP (Camper's chiasm), rotating 180° to insert onto the proximal half of the MP. The tendon to the little finger may be deficient or absent

Decussates

Digital flexor sheath

The flexor tendon sheath lies from the distal palmar crease to the DIPJ and has two components:

- Membranous: A thin layer that covers the distal tendons in the hand. The closed synovial system forms bursae containing synovial fluid that has an important gliding action and also contributes to the nutrition of the tendon
- Retinacular or fibrous: The condensations over the digital portion of the sheath form pulleys, five annular and three cruciate (Table 21). These maintain the tendon in close approximation to bone for mechanical advantage, without which bow stringing occurs

The A2 and A4 pulleys are the most important and should be preserved if possible. They are broad and lie between joints, whereas the A1 and A3 are thinner and are found at joints. The cruciate pulleys, C1 and C2 lie on either side of the PIPJ, whilst C3 is proximal to the DIPJ. The thumb has three pulleys: A1 at the MCPJ, A2 at the interphalangeal joint (IPJ) and the most important oblique pulley across the proximal phalanx (extension of adductor pollicis attachment).

Nutrition

There is much debate regarding the source of nutrition for the tendons of the hand.

- Perfusion: Blood supply to the tendons comes primarily from the vincula (from the Latin 'vincio' to bind) that have segmental branches from the digital arteries forming a vascular territory. The vascularity is concentrated mainly on the dorsum of the tendon and remains superficial in the endotenon septae
  - Short: Vincula in the angle between tendon and insertions, FDP to neck of MP
  - Long: From periosteum of phalanges to dorsum of flexor tendon, FDP to PP
- Nutrients from synovial fluid can reach the tendon by diffusion. Some propose that finger movements pump fluid into the narrow canaliculi that pass through the tendon. Current thinking is that diffusion plays an important role

5 Annular

Table 21	Position of the five annular pulleys (odd ones over joints)
Pulley	**Position**
A1	Over metacarpophalangeal, most common site of stenosing tenosynovitis
A2	Proximal phalanx (proximal part of)
A3	Proximal interphalangeal joint
A4	Middle phalanx (middle of)
A5	Proximal to the distal interphalangeal joint

Flexor tendon injuries

Flexor tendon injuries have significant functional implications for the patient and must be treated properly.

Zones

The level of flexor tendon injuries is classified into zones (**Table 22**). Note that these are zones of tendon injury and not the level of the skin injury. The two do not necessarily correspond as they depend on the finger position at the time of injury (see below).

Mechanism of tendon healing

Tendons contain few cells, of which it comprises tenocytes, fibroblasts and synovial cells. The paucity of cells and the presence of avascular zones within the synovial areas led to the theory that tendons would not heal well intrinsically and therefore needed extrinsic cells. However, while the collagen bundles are dense, tendons are still metabolically active. The theories of tendon healing are

- Extrinsic: It was initially thought that healing came from fibroblasts that produced peritendinous adhesions. These acted as pathways for cell migration and revascularisation. This was the basis for the immobilisation regimes of the past. By this mechanism, the tendon heals though the traditional stages of wound healing (inflammation, proliferation and remodelling)
- Intrinsic: Tendons bathed in synovial fluid were found to heal well with minimal inflammation. Collagen is produced by tenocytes that act like fibroblasts and can bridge tendon gaps. This type of healing is increased by tendon motion and is the basis for early active motion regimes

Stressed tendons heal better with fewer adhesions. The strength of repair decreases between days 5–21.

Management

The following management techniques are presented in more general terms to include most cases of hand injury. Previous hand injuries including digital nerves, patient hand dominance and occupation/hobbies are important. It is also important to determine the mechanism of injury, position of fingers during injury and if there was pulsatile bleeding or numbness immediately after. The potential for contamination, and the disability according to the patient should also be noted.

Type of injury

- Open: Lacerations or puncture, such as from teeth or glass
- Closed:
  - Crush injuries have a wide zone of injury with possible associated injuries, increased risk of infection, repair failure and adhesions
  - Attrition ruptures from rheumatoid arthritis or fractures such as Colles and scaphoid

Examination

Look, feel and movement of the injured body part.

Inspection

In some cases, the lacerated tendon may be visible in the depths of the laceration.

Zone	Position
Zone I	Between FDS and FDP insertions. Only the FDP tendon is found in Zone I.
Zone II	From the FDS insertion to the A1 pulley. There are two tendons wound around each other within a tight tunnel. Repair is difficult and there is a high risk of tendon adhesion. It was dubbed 'No man's land' (by Bunnell in 1918) for its poor results following repair. Around 50% of flexor tendon injuries occur in Zone II.
Zone III	From the carpal tunnel to the proximal A1 pulley. The lumbricals arise from the FDP tendons in this area and thus also known as the lumbrical zone.
Zone IV	Carpal tunnel: 9 tendons.
Zone V	From the muscle origin to the carpal tunnel.

Table 22 Classification of flexor tendon injuries

However, if the finger was flexed at the time, then the tendon injury may be significantly distal to the skin laceration. In closed injuries, there may be little to see apart from swelling and pain on resisted motion. To aid diagnosis of a tendon injury, there are important clues from examining the resting position of the hand.

- Normal cascade of fingers: Composite flexion increases from index to little finger. If there is a flexor tendon injury, the affected finger will be more extended and thereby disrupting the cascade
- Passive manipulation of the wrist to examine finger movement from the tenodesis effect of antagonistic tendons. This is useful if the patient is unconscious or unwilling to comply with active movement
- Squeezing the forearm flexor muscle bellies should normally increase the degree of finger flexion if the flexors are intact
- Partial tendon injuries are more difficult to diagnose and there is a small risk of converting it to a complete injury during examination. For management see **Table 23**

It is important to exclude other injured structures especially nerves and bones. Expose the entire upper limb and examine systematically:

- Soft tissue: Lacerations and tissue loss
- Circulation:
  - Arterial insufficiency: Pale cold part with loss of turgor and delayed refill
  - Venous insufficiency: Congested part with brisk refill
- Sensation: Denervated fingers are dry and smooth (loss of papillary ridges, and will not wrinkle in water). As a rough screen, test the index fingertip, little fingertip and

dorsal first web. The median, ulnar and radial nerves supply these respectively
- Two-point discrimination (2pd) relates to innervation density and is dependent on cortical integration. A moving 2pd of > 3 mm is a more sensitive indicator of nerve dysfunction than a static 2pd >6 mm
- Vibration and pressure thresholds (Semmes-Weinstein monofilament) are more sensitive
- Bone: Fractures should be described according to location, type (oblique, transverse, comminuted) and deformity (angulation, rotational) – can be detected looking at the finger cascade. Both AP and lateral (or oblique) X-rays of the hands are mandatory, as normal examination does not rule out fractures
- Joints: Passive range of motion (ROM)
- Muscles: Active movements, active ROM and strength testing (MRC). Look at the resting posture and the tenodesis effect with passive wrist flexion/extension

Testing scheme

A simple testing scheme is as follows:
- Make a fist (test active mass motion) then extend all fingers at MCPJ (EDC)
- Abduct (dorsal interossei) then adduct fingers (palmer interossei)
- FDS: Test individually while holding other fingers in extension. PIPJ will flex and the DIPJ will be lax. 15% of individuals do not have a functional FDS to the little finger
- FDP: Fix MP and PP to isolate DIPJ
- Thumb movement: Oppose to each digit, adduction then abduction, flex then extend (lift off table with palm down)

Surgery

Repair of isolated tendon injury is not urgent per se, although early repair helps reduce myostatic shortening of the proximal muscle. Furthermore, not all patients should have their tendons repaired, such as the uncooperative or those with active infection, severe contamination and tissue loss. A failed primary repair is worse than no repair at all. Patient compliance is a mandatory component of good therapy.

Table 23 Treatment of partial lacerations

Partial laceration (%)	Recommended treatment
Up to 25%	Smooth down tendon rants that may otherwise catch in the sheath.
From 25% to 50%	Running 6-0 epitendinous suture.
More than 50%	Core suture and epitendinous suture.

General principles

- Antibiotics and tetanus booster immunisation are administered as indicated
- Early repair. Repair within 1 week will still provide good results, whilst satisfactory results are possible up to 2–3 weeks later. After 3 weeks, tendon grafting may be needed
- Adequate visualisation
  - Tendons are repaired under tourniquet control (100 mmHg above systolic, 250 mmHg adults, 150 mmHg children, placed high on the arm and limited to 2 hours at a time). Exsanguination is contraindicated in tumours and active infection. Elevation is preferred. Complications such as nerve injuries are usually related to direct pressure rather than length of tourniquet time (muscle ischaemia)
  - Incisions aim to maximise exposure of injured parts: Extend lacerations as necessary and start dissection from uninjured area towards injury. All incisions heal with a scar and all scars contract, thus incisions should not cross flexor joints perpendicularly to minimise scar-related joint contracture. Use Brunner's (volar zigzag, but can have greater effect on sensation than others), Bunnell (non-dominant mid-lateral incision, involves significant elevation of soft tissue) or a combination of the two, taking care to avoid injury to neurovascular bundles. Incisions on the contact areas, such as the ulnar side of the little finger or radial side of the index finger, should be avoided
- Handle tendons carefully: Avoid handling uninjured areas and grasp only the end of tendon. Injuring the epitenon will increase the risk of adhesions
- Avoid shortening tendons by debriding minimally. Excessive shortening causes a quadriga effect (incomplete flexion due to shortened FDP tendons reaching maximum flexion too early). A loss of > 1 cm of tendon will severely limit excursion
- The A2 and A4 pulleys can be vented without compromising function, as long

as limited to 25% of both or up to 75% of one. Some advocate L-shaped incisions through the sheath that allow adjustable reapproximation
- Dressings in layers: Tulle dressing, fluffy gauze and crepe in diminishing compression from distal to proximal
  - The safe or protective position is IPJ extension, 70° MCPJ flexion and thumb abduction. This keeps the collateral ligaments taut to avoid shortening, while the thumb position maintains the web space. Wrist extension is not strictly necessary with adequate support from the dressings. A neutral wrist position is favoured. Splinting in slight flexion may be appropriate in the higher risk patient
  - Elevation above the level of the heart

Zone II

If both tendons are injured at the same level, then the FDP should be repaired preferentially and one slip of FDS if possible. There is a risk of late swan neck deformity if the FDS is not repaired, but may be an acceptable sacrifice if space does not permit good gliding after repair of both tendons. Tendon ends may not be immediately obvious, as they may have retracted, especially if the finger was flexed when injured. It can be retrieved by milking or with additional proximal incisions.

Repair techniques are numerous and commonly combine the following:

- Core suture: Usually a permanent 3-0–4-0 monofilament suture such as Prolene or smooth-coated braided Ethibond. Common techniques include the modified Kessler (parallel suture with locking) and the Tajima or Bunnell (criss-crossing) with at least four throws. Forty percent of failures are due to knot slippage. With the Kessler technique, the debate whether more volar placement (less ischaemia) is better than dorsal suture placement (up to 50% more strength but potentially disrupts the dorsal intrinsic vascular system more) persists. There is a trend toward a 4-strand repair as a minimum, although the modified Kessler (2-stranded) remains the most common. Two modified Kesslers placed at right angles to each other can be used to comply with this. Other techniques such as the Strickland 4 strand, 4 strand cruciate and MGH techniques have also gained popularity. Multi (4) strand repairs have been shown to reduce gap formation. However, increasing the strands also increases difficulty of surgery, increases tendon manipulation, increases the risk of damaging the core suture with more needle passes and increases the bulk at the repair site. Increasing the size of suture also increases repair strength, but may increase repair bulk, reduce glide and thus increase the resistance and work of flexion. The knot should be buried to reduce friction. External knots can be buried in the tendon substance via a small cut that is sutured up with fine sutures

- Epitendinous suture: Usually a 5-0/6-0 monofilament continuous suture. This provides up to 20% of total repair strength. Starting the epitendinous suture on the back wall as a running locking suture (or simple or inverting mattress) first before the core suture may help to keep the tendon ends together and reduce handling (outside Zone II, the epitendinous suture is less important)
- It is vital that Zone II injuries are repaired meticulously; otherwise there is a high incidence of adhesions and failure. The repaired tendon should be able to pass smoothly under pulleys at the end of surgery

Failure is often related to inadequate tensile strength (inadequate number of strands), gliding resistance and gap formation (leading to adhesions whilst immobilised).

Zone I

If there is > 1 cm of distal stump remaining, the tendon can be repaired conventionally but may be hampered by a tight A4 pulley. If the stump is shorter, the tendon can be reattached via sutures passed through drill holes in the DP and tied over a button on the fingernail. Alternatively, it may be repaired onto a Mitek bone anchor inserted on the DP. Tendon injuries due to avulsion injuries may have a variable bone fragment involved that determines how far proximally the tendon retracts (**Table 24**). These avulsions can be classified according to the level of retraction.

Other zones

These are simple repairs by comparison. Better results are possible in Zone III and Zone V.

- In Zone III, it is important to avoid suturing the lumbricals into the tendon repair
- Zone IV injuries may also have injuries to the median nerve and arteries
- Zone V tendon injuries tend to be multiple (spaghetti wrist) and there may be problems matching up the tendon ends. These should be repaired early to avoid shortening

For treatment of partial lacerations, see **Table 23**. If left there is a risk of late rupture, whereas repair may impede vascularity or increase adhesions.

Table 24 Classification of avulsion injuries (Leddy)		
Avulsion injury type	Size of bone fragment	Position of proximal tendon
Type 1	No fragment	Tendon end lies in the palm and all blood supply has been severed. Early surgery (within a week) is advised. Sheath scarring is likely.
Type 2	Small fragment	Tethered by long vincula. The end is usually near the PIPJ, there is loss of active flexion at DIPJ, pain, swelling and tenderness. While surgery can be delayed up to 6 weeks because the blood supply is intact, early reinsertion is often preferred.
Type 3	Large fragment	Tethered by bone at A4 pulley over MP. These injuries can theoretically be repaired late.

Postoperative care

Splintage   A dorsal extension block splint is used to keep the wrist neutral and the MCPJ 40–70° flexed and IPJ 10–15° flexion or full extension. The trend has been for the amount of flexion in the splint to be reduced. The splint places repaired tendons in a protected, shortened position and preventing full, active extension to alleviate stress on the repair.

Rehabilitation   The key factor in success is patient compliance with the rehabilitation protocol. Patients have to be aware that frequent and regular visits will be needed, and that unrestricted motion and normal use of the hand does not happen until 3 months after repair. Three main protocol groups exist:

1. Active extension associated with rubber band flexion
2. Controlled active motion
3. Controlled passive motion (Duran 1970s, fully passive regime with dorsal block but no elastics)

The Kleinert splint incorporates a dorsal block splint with a spring-loaded roller bar as a pulley system in the mid-palm for maximum DIPJ flexion.

Belfast regime (1989, subject to many local modifications) of early active motion is popular and provides good results, though with an increased risk of rupture (compared to Kleinert, **Table 25**). Although passive motion moves joints, the effect on tendons is unknown and the only proven way of moving tendons sufficiently to prevent adhesions is by active mobilisation. Thus, the trend is to utilise early controlled active motion that aims to facilitate tendon strengthening. This is used in conjunction with a dorsal blocking splint (wrist flexion 0–30°, MCP 50–70° flexion and IP neutral) with active extension and passive flexion to prevent PIPJ contracture.

- After 2–3 weeks:
  - Oedema and scarring increases drag on the repaired tendon, and greater force is needed to move it. The tendon is weakest in the repair phase 5–21 days (ruptures most common 5–10 days). Strength increases gradually after 3 weeks. The repair is protected during the weakest phase, using passive movement to reduce adhesions whilst avoiding excessive loading associated with active motion
- 4–6 weeks: Mobilised tendons will heal faster and stronger and with fewer adhesions by promoting intrinsic healing. Active exercises with active tendon gliding can be used when the tendon is stronger.
  - No forceful use of hand is allowed until after 8 weeks
  - Unrestricted use is allowed after 12 weeks, including driving   3 months
  - Full tensile strength is gained at 8 months   8 months

When not contraindicated, early controlled mobilisation is of clear benefit. The trade off is better tendon excursion for a higher rate of rupture.

Complications   Overall, better results are expected if the injury is outside Zone II (85%, compared to 80% in Zone II) and poorer results if there are other injuries such as fracture or nerve transection. The most common complication is adhesion, causing stiffness that may lead to flexion contractures. The risk of adhesions is increased particularly by trauma to the tendon and sheath, as well as prolonged immobilisation. Other complications include

- Rupture: Especially at postoperative days 7–10, but can be as late as 6 weeks. Patient education is vital as rupture commonly follows inadvertent strong gripping/liftings

Table 25 Outcomes for the Belfast and Kleinert regimes		
	Belfast regime	Kleinert regime
Risk of rupture	10%	5%
Good result	>80%	>70%
Contractures	Fewer	More
Patient acceptance	Compliance higher due to more supervision	Lower compliance

- Delayed commencement of active motion rehabilitation (after day 5) increases the risk of rupture. Between 5–21 days the repair strength is dependent on the suture, as the actual tendon strength (fibrin/clot) reduces
- Injury to neurovascular bundle and other tourniquet related injuries

- Infection is rare. The role of prophylactic antibiotics is unclear. Irrigation and debridement are the most important
- Chronic regional pain syndrome
- Excessive shortening causing quadriga effect with incomplete flexion of uninjured fingers

Further reading

Ruchelsman DE, Christoforou D, Wasserman B, et al. Avulsion injuries of the flexor digitorum profundus tendon. J Am Acad Orthop Surg 2011; 19:152–62.

Related topics of interest

Ganglia

Ganglia are the most common soft tissue tumours in the hand and are more common in women. They may be caused by mucinous degeneration or embryological remnants of synovium in the joint capsule, where there is often a tenuous and tortuous connection between the sac and the underlying joint. This has been theorised to be either of articular origin, spreading to the tissues, or of extraarticular degenerative origin that then communicates with the joint.

Ganglia transilluminate, unless deep. They are not true cysts as the lining is not composed of cells, but instead compressed and degenerative stromal tissue. Indications for treatment include discomfort, restriction of work/hobbies and cosmesis. Most ganglia resolve spontaneously (50% in adults after 5 years, 75% in children) and complications include excision include recurrence, scar tenderness or numbness and joint stiffness.

Common locations

- Dorsal wrist (60–70%): These arise from the scapholunate ligament and there is usually a pedicle between EPL and EDC. Treatments include
  - Aspiration (seeing the clear fluid can often reassure patients): Up to three times as there is evidence to show no benefit beyond this. Injecting intralesional steroids or hyaluronidase after aspiration does not seem to have clear benefits over aspiration alone. Sclerosants are no longer used since the discovery of potential joint connections
  - Surgery: A 40% recurrence rate is commonly quoted, but is extremely variable (as low as 1%). Complete excisions (cyst, pedicle and cuff of joint capsule) have lower recurrence rates

- Volar wrist (20%): These arise from scaphotrapeziotrapezoid (STT) joint. They usually pass superficial and radial to flexor carpi radialis and are closely related to radial artery (which is at risk during aspiration/injection/surgery). A preoperative Allen's test is advisable. These do not respond well to aspiration and usually require excision
- Flexor sheath (10%): These present as an immobile tender mass at A1 pulley, most commonly of the middle finger. They do not move with the tendon, distinguishing them from trigger finger nodes. They are excised with a small portion of the pulley. Aspiration may be more successful than in other areas
- Mucous cysts at DIPJ: These are often found in older patients who may also have osteoarthritis with osteophytes. The earliest sign is often longitudinal nail grooving. They should be excised and traced back to the joint capsule. Flap/graft coverage is frequently needed
- Synovial cysts: These are true cysts and are found in relation to joints, formed by herniation of synovial membrane through the joint capsule. They are less common, usually associated with rheumatoid or osteoarthritis, but may occur in other conditions. The underlying cause(s) may be increased synovial fluid secretion due to joint inflammation and or capsular weakness. The results of surgery (excision with neck ligation and capsular defect repair) may be improved by reducing joint inflammation and thus fluid production. These include splintage, long-acting steroid intra-articular injection, or in selected patients, joint obliteration/excision

Further reading

Dermon A, Kapetanakis S, Fiska A, et al. Ganglionectomy without repairing the bursal defect: long-term results in a series of 124 wrist ganglia. Clin Orthop Surg 2011; 3:152–56.

Related topic of interest

- Rheumatoid arthritis and osteoarthritis

Groin dissection

Malignant disease is one of the most common causes of lymphadenopathy in adults. The practice of routine elective dissection in melanoma patients has been superseded by selective use of lymphadenectomy, either in those with positive sentinel nodes or clinical lymphadenopathy.

Femoral triangle

The femoral triangle or trigone of Scarpa, is bounded by the inguinal ligament (which lies above the level of the groin crease) above, the medial border of sartorius and the medial limit of adductor longus.

During a groin dissection

The common femoral artery lies at the mid-inguinal point (distinct from the midpoint of the inguinal ligament that marks the position of the deep inguinal ring). The superficial branches (superficial circumflex iliac, superficial epigastric and external pudendal) are ligated, sparing the deeper branches.

The long saphenous vein is ligated twice. The first is at the inferior aspect and other at the saphenofemoral junction (SFJ). The long saphenous vein (LSV) may be preserved unless it is grossly involved. The venae comitantes are variable in pattern.

- The superficial nodes that lie above the fascia lata are arbitrarily split into groups by the SFJ: vertical (lower limb), medial (abdominal wall and perineum) and lateral (buttocks and flank)
- There are few deep inguinal nodes except for Cloquet's node, which lies at the highest point of the superficial dissection. They communicate with the superficial nodes at the saphenous opening via the cribriform fascia. A pre-pubic node may be present that is involved in cancer of the penis/clitoris. The obturator nodes are removed en bloc during a deep iliac dissection

Controversy exists regarding the need for deep lymph node dissection. There are few randomised prospective trials showing consistent differences but retrospective data suggests that the risk of deep nodal involvement is correlated with an increasing number of superficial nodes. Those with deeper nodal involvement tend to have worse outcomes.

The elective approach is often Cloquet's node involvement dependent. This criterion is specific but not sensitive (50%). Based on current evidence, deep node dissection is not always necessary and indications for deeper surgery are relative rather than absolute. These include the presence of biopsy-proven deep nodes (including Cloquet's node), suspicious deep node involvement on imaging or presence of grossly enlarged or multiple superficial nodes.

Imaging

- Ultrasound, CT/MRI
- Lymphography has been superseded by newer techniques. Lymphangiography with oily dye may be useful as quality control check at the end of operation, but not commonly used

Preoperative preparation

- Bowel preparation and low residue diet
- Shaving just prior to surgery and prophylactic antibiotics

Incisions

Various incisions for access have been described but should incorporate the FNA tract where possible. The risk of tumour seeding is very rare but has been reported.

- Vertical incisions generally allow better access to the nodes including the suprainguinal nodes, but there are concerns about the vascularity of the skin flaps, particularly the medial side. Variations include a lazy 'S' incision placed two fingerbreadths medial to the ASIS
- Horizontal/ oblique: This runs parallel to the inguinal ligament, although may be curvilinear. The flaps have good vascularity but will need significant retraction at the risk of skin edge necrosis. An additional distal incision may be used to reduce soft

tissue damage, particularly in the obese
- T-shaped incisions: These allow good access but risk T-junction breakdown

Technique

- Leave a fat layer (> 2 mm) on the underside of the skin flaps. Avoid over-retraction, especially since the skin over enlarged nodes may already be thinned
- Dissect from lateral to medial over sartorius to find the femoral nerve, preserving the lateral cutaneous nerve (usually at the lateral limit of the dissection), if possible. The muscle fascia is taken along with the block dissection. Clamp and ligate tissues especially around the LSV to reduce seroma (no strong evidence for this)
- Closing skin with excessive tension will tent it up creating a dead space. Skin grafts may be used if necessary. Two large drains are inserted and kept until < 25 ml/24 hours per drain. Patients can go home with them if taught self-care. Prolonged drainage is expected. Alternatively, serial seroma aspiration can be used if the drains are removed earlier
- It is usually possible to ambulate on the second day, while maintaining compression over the operated site for at least 6 weeks

Complications

- Seroma
- Wound infections/necrosis
- Lymphoedema

Further reading

Robinson AJ, Brown AP. Tumour seeding in a case of malignant melanoma due to fine needle aspiration of a lymph node. J Plast Reconstr Aesthet Surg 2010; 63:e571–72.

Related topics of interest

- Melanoma

Gynaecomastia

Gynaecomastia (a term first used by Galen) is the enlargement of the male breast. It can be a source of embarrassment and in some cases may be painful. Most cases are due to a variety of subtle hormonal factors and are potentially reversible. Sometimes it may indicate severe underlying disease, such as malignancy of the testes, pituitary or breast.

In gyaenecomastia, the glandular tissue is purely ductal. The periductal tissue has no true acinar development and excess fat may be present. Pseudogynaecomastia is a purely fatty breast with no increase in glandular tissue, also termed 'lipomastia'. Figures regarding the frequency and incidence of the condition are widely variable, reflecting the lack of standard definitions for the condition (e.g. some use >5 cm, others 2 cm), but it is common. The age of onset is important in determining the most likely cause of the enlargement.

- Physiological: The majority of these are pubertal but also includes neonatal (due to excessive maternal oestrogens and usually disappears within weeks) and senile gynaecomastia
- Pharmacological: Drug-related gynaecomastia (10–20%)
- Pathological: This includes neoplasms, particularly those that increase hCG (non-small-cell lung, gastric, renal cell carcinomas and hepatoma), liver and renal diseases, and gonadal failure. Together they constitute up to 40% of cases

Overall, the most common identifiable causes are pubertal, drugs, liver disease, lung carcinoma and hyperthyroidism. The majority of cases are idiopathic and self-limiting.

Pubertal gynaecomastia (40–65%)

Pubertal gynaecomastia may be due to a sex-hormone imbalance or tissue hypersensitivity to them. Increased oestrogens induce ductal epithelial hyperplasia, ductal elongation and branching, and an increase in vascularity in a similar manner to female breast tissue. Oestrogens in males (oestrogen and oestradiol) are mostly derived from the peripheral conversion of testosterone and androstenedione via the aromatase enzyme found in the skin, muscle and fat.

Pubertal gynaecomastia is typically asymmetrical and may be tender, distinguishing it from most other causes. A small amount of breast hypertrophy accompanying the adolescent growth spurt is common (up to two thirds of 14-year-old males) and may even be regarded as physiological or normal. The condition resolves spontaneously within a few years in 75% of cases. By age 17, the incidence is reduced to approximately 8%. Gynaecomastia is less likely to resolve spontaneously if the patient is obese or if the breasts are larger than 4 cm in retroareolar thickness.

Most cases do not warrant extensive investigation and only considering surgery for non-resolving cases may be the most appropriate option. Cases with a marked increase (>4 cm) have a secondary cause in 20%, thus endocrine evaluation is indicated. Those with simple gynaecomastia do not have an increased risk of breast cancer (except in Klinefelter syndrome where it is increased by 20–60 times).

Prepubertal gynaecomastia

Gynaecomastia at this age (includes infants) is of greater concern and warrants evaluation by a paediatric endocrinologist. Investigation may reveal

- Reduced testosterone: Klinefelter syndrome (XXY) – Typically tall, with reduced secondary hair and small genitalia. Hyperthyroidism and congenital adrenal hyperplasia are other possible causes
- Raised oestrogen: Testicular tumours (functioning and secreting, such as Sertoli cell or Leydig cell tumours), true hermaphroditism

Adult gynaecomastia

Adult gynaecomastia is usually due to excess fat with or without glandular hypertrophy. It often occurs in healthy men and routine endocrine screening of patients in this category tends to be neither cost-effective nor revealing.

The pharmacological agents commonly responsible can be recalled with the mnemonic 'Some Men Can Develop Rather Excessive Thoracic Diameters' that stand for Spironolactone, Marijuana, Cimetidine, Diazepam, Reserpine, oEstrogen, Theophylline and Digoxin.

- Drugs are the most common identifiable cause of gynaecomastia in men over 40 years of age. Cimetidine and spironolactone inhibit testosterone synthesis. Digoxin has oestrogenic activity. Alcohol, steroids, tricyclic antidepressants and diazepam work though unknown mechanisms. The evidence on marijuana is contradictory
- Abnormal liver function or mild cirrhosis with reduced oestrogen clearance
- In hyperthyroidism, there is reduced ↓ circulating testosterone due to increased plasma binding

Classification

Simon classification (1973) – Grades of gynaecomastia

(handwritten: Simon 1973)

- I   Minor, but visible enlargement as a localised button with no skin excess
- IIA   Moderate diffuse enlargement with no skin excess
- IIB   Moderate diffuse enlargement with minor excess of skin
- III   Marked enlargement with significant excess skin, simulating a female breast

Webster classification (composition and treatment)

Composition	Treatment
Glandular	Excision
Fatty-glandular	Liposuction and excision
Simple fatty	Liposuction

Management

Focus of history:

- Time of onset: If present < 1 year, medical therapy may be an option
- Drug history
- Symptoms suggestive of systemic disease or malignancy. Gynaecomastia with headache and visual disturbance indicates a pituitary tumour until proven otherwise

Examination should aim to ascertain the presence/absence of:

- ⊙ Thyroid disease
- ⊙ Genital problems and testicle size assessment, signs of feminisation or eunuchoid
- ⊙ Lymph nodes

Investigation

Blanket endocrine screening in adult patients is unrewarding. The following may be directed by the history and examination:

- Liver function test (LFT), renal function test
- Testosterone, oestrogen, dehydroepiandrosterone (DHEA) and luteinizing hormone (LH) levels in suspected feminisation
- Thyroid-stimulating hormone (TSH) and free thyroxine (fT4)

The sign of breast cancer is a hard eccentric lump with or without skin dimpling. FNA of simple gynaecomastia is very painful, unrewarding and to be avoided.

Treatment

Non-surgical treatment

It may be advisable to observe early or mild cases to allow for the possibility of involution, but this practice must be tempered by the social and emotional factors of the patient. Obesity is often associated with a fatty breast that may benefit from weight loss but the effectiveness of weight loss in adolescents is very variable. Studies on medical treatment do have shortcomings in their lack of controls and long-term follow-up.

- Correct reversible causes: This is successful in more than half of drug-related cases and in the majority of pathological cases.

- Depending on the case, medication may help but in general the results of hormonal therapy are often disappointing unless treated early before fibrosis occurs
  - Clomiphene (50–100 mg daily for 6 months) is a non-steroidal with a weak anti-oestrogenic effect. The response is variable (20% complete, 50% partial), though side effects are rare (rash, visual disturbance)
  - Dihydrotestosterone (cannot be broken down to oestrogens) is useful in gonadal failure
  - Tamoxifen is an antioestrogen that has been widely used in females but its long-term effects on young males are unclear. A 2–4 month course can be 80% effective with recent onset of disease, although it may improve pain more than reduce bulk
  - Danazol inhibits oestrogen production and has androgenic side effects. A 6-week course is 80% effective. Weight gain is the most significant side effect

Surgical treatment

Surgery should be used cautiously in adolescents or the obese. Approximately 15% of patients proceed to surgery. The choice of treatment is related to the severity of the enlargement and skin excess. Particular attention should be paid to contour deformities and scars. Incisions are not to be placed on non-areolar skin, if possible. Endoscopic excision through an axillary incision may be suitable for selected cases. Diode laser-assisted liposuction has recently been shown to be effective treatment (Trelles 2013).

Cases of minor enlargement (Simon I and II) do not need skin excision. Liposuction is the first choice unless very glandular. Residual glandular components are often retroareolar and can be excised through a classical Webster inferior periareolar

Webster inferior periareolar

incision. Approximately 1 cm of retroareolar tissue should be left attached to the NAC undersurface and the edges feathered smoothly to reduce the risk of retraction and a saucer deformity. Unevenness of the skin surface may result due to either undermining too close to the skin or fat necrosis.

Primary excision for moderate enlargement is prone to the dish deformity, although tapering the edge with liposuction may reduce this. The firm breast bud is not amenable to conventional liposuction but power-assisted (mechanical), ultrasound-assisted (Vaser) or laser-assisted (Smartlipo) liposuction may work better. A planned two-stage approach to take advantage of the significant skin contraction especially in the young is common. Liposuction is performed first and the residual skin excess is then excised after 6–12 months. The ultrasound-assisted and laser-assisted techniques claim greater skin contraction, which may eliminate the need for the second stage.

Circumareolar doughnut mastopexies with a periareolar Gore-Tex purse string suture can be used to compensate for moderate skin excess. With larger degrees of skin excess, incisions through non-areolar skin are inevitable.

- Breast reduction type incisions may be used, but to be avoided unless absolutely necessary
- Male-specific techniques: The aim is for a flat chest
  - Letterman technique: Skin and parenchymal excision, nipple transposition on medial pedicle
  - Horizontal ellipse +/– with 7–8 cm superior pedicle

Postoperative seromas and haematomas are relatively common. Extensive surgery warrants placement of drains. A pressure dressing is worn for two weeks with dressing changes as required.

Further reading

Qutob O, Elahi B, Garimella V, et al. Minimally invasive excision of gynaecomastia – a novel and effective technique. Ann R Coll Surg Engl 2010; 92:198–200.

Related topics of interest

- Breast reduction
- Liposuction

Hair removal

Excessive hair is a common cosmetic problem that can affect healthy individuals. The normal amount of hair for an individual is related, in part, to their ethnicity. Cultural factors determine its acceptability.

- Hirsutism is excessive growth of hair in females in a male pattern. Most cases show a genetic predisposition, and the problem is usually androgen hypersensitivity rather than oversecretion
- Hypertrichosis is excessive growth of hair in a non-androgenic distribution that is above normal for the age, sex and race of the patient. It can be congenital or acquired. Drugs that frequently cause this are cyclosporin, phenytoin and minoxidil

Excessive hair may also be due to hormonal disturbances. Hyperandrogenism is most common and can be from exogenous or endogenous sources (ovarian or pituitary). Examples include congenital adrenal hyperplasia and polycystic ovary syndrome. Idiopathic cases may bear a subtle hormonal overactivity or hypersensitivity. Patients with a suspected hormonal aetiology should be referred appropriately, before any treatment.

Hair cycle

Hairs grow and rest in cycles. Hairs from different body areas display different cycle lengths and not all hairs in an area will be in identical phase.

- Anagen: Growth phase with 85–95% of hairs in it at any time. Hairs grow at 0.3–0.4 mm per day. The length of anagen influences the length of the hair, whilst the anagen to telogen ratio influences the amount of hair, which is also subject to a number of intrinsic and extrinsic factors. Anagen lasts 3 years
- Catagen: This is a transition and regression phase with 5% of hairs in it at any time. It lasts 3 weeks
- Telogen: This resting phase has 10% of hairs in it at time. Hairs in telogen are less susceptible to laser effects. Hair is ejected (exogen) leaving a hard white nodule at the proximal shaft. The proportion of

follicles in this stage (and the length of time) will determine the number and frequency of laser treatments required to achieve near-complete hair removal. Up to 100 telogen hairs are lost each day with approximately the same number entering anagen. Telogen lasts 3 months.

Methods of hair removal

Shaving

This is simple but needs to be repeated every day or so with risks of cuts, irritation and developing ingrown hairs. Contrary to popular myth, shaving does not increase the number of hairs.

Depilation

Thioglycolates (usually in combination with sodium hydroxide) are used to disrupt the disulphide bridges in keratin, resulting in the hair breaking above the skin surface. Allergies, irritation or chemical burns can occur.

Epilation

This involves removal of the entire shaft by various means. The long-term effects on hair growth are unclear, but hairs may become finer with repeated damage to the matrix.

- Waxing is one of the most effective method and effects can last for several weeks. It is more effective when performed by experienced practitioners. Honey is used in a similar way
- Plucking by hand with tweezers or with machines is similar in principle. Threading is a method of avulsing finer hairs
- Electrolysis works by ablating follicular germ cells by insertion of fine needle electrodes into the follicle. It is time-consuming, as it has to be done individually for each follicle. There is a theoretical risk of causing infection
  - DC current: Galvanic electrolysis causes chemical damage by generating sodium hydroxide at the cathode
  - AC current: Thermolysis is thermal damage due to vibrational energy. Most

modern equipment uses this mode alone or in combination with a galvanic mode. The caustic damage is greater when combined with heat

Temporary reduction of hair

Eflornithine hydrochloride (Vaniqa) is applied as a cream and by irreversibly inhibiting ornithine decarboxylase. It reduces hair growth after several weeks of use and is licensed for use in the UK to treat facial hirsutism in women. Dianette, acting via androgen suppression, is the only other licensed drug for hirsutism in UK. It is much cheaper, but contraindicated in those with a risk of thromboembolic disease. It is effective in 50% of patients and as it does not actually remove hair but slows down its growth, it has to be combined with the hair removal techniques described above. Hair will return (in about 8 weeks) when the treatment is stopped. Side effects such as mild acne, rash, pseudofolliculitis barbae, irritation and dryness are rare, with only 2% of patients stopping treatment for these reasons.

Laser hair removal

Lasers have proved to be very useful in hair removal. The pluripotent cells responsible for hair growth are in the bulge/bulb region that lies 4 mm below the skin surface (not exclusively as recent labelling studies have shown). These cells are destroyed by heat conducted from the melanin in the follicle (the chromophore). Only hair follicles in the anagen stage are vulnerable to laser energy (an oversimplification), and since hair follicles are at different stages of the hair cycle, laser treatment must be repeated. Laser treatment also tends to prolong the telogen phase. The hair colour needs to be much darker than the surrounding skin colour for lasers to be most effective. It is consequently least effective on fine vellus or white hairs.

Pretreatment preparation

- Patch testing is important to determine the optimal fluences to be used. There should be hyperaemia, mild swelling and some pain with an effective dose
- Topical anaesthesia is usually needed

- Use of sunscreens +/– bleaching. Sun tanning before laser treatment should be avoided as this reduces the contrast between skin and hair
- Avoid other forms of hair removal, such as plucking and waxing, up to 4–6 weeks prior, to maximise hair follicle damage. Shaving is acceptable

Upon exposure to laser light, there is heating of the melanin-containing shaft, follicular epithelium and matrix (600–1100 nm). However, there is also competing melanin (and haemoglobin) in the epidermis. In the past, a hyperpigmentation was frequent concern, especially with darker skin. Modern machines with longer pulse widths and longer wavelengths are safe enough to be used on most skin types, although caution is still required with darker skin types.

- Pulse width is important. The thermal relaxation time (TRT) of a hair follicle is estimated to be 10–100 minutes. However, some of the targets are not pigmented and are at a distance from the melanin, such as the follicular stem cells in the bulge. Therefore, laser hair removal often involves matching pulse widths, not to the TRT but to the thermal damage time (TDT). This means deliberately using longer pulses to allow better distant damage
- Fluence is also important but is dependent on patients' skin pigmentation. In practical terms, the largest spot size and highest tolerable fluence is used
- Longer wavelengths allow better skin penetration and offers better protection for epidermal melanin. It is however, less effective at removing hair than shorter wavelengths

Laser systems

The majority of hair-removal lasers utilise wavelengths in the red or near infrared spectrum, with cooling systems (cryogen or contact cooling). Early techniques, such as Q-switched lasers with carbon powder as an exogenous chromophore, Argon or pulsed dye lasers (PDL) are not in common use any more for this purpose.

- Long-pulse ruby (694 nm): Less commonly used

- Long-pulse Alexandrite (755 nm): Effective but safe only on pale skinned patients
- Long-pulse diode laser (810 nm): Safe for light to medium skin types
- Long-pulse Nd:YAG (1064 nm): Safe for darker skin types
- Intense pulsed light (IPL 500–1200 nm): Tends to result in more post-inflammatory hyperpigmentation (PIH) and evidence for long-term reduction is lacking

Long-term studies on the effectiveness of laser hair removal are lacking with inadequate evaluation of hair regrowth being the primary problem. In general, efficacy is improved with repeated treatments. The best evidence for hair removal lasting > 6 months exists for Alexandrite and diode lasers (about 50%, Cochrane review 2009). Lasers have also been used with some success for pseudofolliculitis barbae (ingrown hairs).

Effects of laser

The effects of laser on hairs can be described as follows:

- Temporary total loss: Lasts 1–3 months i.e. telogen
- Permanent reduction (not total): Significant reduction in the number of terminal hairs after a given treatment, which is stable for a period of time longer than the complete growth cycle of hair

follicles at the given body site (FDA definition). An additional 6 months may be required to judge the results, to allow time for damaged follicles to recover and re-enter the cycle

The commonest complication is hyperpigmentation that may last for several months. Significant scarring is rare. Patient satisfaction is usually good, but 100% efficacy rates or zero regrowth rates are unrealistic. In reality,

- Individual responses cannot be predicted. Many have a good results but some will have poor results
- Usually 2–3 treatments are required to catch the majority of hairs in the anagen phase, but some regrowth is possible. On average, an 80% clearance is expected
- Effective painless treatment (without anaesthesia) for permanent hair removal does not yet exist. Permanent damage to the follicles only comes at energies that cause pain. Otherwise, the follicles are simply pushed into the resting phase (telogen) for a period of dormancy before returning. Sublethal laser energy may alternatively cause regression of the terminal hair or vellus (miniaturisation), giving the appearance of apparent hair loss

Further reading

Lapidoth M, Dierickx C, Lanigan S, et al. Best practice options for hair removal in patients with unwanted facial hair using combination therapy with laser: guidelines drawn up by an expert working group. Dermatology 2010; 221:34–42.

Related topic of interest

- Lasers: principles

Hair restoration

Alopecia areata

This affects men and women equally. The exact mechanism is unclear but involves T-cell autoimmunity, as evidenced by the perifollicular lymphocytic infiltration. The pathogenesis is likely to be multifactorial with a genetic predisposition and as yet, an unidentified environmental trigger(s). There are associations with atopic dermatitis, vitiligo, thyroid disease and Down's syndrome. The relationship to stress is unclear. It mostly involves the scalp in patches, with the underlying skin otherwise normal in appearance. Variants include alopecia totalis (AT, whole scalp) and alopecia universalis (AU, all body hair).

The natural history is unpredictable and though the rate of spontaneous recovery is high, recurrences are also common. This makes assessing the effectiveness of treatment(s) difficult to judge. It is common to test treat half the area first. Differential diagnoses include tinea capitis, trichotillomania, traction (hairstyle), cicatricial (post infective) and syphilis (moth-eaten appearance). The condition is usually asymptomatic, with only 1 in 7 suffering burning sensations. The exclamation point (hair tapering proximally) is a pathognomonic feature. Some patients have nail changes, especially pitting.

Treatments

The most common options are:

- Intralesional steroids
- Minoxidil (5% twice daily): Effects are seen after 3 months, but alopecia will relapse when minoxidil is stopped
- Topical immunotherapy: Weekly squaric acid dibutylester (SADBE). The precise mechanism of action is unknown
- Anthralin (an antipsoriatic) may be useful in children
- PUVA (either topical or systemic) can be used, although there is a small risk of cancer development. It is often the non-surgical option of last resort

Telogen effluvium

Effluvium is Latin for 'flowing out'. Telogen effluvium is a non-scarring alopecia associated with diffuse hair shedding. There is usually spontaneous recovery over 6 months. The rate of normal hair loss is approximately 100 hairs per day with a shift into telogen stage. Stress alone may cause up to 70% of hairs to enter telogen. This is evidenced by increased shedding 2 months after the inciting event, and the typical club-shaped root appearance (white bulb and lack of gelatinous sheath). The classic example is postpartum alopecia. Other reported causes include severe illness, high fever, crash dieting or medication, especially antidepressants. The condition is usually acute (sometimes chronic) and affects the scalp most often, but is not restricted to it. There is little to see on examination, as there are no areas of total alopecia. A gentle hair-pull test (4 or more hairs, greater than 25% telogen hairs) is strongly suggestive of the diagnosis. Biopsy is rarely necessary and even so, the histological changes can be subtle.

Usually no treatment is required, other than cessation of identifiable causes. Minoxidil is often used but it may be of greater psychological benefit than physical.

Male pattern baldness

Male pattern baldness (MPB, androgenetic alopecia) affects up to 70% of white males and is related to androgens (dihydrotestosterone, DHT). The degree of loss appears to be genetic as the most important determinant is family history. In most cases, it behaves as a dominant sex-linked autosomal condition. Hair loss starts at puberty and proceeds at a variable rate. The defect is in the follicle rather than the skin. The frontal scalp follicles have higher levels of DHT, 5-a-reductase and receptors, in the presence of normal circulating plasma testosterone and oestrogen levels. DHT causes a progressive miniaturisation of terminal follicles due to a shortened anagen phase and reduction in size of hair matrix.

MPB is most often staged according to Hamilton or its modification by Norwood. It is important to assess the likely final pattern of MPB, as this will impact the choice of treatment. With hair transplantation, it is imperative to avoid taking donor follicles from areas of likely future loss. Transplantation in patients destined for major baldness may result in a halo of baldness around grafted areas as the loss progresses. At this point, there may be insufficient donor hair available to treat this problem. It is important to anticipate likely long-term results.

Management

The diagnosis is clinical and investigation is usually unnecessary (except in females, where androgen screening and thyroid hormone testing should be considered). Medical treatments generally take at least 3 months for effects to be seen.

Medical treatments

- Topical treatment: Minoxidil (Rogaine and Rogaine Extra Strength are 2% and 5% minoxidil respectively. It is branded as Regaine in Europe and Asia, and is also available generically). It is applied twice daily but is messy to use and may cause skin irritation (more common with 5% preparation). Different applicators are available, such as the dropper, sponge and spray. Minoxidil is a vasodilator (relaxes arteriolar smooth muscle by acting on potassium channels to reduce calcium entry into cells), originally used to treat high blood pressure. Loniten, the oral preparation version, is still used for hypertension. It also has a direct mitogenic effect but no anti-androgen properties. Meaningful hair growth is seen in one third of patients, with a 50% response rate at best. Overall, the effects are limited, short term, and continued use is required. It does not work on completely bald areas. However, it prolongs the anagen and shortens the telogen phases and converts intermediate hairs to terminal hairs. It is generally regarded as first-line treatment and can be combined with oral medication such as tretinoin for synergy

- Oral treatment: Finasteride (Propecia 1 mg, Proscar 5 mg) is an anti-DHT compound that was developed from treatments for benign prostatic hypertrophy. It inhibits 5α-reductase (Type 1 inhibitor) preventing the conversion of testosterone to DHT. It is regarded as the best medical treatment, if tolerated. The adverse effects include a 1–2% rate of decreased libido and impotence. There is some evidence for low dose regimes (< 1 mg daily) being effective. It primarily retards loss, but may increase hair growth in some patients. Response rates of 77% (15% placebo response rate) have been reported. However, the effects are temporary and it is expensive. The most commonly prescribed anti-androgen for MPB is spironolactone. This is an androgen receptor antagonist that similarly slows hair loss but does not seem to stimulate regrowth. It is often prescribed for androgenic loss in females

There are many non-approved medications that are used to reduce hair loss, such as cimetidine, progesterone, cyproterone acetate and herbal remedies, which are largely unproven.

Surgical treatments

Individual patients often benefit from a combination of techniques.

- Scalp reduction to remove bald skin thus reducing the area that needs transplanting and helps to conserve donor sites. Various excision patterns have been described, with sagittal ones being most efficient due to laxity lying primarily in this plane. Alternatively, inverted-Ys can be used, with each limb excised as an ellipse. Significant undermining may be needed

- Flaps with or without tissue expansion to move hair-bearing skin *en masse*. The major advantage of bilateral advancement transposition flaps with tissue expansion over Juri flaps (temporoparietooccipital, TPO) is that the hair grows anteriorly rather than posteriorly, hiding the scar.

The Juri flap needs to be delayed and often requires revision
- Tissue expansion although effective, may not be tolerated due to the cosmetic deformity of having inflated expanders. Some use intraoperative expansion (or slower expansion under LA over several hours) to improve alopecia reduction
- Transplantation (see below)

Transplantation

Initial attempts at hair transplantation used biopsy punches to transfer 3–4 mm patches of hairy skin with 30–40 hairs to bald areas whilst the donor areas were left to granulate. This gave reasonable results but was liable to produce a 'tufted' appearance that was more obvious in patients with black straight hair and pale skin. The technique has since been refined but remains time-consuming. There should preferably be at least two assistants for the surgeon/implantor.

- The concept of donor-recipient dominance is used to explain the phenomenon of occipital hairs growing in frontal alopecia areas. The hairs from the occiput have fewer enzymes and therefore are less susceptible to hormonal influence, making MPB a donor dominant condition. Hairs transplanted into an area of MPB, will grow as it would in its original site (the permanent donor rim)
- Recipient dominant: Diseased recipient scalp (active scarring conditions such as lupus and lichen) will destroy follicles. Treatment is required before transplantation can be successful. Transplantation can be performed when the disease is in the quiescent phase, but the results are suboptimal. Similarly, alopecia areata and females with diffuse type baldness are not good candidates for transplantation

Hair transplantation can be performed under a GA or LA and sedation. LA with adrenaline is used to block occipital and supraorbital nerves, and tumescent solution is then injected into the donor and recipient areas (100 ml of 0.25%). After trimming hair to about 1 cm long, the donor hair is usually taken as 0.75–1.5 cm strips (some use multibladed knives) from the occipital area below the level of the top of the ears. The strip is harvested down to the fatty layer but not through the galea, and is subsequently dissected into smaller sections under magnification. Donor site closure (with or without trichophytic closure techniques) usually leaves acceptable scars. Fascial subtunnelling and imbrication (overlapping of fascial edges) may help for wider (> 1 cm) donor sites.

Number of hairs in grafts
- Standard: Punch grafts 3.5–4.5 mm with 8–30 hairs in each
- Minigrafts: 3–8 hairs, small or larger subtypes, harvested by sectioning strips or less commonly small punches
- Micrografts: 1–3 hairs harvested by sectioning strips

Follicular units
- Follicular unit grafts: Hairs grow naturally in follicular units, which are groups of 1–4 terminal hairs and 1–2 vellus hairs and glands. Follicular grafting implants these units into needle tracts or slits with 20–30 grafts/cm^2. The density can be increased with further sessions. Natural results are produced from the first session. Minigrafting tends to produce an initial artificial appearance, until after further treatments are instituted. A criticism of the technique is that it trims away non-hair bearing skin, which may be perceived as inefficient use of the donor
- Follicular unit extraction (FUE). Hairs are extracted with a narrow calibre punch that only cuts the epidermis. The follicular unit is then extracted by pulling on hair with forceps. This 'blunt dissection' aims to reduce hair transection and the donor heals by secondary intention. The procedure is more time consuming, costs more and follicular units can still be damaged with poor technique. Since contiguous follicles cannot be harvested (to avoid scar coalescence), it is actually less donor efficient

Classically, the best results have come with multiple sessions of mixing mini/micrografts placed into slit/holes in a regular pattern (organised disorganisation, rather than a truly random pattern). The current trend is to use follicular units for all areas with megasessions (thousands of grafts) at a single sitting. Although the latter is less efficient in its use of hairs and manner of increasing hair density, it tends to produce better results.

Placement

- Stick and place technique: A puncture is made with an 18–22G needle just before placing the graft, as the hole stays open for only a few seconds. It is less traumatic and a favoured technique but can be difficult to master. Grafts should not be buried and if in doubt, they are better slightly above the skin level than slightly below
- Slit grafting: A slit (1–2 mm long) is made with a blade. It is a simple method and allows 1–3 hair micrografts or follicular units to be placed, but more liable to compression. In addition, it does not remove alopecia and therefore the overall hair density is lower compared to needles that remove 1–2 mm of bald scalp. There is however, less handling of the grafts due to greater space. There is theoretically less pain and bleeding, as well as fewer problems with inclusion cysts

Postoperative care

- Hydrogen peroxide is useful to remove blood at the end of the procedure. Saline sprays or creams and ointments may be used, or may be left to dry. It is common to inspect the treated area after 1–2 days, along with gentle cleansing
- Grafts appear to grow immediately postoperatively (false growth) but there is shedding after a month when telogen phase is reached. Then, there is regrowth at a rate 1 cm or more per month and is stable by about 9 months to 1 year. Whilst most transplanted hairs will survive, some will die and minor top-up revisions may be required
- During the early regrowth phase (1–3 months), pustules may form with pseudofolliculitis and inclusion cysts (can incise). Some numbness is to be expected. Rarely arteriovenous (AV) fistulae may form, but they often resolve spontaneously after 6 months

Further reading

Rose PT. The latest innovations in hair transplantation. Arch Facial Plast Surg 2011; 366–77.

Related topics of interest

- Scalp reconstruction
- Tissue expansion

Hand infections

Principles of treatment include:

- Rest: Reduces spread of infection and improves comfort
- Heat: Enhances local circulation. Moist heat is preferred and in mild/moderate infections, 10 min of dependent soaking in warm solution is beneficial and outweighs the disadvantage of not elevating. However in severe infections, the arm should be kept elevated
- Elevation: Above the right atrium as reference point, reducing oedema

Cellulitis

This is a superficial spreading infection (*Staphylococcus aureus* or *Streptococcus pyogenes*) that can be associated with lymphangitis and lymphadenopathy. Penicillin-based agents or a first generation cephalosporin is usually sufficient, but may vary according to local resistance patterns.

Paronychia

- Acute paronychia: Infection of the tissues around the nail is often due to microbial inoculation. Eponychia refers to infection of the proximal nail fold. In addition to *Staphylococcus,* there may also be anaerobes from oral contamination. If conservative therapy is unsuccessful, then surgical drainage may be required. The edges should be trimmed to keep the cavity open while it heals by secondary intention. The nail plate does not require removal unless infection has tracked around it, which is unusual
- Chronic paronychia is usually due to *candida* and often requires removal of the nail plate for adequate debridement. A trial of topical gentian violet may be effective treatment alone or to obtain quiescence prior to surgery (Merritt 2008)

Felon

This is a painful pulp infection from a 'compartment syndrome' caused by increased pressure within the many fibrous septae that compartmentalise the pulp. Drainage is indicated if conservative treatment fails. Septae are divided and a continuous irrigation system is often advisable (and better than intermittent irrigation).

Felons can be difficult to differentiate from herpetic infections. With the latter, there is typically 2–3 days of prodromal pain before the small multiple lesions form. These subside spontaneously after 2 weeks (20% reactivation). Treatment is primarily supportive although aciclovir can be considered for the immunocompromised patient. Surgery is contraindicated and only adds to the damage.

Tenosynovitis

This is often due to a penetrating injury (*Staphylococcus).* The classic cardinal signs of tenosynovitis (Kanavel's signs) are:

- Severe pain with passive extension of the digit (most sensitive).
- Flexed finger position at rest.
- Fusiform finger swelling.
- Painful palpation along the tendon sheath.

If left untreated, can lead to adhesions (stiff non-functional finger), tendon necrosis and finger loss. Rapid surgical drainage in combination with intravenous antibiotics is the standard of care. This can be achieved through marsupialisation with Brunner incisions and sheath washout, or a more limited approach with a proximal incision in the distal palm to introduce a small irrigation cannula with a small distant incision for outflow. Multiple returns for inspection and/or debridement may be necessary.

Bite wounds

- *Pasteurella canis, Pasteurella multocida* in dog or cat bites (cat scratch fever is usually caused by *Bartonella*) may seem deceptively innocuous with small puncture wounds. Deep seeding of infection and concomitant deep degloving injuries may be present, especially from large dogs with a powerful bite

- *Eikenella corrodens, Streptococcus, Staphylococcus* and anaerobes are common in human bites. Patients often present late and may not freely volunteer the full history. Urgent standard debridement and irrigation is required and wounds left open

Most bite wounds contain multiple organisms. Antibiotics will work best if given (in order of decreasing effect) within 4 hours of wounding, at time of debridement or within 4 hours of debridement (small effect but still significant). Antibiotics are of little use in chronic wounds (more than 24 hours old or have evidence of granulation tissue). Depending on the locality, rabies may need to be considered with animal bites (dogs, cats, skunks, bats or raccoons). A Cochrane review concludes that co-amoxiclav is a good first line treatment in bite injuries.

Mycobacterium marinum

Also known as 'fish tank' disease, this may affect those working with warm fresh or seawater (mycobacterium thrives at $31°C$). Being fishermen or swimming pool staff is an occupational risk factor. A high index of suspicion is required in patients who present with a granuloma or chronic inflammation around a laceration. Cultures will take 6 weeks (metabolically fastidious) and thus empirical treatment is usually commenced before definitive diagnosis. Severe disease requires rifampicin and ethambutol combination therapy, whereas milder disease can be treated with cotrimoxazole.

Aeromonas hydrophila

This is a Gram-negative rod-shaped bacterium found in fresh water and is resistant to penicillin. It may be found in leeches and antibiotic prophylaxis with use of medicinal leeches is recommended.

Further reading

Kuvat SV, Bozkurt M, Kapi E, et al. Our treatment approaches in head-neck injuries caused by animal bites. J Craniofac Surg 2011; 22:1507–10.

Related topic of interest

- Leeches and maggots

Head and neck cancer principles

Ninety-five per cent of head and neck cancers are squamous cell carcinomas (SCCs). The mucosa can be conceptually viewed as being 'sick', with synchronous tumours occurring at a rate of 5–15% and metachronous tumours appearing at a rate of 5% per year (to eventually exceed the risk of recurrence of first primary).

Smoking is the greatest risk factor, especially those with > 20 pack years. Tobacco-associated head and neck tumours are rare before the age of 50 years. Smoking cessation may reduce the risk of head and neck cancer as well as lung cancer (but not laryngeal cancer). Metachronous cancers occur in 40% of patients who are smokers, compared to 6% in those who are not. Alcohol is not a strong carcinogen on its own, but potentiates the effect of tobacco.

Surgery is the best option for local control. For early stage disease, single modality treatment with either surgery or RT has similar rates of disease-free survival (60–90%). For locally advanced but resectable disease,

- Combined surgery and RT is optimal but provides cure only in the minority (< 30% 5-year survival). Chemotherapy and RT can have similar survival rates whilst avoiding or delaying radical surgery, but may impact on outcome of salvage surgery
- In recurrent disease, the chemotherapy response rate is 1/3 but it lasts for only 3–6 months. Note that a response is not equivalent to survival or cure
- Clinically obvious neck disease: Combined surgery and RT
- Distant metastasis: Chemotherapy for palliation

Surgery

Surgery allows for the control of margins and provides tissue for pathological study. Margins of 1–2 cm are common (80% recurrence rate with margins < 0.5 cm), and may be deforming with functional consequences. Residual microscopic disease may still be present as surgery can debulk 99% of the tumour mass, whereas RT reduces the tumour by approximately 25%. In general, salvage surgery post-RT is better than salvage RT post-surgery. The best treatment for incomplete margins is re-excision.

Node spread (from primary to node) is embolic and therefore *en bloc* excisions are not absolutely necessary. Node-to-node spread may be partly due to permeation.

Radiotherapy (RT)

The advantages of RT are less deformity than surgery and the ability to eliminate microscopic tumour. It is well established that the use of RT increases survival rate in cases of head and neck cancer. However, it cannot (usually) be used twice and may delay surgery if used inappropriately. A fairly hectic schedule must be adhered to, usually 55-70 G over 6–8 weeks (1 Gray is 1 Joule of energy per kg of tissue and equals 100 rads). Side effects include

- Early: DNA damage and cell death in dividing cells that is related to overall treatment time, such as mucositis and xerostomia
- Late: Microvascular damage that is related to fraction dose-dependant, causing decreased vascularity, fibrosis and telangiectasia

Trials have shown much better locoregional control with postoperative RT. It is common to commence adjuvant RT 3–6 weeks after surgery. Although it has been administered as early as 1 week with no adverse effects on healing, this may be impractical. In trials of pre and postoperative RT in patients with hypopharyngeal carcinoma, the high rate of postoperative mortality in patients who had had preoperative RT caused the trial to be stopped early. Performing surgery 5–17 weeks after RT may be optimal, possibly during the window between the early and late effects. Fractionation aims to increase the total dose of radiation (thus higher rate of tumour kill) whilst reducing late damage to normal tissues. Compared to conventional RT, fractionation results in better locoregional control and function, but at the expense of lower acute tolerance (though no difference in late side effects).

- Hyperfractionation: The dose per fraction is reduced but the fraction number and total dose increased
- Acceleration: The overall treatment time is reduced but with similar total dose and dose per fraction
- Split course

There are some reported strategies to reduce acute and chronic side effects of adjuvant therapy, such as amifostine (cytoprotective adjuvant) and growth factors such as granulocyte colony-stimulating factor G-CSF (early studies showed that it reduced post RT oral mucositis).

Chemotherapy

Chemotherapy can be given neoadjuvantly, adjuvantly or simultaneously with RT. It may also play a role in palliation. On average, there is a 20% response rate from single agents (methotrexate, cisplatin, 5-FU). The combination of cisplatin and 5-FU produces an 80% response rate when used as first line and a 45% response rate for recurrences. However, there is little effect on overall survival. Side effects also increase with combination therapy. There have been many trials on chemotherapy but optimal schedules remain unclear.

Chemotherapy impairs wound healing. It should be avoided within one week of surgery. Conversely, surgery should be postponed until the white blood cell count has returned to normal.

Neoadjuvant vs adjuvant

Adjuvant chemotherapy means that definitive surgery/RT is performed first, but it may affect chemotherapy delivery through altered blood flow. Neoadjuvant chemotherapy refers to chemotherapy given prior to definitive surgery/RT. The theoretical advantages of neoadjuvant chemotherapy are

- It reduces the risk of developing drug resistance
- It gives a better response (fraction of drug-resistant cells increased with tumour size)

- It reduces the size of tumour/nodal disease and enhances local control

Improved response rates are reported but with no significant overall reduction in recurrence. Although trials have shown that it is feasible to give aggressive treatment to ill patients (meta-analyses show 6.5% toxicity), there is no real survival benefit in advanced cases when compared to the traditional combination of surgery and RT. Trials have also demonstrated more local recurrences but fewer metastases. This delay in appearance of metastases is responsible for the early survival advantage, but this disappears by the fifth year. While neoadjuvant treatment may not increase cure rates, it may show benefit in organ preservation, such as allowing Stage III and IV laryngeal cancer patients to keep their voice for longer until salvage surgery is needed.

Common criticisms of the use of neoadjuvant chemotherapy include the delay of definitive treatment (surgery or RT) and the potential increase in adverse effects of subsequent RT/surgery. Studies to date have not shown this to any significant extent.

Chemo-irradiation

Chemo-irradiation: The (theoretical) rationale for simultaneous administration of chemotherapy and RT is synergy and a decrease overall treatment time. This comes at the cost of increased local toxicity, including an increase in plate complications in bone reconstructions. Current indications for primary chemo-irradiation are nasopharyngeal carcinoma (NPC), organ preservation in laryngeal carcinoma and recurrence after surgery. Alternating courses of RT and chemotherapy may theoretically reduce resistance and side effects but prolongs the total treatment time.

Chemoprevention

Chemoprevention is not yet a reality.

- Treat premalignant conditions such as leukoplakia (5% risk of malignant change). The data on the role of carotene is contradictory whilst studies with bleomycin and vitamin A are inconclusive
- Prevent second primary (5% risk per year): Evidence of reduced risk of a

second primary (4% vs. 24% in placebo) or recurrence using retinoids (13-cRA) was seen in early studies (Hong 1993) but have been difficult to confirm in larger studies. There is a discontinuation rate of up to 33% due to the side effects

- High-risk population: There is no evidence of benefit from prophylactic vitamins, retinoids or carotene. Beta-carotene (that was taken during cancer prevention trials undertaken based on early 1980s epidemiology) may increase risk of lung cancer in smokers and those with asbestos exposure. A Cochrane review (2007) demonstrated a 1–8% rate of increased mortality, although the methodology of these studies have been disputed

Further reading

Masuda M, Wakasaki T, Toh S, et al. Chemoprevention of head and neck cancer by green tea extract: EGCG-the role of EGFR signaling and lipid raft'. J Oncol 2011/540148.

Related topic of interest

- Oral cancer

Healing

The main phases of healing (with some overlap) are in simple terms:

- Haemostasis: Bleeding is halted through a combination of fibrin filling the void, the platelet plug and vasoconstriction
- Inflammation:
  - Early: Complement activation and neutrophils arrive by diapedesis (numbers peak at 24 hours). Neutrophil functions include phagocytosis and release of cytokine and proteases that remove dead tissue. They are not essential for wound healing
  - Late: Macrophages derived from blood monocytes arrive later (day 2–4) and are the most important cells in the healing process. They aid debridement by phagocytosis and production of collagenases, but are also important regulatory cells for the transition to the proliferative phase, and also secrete growth factors (promoting angiogenesis, fibroplasia, and stimulation of keratinocytes). Lymphocytes arrive last, in limited numbers, but their exact role in healing is unclear
- Proliferation: See below. The normally quiescent fibroblasts are activated
- Remodelling: This is longest phase and can last for a year or more. Strength is increased as the collagen remodels. Matrix metalloproteinases (MMPs) are required for collagen degradation

Inflammation with haemostasis (day 0–4)

Haemostasis

- Vasoconstriction
- Collagen activates clotting cascade and fibrin deposition leads to formation of a platelet plug. Fibrin is an essential component of healing
- Platelets release thromboxane A2, PDGFα (vasoconstriction) and TGF-β from alpha granules, which attract inflammatory cells.
- After haemostasis, there is vasodilation with increased vascular permeability

Proliferation (day 4 to 3–4 weeks)

- Epithelium: If the basement membrane is intact, then the basal layer restores continuity within 2–3 days. However, if the basement membrane is destroyed then cells at the edge of wound migrate and proliferate under the control of TGF-α and epidermal growth factor (EGF) from macrophages and platelets, and keratinocyte growth factors from fibroblasts. The dissolution of anchoring junctions and reorganisation of cytoskeleton increases keratinocyte mobility. The epithelium begins to stratify once a 1–2 cell layer is re-established and contact inhibition occurs. The rate of epithelialisation is increased by a moist environment and slowed by presence of a dry eschar
- Blood vessels/angiogenesis: TNF-α from migration of capillaries into wound bed
- Connective tissue (granulation tissue) formation and collagen deposition requires nutrients from well vascularised tissue. Fibroblasts migrate (under influence of PDGF, EGF, TGF-β from platelets and macrophages), become activated and then proliferate. Peak fibroblast numbers occur at day 7 and the total collagen content increases for a month afterwards

Remodelling (3 weeks onwards)

This is the most important phase clinically, as wound connective tissue, especially collagen, is not initially deposited in an organised way. As the wound matures and gains strength, the collagen is remodelled but is never as organised as unwounded tissue. Strength is never restored to 100% of normal, but plateaus at 80% at 8 months. Wounds have little strength in the first 2–3 weeks, and are almost weakest at the time of suture removal.

Collagen is a trimeric (2+1) protein chain that is can form fibres, fibrils, and bundles with many subtypes. Vitamin C is important for hydroxylation of proline in collagen. This is necessary for cross-linking the triple helix, which is in turn required for its stability. Hydroxylated proline in collagen is also necessary for its export from the cell.

- Early wound collagen is thinner and lies parallel to the skin. Later on, the collagen becomes thicker and lies along stress lines and so increases wound tensile strength.
- Initially, type III collagen production is high in the wound. Type I collagen then gradually replaces type III, until a pre-injury ratio of 4:1 is achieved
- Myofibroblasts cause wound contraction and reduce the wound size (not the same as a contracture which is excessive scar contraction across a mobile surface)

Factors affecting wound healing

Local factors

- Infection: $> 10^5$ organisms per gram of tissue (or lower concentrations of β-haemolytic *streptococcus*) will prolong the inflammatory phase. Taking swabs of open wounds is generally pointless. Colonisation does not equate to infection and would not normally inhibit wound healing
- Ischaemia: Energy in the form of glucose and oxygen is required for proliferation as well as activity of fibroblasts and neutrophils
- Foreign bodies (or necrotic tissue) prolong inflammatory phase, are obstacles to healing, and nidi for bacteria
- Oedema compromises tissue perfusion and leads to capillary closure
- Hydration increases rate of epithelialisation, hence the rationale for the use of occlusive dressings

Systemic factors

Diabetes

Recent evidence suggests that the effects are not simply due to microvascular disease.

- Increased glucose levels impair cellular function, whilst sorbitol by-products are toxic. Reduced insulin levels may also have a role
- Increased dermal vascular permeability leads to accumulation of pericapillary albumin (a barrier)
- Non-enzymatic glycosylation inhibits protein function and makes them less soluble/degradable. Glycosylated haemoglobin has greater oxygen affinity, which reduces oxygen delivery to tissues
- Impaired neural function: Peripheral neuropathy affects protective reflexes

Nevertheless, if the wound is well vascularised and the glucose levels well controlled, then surgical wounds should still heal adequately. The diabetic foot is a challenge and off-loading is very important (air cast and immobilisation). Some countries prohibit the use of topical antibiotics in diabetics (due to problems with resistance) though antiseptics can still be used. Systemic antibiotics should only be given for clinical infections. Haemolytic streptococcal and synergistic infections should be treated aggressively.

Hypothyroidism

There is some evidence that hypothyroidism decreases fibroblast function and wound strength (based primarily on animal studies).

Age

The elderly tend to have more comorbid factors affecting healing but there is also some age-specific reduction in wound healing. Although this tends to be more quantitative than qualitative, certain aspects of wound healing may be delayed or prolonged.

- Foetal healing is a phenomenon that occurs up to the third trimester. There is quicker healing with less acute inflammation, less angiogenesis and faster epithelialisation. It is scarless with respect to skin and bone, but muscle, tendon and gut wounds still tend to have scars. With fetal healing, there is more regeneration than repair. It is not true regeneration per se, but rather a well-organised matrix with type III collagen, rich in HA and glycosaminoglycan (GAG). The exact mechanism is not fully understood but it may be related to the warm sterile environment, growth factors, and thus minimal inflammation. The extracellular matrix (ECM) is also different as it is rich in HA, unlike in the adult

Perfusion

- Local causes: Pressure (> 32 mmHg), arterial insufficiency, venous insufficiency, protein extravasation (forms a barrier) and oedema that increase diffusion distances
- Generalised: Major trauma, including burns and sepsis that provokes a major systemic inflammatory response with circulating cytokines and mediators including TNF-α. The aim of treatment is to maintain the normovolaemic state but peripheral vasoconstriction can persist for up to 60 hours, even after normalisation of blood pressure
- Prolonged generalised hypoperfusion may lead to organ failure: gut (bacterial translocation), liver (low protein), renal (uraemia and metabolic acidosis) and lungs (hypoxaemia). Reperfusion may cause further damage

Nutrition

There is no simple and singly reliable method of assessing nutritional status. Criteria used for this includes

- Clinical: Recent weight loss, signs of loss such as muscle wasting, loss of fat and oedema
- BMI: <18.5 implies nutritional impairment, while a BMI < 15 is associated with significant mortality
- Skin fold thickness
- Biochemical markers: Transferrin, retinol binding protein and most commonly, prealbumin. Prealbumin (170–450 is the normal range) has a half-life of 2–3 days and is thus a better measure of protein nutrition than albumin (half-life of 20 days, and may be reduced by sepsis/inflammation itself). Some studies show that closure of surgical wounds is more successful if the albumin is > 30
- Nutrition Risk Index = (1.519 × albumin g/L) + 0.417 × (present weight/usual weight × 100). A score of < 100 indicates malnutrition
- Lymphocyte function and body nitrogen are useful in research only

Glucose is the main fuel for wound repair. Protein malnutrition, especially arising from deficiencies of arginine and methionine, will compromise wound healing. The septic or post-traumatic patient is hypermetabolic, and stores of body fat and muscle are quickly lost in order to maintain blood glucose levels.

- Glutamine enhances cellular lymphocytes, macrophages and neutrophils
- Micronutrients may be important but warrant replacement only in deficiency
  - Zinc: Re-epithelialisation and collagen synthesis
  - Vitamin C for collagen
  - Copper, selenium, manganese, magnesium, calcium and iron are collagen cofactors in collagen synthesis

Nutrition can be supported by various means. NICE recommends support for patients with reduced intake for more than 5 days, or those with poor absorption, high losses or increased requirements.

- Oral supplements: Over and above normal hospital diet, is simple and relatively effective
- Enteral feeding (nasogastric/jejunal/PEG tubes) for those with inadequate oral intake or other problems, such as swallowing disorders. It is cheaper and safer than parenteral feeding and numerous studies have shown benefit
- Parenteral feeding (peripheral or central) is reserved for those with a non-functioning gut. Some trials show that preoperative TPN reduces complications but not mortality in malnourished patient. There is less support for the use of postoperative TPN and may actually be harmful (see Burns)

The best evidence of benefit for immuno-nutrition is with glutamine (better given enterally than parenterally). Arginine and omega-3 fatty acids may have mixed effects.

Smoking

Smoking is detrimental to the surgical patient and there are higher graft failure rates, decreased healing and increased infection rates with it. It is particularly risky in operations that leave tissue of vulnerable viability such as replants or where extensive undermining is performed, such as facelifts. The mechanism(s) are multifactorial. Nicotine is a vasoconstrictor and inhibits cellular proliferation, cyanide inhibits oxidative enzymes and carbon monoxide decreases oxygen carrying capacity. There is also increased platelet aggregation, blood viscosity and decreased collagen deposition.

- 10 min of smoking reduces subcutaneous PO_2 for 1 hour
- 1 cigarette causes vasoconstriction for up to 90 minutes
- 1 cigarette reduces the blood flow to the arm by 42% for 1 hour (Chang 2004)

Patients should stop smoking at least 2 weeks before surgery (for vascular effects), but a 4 months abstinence is required for its wound healing effects to abate. Urinary nicotine levels can be used to monitor compliance. Some studies have shown that perioperative oxygenation can improve healing.

Steroids

Steroid administration causes a global inhibition of cell growth and cellular response to injury.

- Decreased collagen production by fibroblasts
- Reduced phagocytosis by macrophages and neutrophils
- Decreased epithelial regeneration and proliferation

Vitamin A reverses most steroid effects on inflammation, with the notable exceptions of infections and wound contraction. Vitamin A is one of the exceptions to the rule that supplementation is not required when no deficiency exists.

- In contrast, vitamin E has not been shown to have any beneficial effects on wound healing and large doses may actually inhibit healing (decreased collagen accumulation and wound tensile strength)
- Chronic deficiency of vitamin C reduces wound tensile strength, but taking large doses does not improve healing

Radiation and chemotherapy

Radiotherapy damages the genome directly or via the generation of free radicals.

- In the acute phase there is inflammation, and the skin becomes erythematous and oedematous
- This is followed by thrombosis and fibrinoid necrosis of capillaries that decreases oxygen delivery, while deposition of densely hyalinised collagen contributes further to the state of relative ischaemia
- There is impairment of the fibroblast response in wound healing (which may be permanent) and granulation tissue formation

Chemotherapy suppresses the bone marrow and decreases inflammation as well as the fibroblast collagen response. The effects are transient but are worse if combined with RT. If possible, chemotherapy is delayed until at least 10–14 days after surgery.

Syndromes associated with altered healing

- Ehlers Danlos: Defects in collagen metabolism (lysyl oxidase) commonly affecting type III collagen, but may affect type I and V. Patients have joint hyper-extensibility, tissue fragility and poor healing with wide atrophic scars. Non-essential surgery is relatively contraindicated
- Cutis laxa: Defect in elastin, causing the skin to be thin, stretchable and bruise easily. Necessary surgery can be performed
- Homocystinuria: Autosomal recessive deficiency of cystathionine synthase that is required for methionine metabolism. Consequently, homocysteine accumulates which then initiates the clotting cascade, causes arterial sclerosis, thrombosis, poor perfusion and platelet malfunction. Patients have a high risk of developing cardiovascular disease
- Osteogenesis imperfecta: Defective collagen type I gene. Scars are typically wide

Adjuncts to healing

- HBOT effects are controversial
- NPWT removes interstitial fluid and oedema to improve oxygenation, removes deleterious inflammatory mediators, reduces bacterial counts and speeds up formation of granulation tissue
- Growth factors: Some are commercially available, such as PDGF, GM-CSF and KGF2
- Bioengineered skin: Apligraf when placed in chronic wounds leads to outgrowth of previously dormant keratinocytes at wound edges
- Electrostimulation with DC or pulsed current at low frequency or high voltage, pulsed EM field
- Hydrotherapy: Debridement, warmth and physical therapy
- Lasers: Low energy laser treatment at wavelengths of 680–890 nm as a biostimulant may increase the cellular activity of fibroblasts and keratinocytes. It may have a role in lymphoedema treatment
- Ultrasound (20 kHz) has been used in venous ulcers and pressure sores but with inconsistent results

Further reading

Guo S, Dipietro LA. Factors affecting wound healing. J Dent Res 2010; 89:219–29.

Related topics of interest

- Cleft palate
- Facial lacerations
- Flexor tendon injuries
- Hyperbaric oxygen
- Lymphoedema
- Vacuum wound closure

Hidradenitis suppurativa and hyperhidrosis

Both terms are derived from the Greek word for sweat, '*hidros*'.

Hidradenitis suppurativa (HS)

HS has been estimated to affect up to 1 in 50–300 of the general population. The aetiology is unclear but the primary event is follicular occlusion of apocrine gland ducts due to the formation of a hyperkeratotic plug. This leads to perifollicular inflammation and formation of nodules, which may then rupture to form sinuses. These may become infected or resolve spontaneously without surgical drainage. As nodules heal spontaneously in most cases, drainage of non-fluctuant, non-abscess nodules is not mandatory. It is a chronic relapsing condition that leads ultimately to scarring.

- HS is likely with the occurrence of > 4 nodules in the axillae or groins. It may also affect the areolae, inframammary fold, perineum, buttock folds, nape of neck, and periumbilical regions. It is more common in women (three times) where the axilla is most commonly affected, whereas the groin is most commonly affected in men. It is rare before puberty and a premenstrual flare is common, but the exact role of hormones in HS is unclear. Obesity may have an effect by altering sex hormone metabolism, but its physical effects are also contributory. Poor hygiene is not a cause, but may exacerbate the disease. Smoking is a strongly associated factor
- There is an association between HS and polycystic ovarian syndrome (PCOS) and insulin resistance. Arthropathy, chronic inflammatory bowel disease and thyroid disease are associated to a lesser extent
- It may be inherited in an autosomally dominant fashion with variable penetrance in some cases

The most common organism found in the lesion is *Staphylococcus epidermidis,* and can involve a range of bacteria.

Hidradenocarcinoma or SCC is a rare complication, with and estimated risk of 3% over 10 years. Suspicious chronic wounds should be biopsied to exclude other diseases.

Management

Conservative measures include:

- Simple wound dressings, warm compresses
- Weight loss and wearing loose clothing

Drugs

- Antiandrogens, such as cyproterone and Dianette
- Antibiotics (including a mix of topical and systemic) are commonly used though antibiotics are not proven to be of benefit in simple HS without superinfection. There is some evidence for long-term oral antibiotics for extensive disease. Dapsone is sometimes used but its mechanism of action is not well understood. It has sulphonamide-like activity and some anti-inflammatory activity
- Steroids
- Retinoids work well for acne but are less effective on HS as they act by altering gland activity, reducing sebaceous activity, which is not a major problem in HS

Incision and drainage of abscesses and de-roofing of sinuses may be necessary before definitive surgery. For quiescent disease,

- Curettage
- Excisional surgery: Once there is established deep scarring and formation of sinus tracts, resection is the only option. Resection can be limited (hair bearing skin) or wide (with 2 cm margin). The latter has a lower recurrence rate at the expense of a larger wound, but otherwise no significant advantage over limited excision. Wounds tend to have high infection and dehiscence rates compared to non-HS wounds. Complete cure cannot be guaranteed as isolated glands may fall beyond the typical areas. The choice of reconstructive method may affect the

quality of reconstruction, but does not seem to affect the risk of recurrence
- Alternatives to surgery include ablative CO_2 laser with secondary healing over 1-2 months, cryotherapy, RT (rarely used) and IPL

Hyperhidrosis

Hyperhidrosis can be defined as excessive sweating beyond the amount required to cool the body. The complaints are mostly subjective although there may be objective signs such as skin maceration in a minority. It affects up to 0.5-1% of the population with a peak in the third and fourth decades and can cause significant embarrassment.

- Most are idiopathic (sympathetic overactivity of unknown cause) and limited to certain sites: 60% palms/soles, 30% axillae and face. There are no detectable histological differences between the glands of sufferers and normal patients. A positive family history detected in a third of cases
- A specific localised form may result from disruption of nerves with abnormal regeneration, e.g. Frey's syndrome or gustatory sweating after parotid surgery. Cases that do not respond to conservative measures or botulinum toxin may require interpositional surgery
- The generalised form of the condition is rare, tends to present later in life and may be linked to disease processes such as
  - Endocrine: Diabetes mellitus, hyperthyroidism, phaeochromocytoma and hypoglycaemia
  - Drugs: Propranolol, pilocarpine and tricyclic antidepressants
  - Neurological: Syringomyelia, stroke
  - Others: Hodgkin's lymphoma, tuberculosis and chronic alcoholism
- Bromidrosis is the offensive odour caused by the breakdown of apocrine secretions into ammonia and short chain fatty acids by the axillary florae, especially *Corynebacterium* (there is a less common eccrine form, see **Table 26**). Conservative measures include general hygiene, topical deodorants and antibiotics such as clindamycin and erythromycin. Other measures include sweat reduction techniques (see below)

Local treatment

Antiperspirants are often used as first line treatments.

- Aluminium hexachlorhydrate in alcohol is the first choice in most cases. The maximum effect comes from regular application to dry skin. This is postulated to work by aluminium ion mediated damage to the terminal duct lining. It can be combined with steroids or emollients to reduce the irritation and skin drying effect
- Formalin and glutaraldehyde are not as effective, are unpleasant to use and there is a risk of sensitisation with the former
- Local anaesthetics are short acting and liable to show tolerance
- Iontophoresis works by blocking sweat ducts with ions or coagulated surface proteins. The hands (or feet) are soaked in tap water and a weak electric current applied. The addition of anticholinergics such as glycopyrronium into the solution

Table 26 Comparison of apocrine and eccrine sweat glands	
Apocrine	**Eccrine**
These are associated with hair follicles and concentrated particularly in the axillary and perianal areas making up to 10-40% of the sweat glands in these areas. They are inactive until puberty when they begin to secrete pheromones. • No thermoregulatory role • Stimulated by androgens and inhibited by oestrogens • Adrenergic innervation Strictly speaking, the secretion is merocrine (exocytosis) not apocrine (sloughing of top of cell). The sweat they produce also has fatty acids. The odour comes from bacterial breakdown of the organic compounds.	These are found all over the body with increased density in glabrous skin. They lie in the deep dermis and produce a dilute solution of urea, lactic acid and sodium chloride of varying concentration. • Role in thermoregulation • Sweating on the palms and soles is controlled by the cerebral cortex. It responds to emotional stress rather than temperature regulation and therefore will not produce sweat during sleep or under sedation. • Cholinergic sympathetic innervation that is blocked by botulinum toxin.

may increase efficacy. The beneficial effects begin immediately and only last for 3–4 days. It is thus time-consuming and rather inconvenient to use. However it is safe and can be reversed by using adhesive tape to strip away the plugs. It is often a first line treatment and can be combined with other modalities

Systemic

- Anticholinergics are effective but side effects limit their use (dry mouth, blurred vision, difficulty with micturition and constipation). Commonly used medications included Robinul (glycopyrrolate), oxybutinin, clonidine, propantheline and benztropine.
  - Glycopyrrolate solution (0.5–2%): Can also be used topically
  - Topical 3% scopolamine
- Tranquilizers may be used if anxiety is a component or a precipitating factor but side effects may be severe. Beta-blockers have also been used with varying success

Surgery

- Incision and curettage may be useful for the axilla but may cause scarring and sensory changes. Its effectiveness may be due in part, to denervation. It is unsuitable for the palm or sole
  - Subcutaneous liposuction may achieve the same effect with less scarring
  - Excision and grafting: Undermining of the adjacent skin may enhance the denervation effect
  - Thoracic sympathectomy (T1 facial, T2–3 palmar and T4 for axillary sweating) by the transthoracic endoscopic route (requiring lung deflation/pneumothorax with CO_2 insufflation) is the treatment of choice for severe cases but requires GA and the potential complications may be severe
  - Residual pneumothorax, Horner's syndrome, bradycardia and recurrence
  - Compensatory increase in sweating in other areas, especially chest, abdomen and buttocks may occur in around half of the patients and can be severe in 10%. This is the most common cause of dissatisfaction and requests for reversal, which may only be possible if clamp/clips have been used
  - Dryness (anhidrosis) particularly of the face and hands

Botulinum toxin has been a major development in the treatment of unwanted sweating. The effect on sweat glands may be longer lasting than on muscle, possibly reflecting the differences between autonomic and motor nerves. The use of botulinum toxin for hyperhidrosis came from observations of the side effects of hemifacial spasm treatment. Several reports published in 1997 demonstrated beneficial effects lasting 9–14 weeks, with a light decrease in hand grip force in one study. There were no effects on unpleasant odours (adrenergic apocrine glands not affected).

The area to be treated is mapped out, such as with Minor's starch iodine method. Patients should shave underarms and abstain from use of over-the-counter antiperspirants for 24 hours prior to the test and avoid precipitating activities such as exertion within 30 minutes of the test.

- Dry the area and paint with iodine solution (Betadine works). When dry, lightly sprinkle with starch powder (flour) and the hyperhidrotic area will develop a deep blue-black colour over a few minutes
- Each injection site has a ring of effect due to diffusion of up to approximately 1 cm radius (depends on dilution/volume). Ink can be used to mark sites but do not inject through ink to avoid tattooing. White makeup pencil can be used, with each mark rubbed off upon injection
- Inject evenly at a 2 mm depth at a 45° angle. Bevel upwards to ensure intradermal placement (a fluid bleb under skin is seen). Avoid patching gaps before 3 months

The main problems are:

- Injection pain that is not significantly reduced by EMLA. Usually requires injected LA. Nerve blocks are usually not needed for axillary injections but are recommended for the palm. Dermojets (needleless injection system) have been used to reduce pain but usually with lesser effect
- Muscle weakness is uncommon but may

be reduced by injecting intracutaneously rather subcutaneously at the cost of more pain and less efficacy (glands lie deeper)

Further reading

Highton L, Chan WY, Khwaja N, et al. Treatment of hidradenitis suppurativa with intense pulsed light: a prospective study. Plast Reconstr Surg 2011; 128:459–65.

Related topics of interest

- Botulinum toxin
- Parotid gland tumours

Hyperbaric oxygen therapy

During hyperbaric oxygen therapy (HBOT), a patient breathes in 100% oxygen in a chamber (**Table 27**) pressurised to greater than atmospheric pressure. It was once touted as a general panacea to many diseases. At present, there is only evidence to support its use for selected indications, but its precise role is still not well defined.

- Problematic wounds: Osteoradionecrosis, osteomyelitis and NF
- Carbon monoxide poisoning
- Air embolism/decompression sickness
- Failing flaps or grafts

At normal atmospheric pressure, most of the oxygen in the blood is bound to haemoglobin which is 97% saturated, with only a small percentage in solution (3 ml/L at 1 ATM). This increases to 60 ml/L when breathing 100% oxygen at 3 ATM, which is enough to support resting cellular metabolism. The increasing oxygen tension increases the oxygen gradient and improves oxygen supply.

- Local hypoxia may explain why many chronic wounds fail to heal. Subcutaneous oxygen tension levels are usually 10–30 mmHg, but they require 50–100 mmHg for essential processes such as healing, killing of microorganisms and angiogenesis. Dividing cells require 30–50 mmHg. HBOT provides 800–1100 mmHg
- In normal tissues, there is a rapid vasoconstriction that compensated for by the increased oxygen supply. However, the microvascular blood-flow in ischaemic tissues is improved, which also reduces tissue oedema
- The oxygen tension plateaus at about 90% of normal tissues after about 20 sessions and drops further to 90% of peak after a few years

The increased oxygen gradient may
- Promote the formation of an oxygen-dependent collagen matrix for angiogenesis
- Reduce oxygen free radicals which would otherwise oxidise proteases and membrane lipids
- Possibly inhibit bacterial metabolism of anaerobes in particular. It may also enhance the oxygen-dependent peroxidase antibacterial mechanism in white cells and reduce pseudomonas and clostridial α-toxin
- Induce PDGF receptors and VEGF release

The major use of HBOT is to improve wound healing, although the proposed mechanisms have not been fully elucidated. There is evidence that HBOT is beneficial for treatment of the osteoradionecrotic mandible when compared to treatment with penicillin (Marx 1985).

- There have been four RCTs investigating the use of HBOT in diabetic ulcers that demonstrate a reduction in the number of major amputations, although the patient numbers were small. Medicare (US) will reimburse costs of HBOT for diabetic ulcers not responding to 30 days of standard treatment. Kranke's 2004 Cochrane review showed that the number needed to treat to avoid an amputation was 4
- Venous ulcers: A RCT demonstrated benefit after 6 weeks but Kranke concluded that there was too little data to make recommendations. Kloth (2002) rated it class C evidence (vs. B for diabetic ulcers)

Table 27 Types of hyperbaric chambers	
Chamber type	Notes
Monoplace chamber	Cheaper and portable, as it can be moved, although with difficulty. Patient lies on a narrow bed. It uses 100% oxygen at approximately 2.5 ATM hence face masks are not needed. 'Air breaks' are given every 30 min to reduce CNS toxicity (seizures).
Multichamber	It can accommodate 12 or more people with an airlock system that allows staff to enter and leave. Pressures can go up to 6 ATM. Uses compressed air and patients breathe oxygen via masks.

- There are no RCTs examining the use of HBOT in arterial insufficiency or pressure sores
- The benefit in burns is equivocal

Complications

Hyperbaric oxygen therapy is relatively safe as long as the pressures remain below 3 ATM and treatment times are less than 120 min per sitting. Untreated tension pneumothorax is one of the few absolute contraindications. Relative contraindications include patients with impaired pressure equalisation and those with cardiac disease. The most common problem is mild ear popping or discomfort that lasts up to 2 hours, although fatigue and headaches may also occur.

- Myopia due to reversible lens deformation is common and may last for weeks to months
- Barotrauma to the middle ear/tympanic membrane or lung especially with repeated treatment is found in up to 15–20% of cases. These can be minimised by thorough pre-treatment assessment
- Oxygen toxicity (fits, respiratory failure) is rare with sessions < 2 hours and usually do not cause permanent damage. Diabetic patients may be more prone to developing this due to increased levels of glutathione peroxidase
- Fire hazard: Restricts the use of some equipment
- Claustrophobia

Overall, the greatest hurdle to the wider use of HBOT is the lack of availability of chambers and the relatively high outlay required for hardware, maintenance and manpower. However, there are overall savings to be made from reduced hospital stay and community care, as a large portion of the health budget is consumed by chronic wound care.

Further reading

Feldmeier JJ. Hyperbaric oxygen for radiation injury: is it indicated? Curr Oncol 2011; 18:211–12.

Related topics of interest

- Necrotising fasciitis
- Osteoradionecrosis

Hypoplastic facial conditions

There is a range of conditions associated with facial hypoplasia and reconstruction is typically complex, involving many operations.

Treacher–Collins syndrome

Treacher–Collins syndrome (TCS or mandibulofacial dysostosis) is associated with bilateral first and second arch abnormalities. The TCOF1 gene on chromosome 5 is implicated and inheritance of the condition is autosomal dominant with variable penetrance. Clinical expression is highly variable with minimal forms possible but the severity may increase with subsequent generations. It occurs in approximately 1 in 10,000 births and nearly half are due to a new mutation. Isotretinoin use and advanced paternal age has been implicated but consistent predisposing causes have not been found. Prenatal diagnosis by chorionic villus sampling or amniocentesis is available.

- Treacher was a British ophthalmologist who described children with notched lower eyelids and hypoplastic zygomas, although Berry's description 11 years earlier in 1889 was more detailed. An alternative name of Franschetti's syndrome is often applied to the complete form

Affected children have the distinctive features with a convex shaped facial profile due to the hypoplastic maxilla. The typical appearance resembles a sad fish. It has also been described as a confluent Tessier 6,7,8 cleft. The IQ is normal and any developmental delay present may be related in part to hearing loss. Nager and Miller syndromes show similarities to TCS with additional limb anomalies.

- The hypoplastic midface is the central feature. The maxilla is projected and narrow. An OMV facial radiograph demonstrates the dysplastic zygoma and absent arches, which lead to deficiency of the inferolateral orbital rim. Mandibular

(and TMJ) hypoplasia in combination with choanal atresia and a narrowed retropharyngeal space can cause severe airway compromise at birth. There is a facial convexity, an Angle Class II bite and a long retrusive chin

- Sleep apnoea is a common problem. The airway problem may be managed simply by nursing prone, but some may require a tracheostomy or formal mandibular surgery with or without distraction osteogenesis
- There may be macrostomia, with blind fistulae between mouth and ears
- Eye and ear abnormalities:
  - Coloboma, loss of medial lower lashes, antimongoloid slant due to the dystopic lateral canthus, strabismus and hypertelorism. There is a lack of lower lateral orbital support due to the abnormal zygoma
  - Microtia, cryptotia, narrow ear canals, middle ear abnormalities. The majority (95%) have hearing loss that is usually conductive
- Prominent nasal dorsum and long sideburns. There is an association with cleft lip/palate. In its absence, a high arched palate may otherwise be present. Some have abnormally shaped heads without true craniosynostosis

Treatment is individualised (under a multidisciplinary team) but a typical sequence of elective surgery is

- Cleft palate surgery at 6 months
- Lower eyelid and zygoma surgery at 3–5 years
  - The coloboma can often be treated with a laterally based hemi-Tripier upper lid flap and lateral canthopexy, but aesthetic results are usually disappointing
  - The zygoma and orbital floor is usually grafted, preferably with split calvarial bone. Calvarial bone should be harvested from the non-dominant hemisphere to theoretically minimise functional consequences if inadvertent

brain damage is inflicted during harvest. Temporal flaps may be used to augment or cover the bone, but the amount of muscle available is small and the donor depression is often noticeable. Use of vascularised bone has not been promising and with local flaps in particular, it is difficult to maintain the blood supply whilst optimising fit. Similarly, alloplastic reconstruction is also usually disappointing. Continued differential growth of the midface and zygoma may cause a dynamic relapse of the deformities that necessitate further surgery. For this reason, Posnick advises against reconstruction before the age of 5

- The broad nose bridge is usually treated with open rhinoplasty and osteotomies
- Mandibular retrognathia and malocclusion is treated at age 4–5. Augmentation is achieved by vertical sagittal osteotomy and bone grafting or distraction. Other procedures include Le Fort I osteotomies and genioplasty. Some surgeons delay this surgery until late adolescence
  - Classification as per the Mulliken modification of Pruzansky (hemifacial microsomia), and treated similarly
- Microtia: Ear reconstruction from 7–8 years onwards, depending on the technique chosen. BAHA (or Vibrant Soundbridge) should be fitted early. There is no value in middle ear reconstruction

Hemifacial microsomia

There are a number of alternative terms for this relatively common craniofacial condition that occurs at a rate of 1 in 3500 (the second most common after cleft lip/palate). These include craniofacial microsomia, otomandibular dysostosis and first or second branchial arch syndrome. The condition may be related to stapedial artery thrombosis/haematoma (which has been reproduced in monkeys with thalidomide), which may account both for the variable

extent, as well as the involvement of structures not derived from the first or second arch.

Most cases are sporadic with a variable degree of clinical expression. The overall risk of passing on the condition is 3%. It resembles TCS and although bilateral in 10%, it can be distinguished from it as it is usually asymmetrical. The term hemifacial microsomia (HFM) and Goldenhar syndrome are used interchangeably, although it is more accurate to think of HFM (the condition) as a feature of Goldenhar (the syndrome). Less than 5% of patients with HFM will have the other characteristic features of Goldenhar's syndrome (oculoauriculovertebral syndrome), with benign growths around the eye (epibulbar dermoids), coloboma, accessory ear appendages, and vertebral anomalies (e.g. fused or hemivertebrae) particularly in the neck, and rib anomalies. The classical facial features of HFM can be summarised by the acronym OMENS (see **Table 28**) which was used primary as a scoring/record-keeping system. HFM can be classified by

- Pruzansky classification of the mandible abnormality (see below)
- Munro: A clinical system designed to help surgical planning

Mandible

Jaw translation is minimal/tends to translate to affected side on opening and the occlusal plane is canted (higher on affected side). The mandible deformity (affecting the ramus most) is the most obvious and the modified Pruzansky classifies its severity.

The modification subdivides type II deformities according to the TMJ anomalies.

I. Mild hypoplasia. Absent glenoid fossa, small condyle and hypoplastic muscles of mastication. Overall morphology is maintained

II. A: Condyle small and cone shaped. TMJ functional
B: No condyle. Masseter and medial pterygoids are rudimentary. TMJ non-functional

Table 28 Facial features of hemifacial microsomia*		
	Problem	Treatment
Orbit	Distorted small orbit with micro/anophthalmia. Some have ophthalmoplegia and epibulbar dermoids.	Advancement.
Mandible	The mandible is variably affected but there is usually hypoplasia leading to tilted occlusion and chin deviation. TMJ deficiency is present.	Reconstruction with bone or costochondral grafts or distraction techniques.
Ear	Microtia, conductive hearing loss. The external ear deformity does not correlate with the hearing loss. Preauricular skin tags and parotid hypoplasia. The hypoplastic zygoma and arch shortens the distance between the eye and the ear.	Staged reconstruction, hearing aids.
Nerve	Facial nerve palsy (marginal mandibular branch in 25%). There may be CNS anomalies such as hypoplasia of corpus callosum or cerebrum.	May need two-stage operation with sural nerve grafting and muscle transfer. Nerve transfer works better when done early, (1 year old).
Soft tissue	Deficiency of fifth and seventh nerve muscles and oblique lip. Macrostomia due to a cleft lateral lip is uncommon.	Flaps for soft tissue augmentation. Cheek may need bone augmentation. Commissuroplasty. Macrostomia should be corrected in the first few months

* (this is **not** the OMENS classification by Vento, which as a scoring system is based on orbit size and position, mandible deformity, ear anomaly, facial nerve branch and soft tissue deficiency).

III. Absence (or subtotal absence) of ramus and TMJ. The muscles of mastication, including the temporalis are either rudimentary or absent

The HFM deformity generally regarded as being non-progressive (though this has been challenged again recently). The timing of surgery does not change the disease. Mandibular surgery is often required, while there is a variable need for surgery to the cranium, orbit and zygoma, which have traditionally been treated with osteotomy and bone grafting. Early surgery does not seem to reduce teasing, as the remaining deformities are significant. Hence, most surgeons prefer to wait for skeletal maturity before operating. OPG and CT scans are required for treatment planning.

- Le Fort I with resection of contralateral maxilla and bone grafting of ipsilateral, to straighten maxillary cant
- Sagittal split mandibular osteotomy with resection to straighten the cant, with genioplasty

- A costochondral graft may be harvested if a TMJ is needed. Some advocate early surgery between the ages of 4–9 but the cartilage graft grows independently from the other side, sometimes more rapidly, causing asymmetry. Another graft with a cartilage cap can be used to simultaneously reconstruct the zygomatic arch and a neo-glenoid fossa for the TMJ
- There will be a need for orthodontic treatment and further bone grafting as the child grows

Distraction osteogenesis offers an alternative for HFM treatment for up to Pruzansky IIAs. It is an extension of the Ilizarov technique that relies on the formation of bone in the gap between the gradually distracted bone ends of a corticotomy. Bone forms at the corticotomy by intramembranous ossification (without a callus). Distraction partly overcomes the soft tissue deficiency by increasing the soft tissue envelope, albeit not uniformly and in a limited extent (as little as 53% for the nasal tip). Distraction is also avoids donor sites and the need for bone grafts.

- Latency (interval from osteotomy to commencing distraction that allows inflammation to settle and osteoprogenitor cells to arrive) 5–7 days in the classic Ilizarov or 10 days in De Bastiani (callotasis). An excessively long wait leads to premature consolidation. Some question the need for a latent period
- Distraction: Generally performed at a rate of 1 mm/day. Some choose to divide this into smaller distractions but at more frequent intervals (1–4 times a day). Motorised distractors may allow continuous distraction. The rate may be adjusted according to the quality of the bone laid down, premature consolidation or nerve palsies (pain, hyperaesthesia then hypothesia). The efficacy can be followed radiologically and maturation is indicated by formation of a medulla within the generated bone
- Consolidation: This holds bones rigidly until bone mineralisation occur, usually at 8 weeks for children and 12 weeks for adults (or 1 month/cm gained). Excessively long consolidation periods may cause disuse atrophy and weakening
- Non-unions can usually be managed by eradication of infection, compression or bone transport for large defects after debridement

The process is time and labour intensive and meticulous planning is very important. It is the only technique capable of producing substantial lengthening of 7–15 cm while simultaneously addressing malalignments and contractures. The distractors can be external or internal. The latter are less common but have the advantages of avoiding external scars, possibly at the expense of reduced vector control and less elongation. Resorbable devices have also been described.

There is at least one complication per patient (up to 30%) on average, but most are minor or transient. Deep infections including septic arthritis, non/malunion or muscle contractures are more difficult to deal with. Pin tract problems are almost inevitable given the long treatment period and any movement of skin or bone relative to the pins increase the risk. Other complications include nerve injuries and joint stiffness/subluxation.

Hemifacial atrophy of Romberg

This is poorly understood, the exact incidence is unclear and the cause unknown. There is evidence of a genetic alteration in the early stages of embryogenesis of the central nervous system. Alternatively, an autoimmune aetiology that causes hyperactivity of brain stem sympathetic centres leading to the atrophy has also been suggested. It resembles a localised form of scleroderma and can be difficult to distinguish from this disease. This may account for the finding of antinuclear antibodies in some cases. There seems to be no strong evidence of genetic inheritance with most cases being sporadic.

The presentation can be very diverse. There is progressive unilateral wasting of the face and forehead that begins before the patient reaches their 20s (average 9 years old) and lasts for 9 years on average before burning out, leaving hypoplasia and atrophy. It affects either side with equal frequency and is only rarely bilateral (5%). The more serious cases tend to present earlier with significant atrophy, although more recent studies have challenged this. The disease primarily affects the subcutaneous tissue and fat (more than the skin or muscle) and appears to follow the distribution of sensory divisions of the trigeminal nerve. Those with skeletal involvement tend to have an earlier onset, but this is not correlated with overall severity.

- *En coup de sabre*: Sharp indentation across face and extending to hairline, with localised hair loss affecting the scalp, eyebrow and eyelash. This upper face involvement may progress to the entire hemi-face in prolonged active disease. Late onset disease tends to involve the lower face more often

- Skin may show atrophic changes, hyperpigmentation or vitiligo. Soft tissue changes are commonly found in upper half of face, whilst bony changes are more common in lower half and may be due to a combination of intrinsic disease in the bone and the restrictive, abnormal soft tissue envelope
- Neurology: Epilepsy, migraine and trigeminal neuralgia
- There may be ocular symptoms

No treatment has been shown to stop the progression of the disease. Surgery is usually postponed until the condition has burnt itself out and has been stable for at least 6 months (usually longer). There have been anecdotal reports of flaps atrophying if transposed while the disease is still active. As a general rule, bony abnormalities are corrected first with osteotomy and bone grafts before the soft tissue is filled in various ways including free flaps. It is advisable to overcorrect to account for subsequent atrophy. Debulking if required is delayed for at least 6 months. Recently, lipomodelling has been used to treat mild to moderate deformities, including during the active period. In addition to soft tissue, bone grafting or alloplastic implants may also be needed while the most severe cases may require osteotomy.

Fibrous dysplasia

This is an uncommon, non-neoplastic disease first described by von Recklinghausen in 1891 that is characterised by the arrest of bone maturation in the woven bone stage with irregular trabeculae. It usually presents as a painless mass causing asymmetry that may displace or compress normal structures. It is progressive until approximately 30 years of age, but rarely beyond. Pain is not uncommon but may appear later in the course of the disease. Bisphosphonates have been effective in relieving pain (though their use has been associated with osteonecrosis). Craniofacial lesions can cause disfigurement and symptoms due to deformation (it can affect the eye, causing blindness and other cranial nerve palsies). Malignant transformation (0.5%) to sarcomas can occur after a mean period of 13.5 years, especially after irradiation.

- Monostotic: Single bone form that is 4 times more common and affects ribs, tibia/femur, cranium/maxilla and mandible most commonly
- Polyostotic (20%): There is a high association with abnormal pigmentation (café au lait spots with irregular borders; those typical of neurofibromatosis have regular borders), hyperthyroidism, rudimentary kidneys and premature sexual development. This association is commonly called the McCune-Albright syndrome

In the past, treatment tended to be conservative with contouring procedures as needed. Although the affected bone does not involute, earlier surgery may possibly result in fewer problems. The currently favoured option is the total excision and immediate reconstruction where possible. However in most cases, the affected bone can only be partly excised (without causing massive deformities). Some have used the excised bone (with or without autoclaving to destroy cells) for grafting with few problems and there is a supposed low potential for recurrence.

Familial fibrous dysplasia is otherwise known as cherubism and characteristically affects the mandible and maxilla. It is a self-limiting and extremely rare condition in children and does not require surgery as it often regresses without residual deformity. The current view is that it resembles a giant cell granuloma more than fibrous dysplasia.

Further reading

Steinbacher DM, Gougoutas A, Bartlett SP. An analysis of mandibular volume in hemifacial microsomia. Plast Reconstr Surg 2011; 127:2407–12.

Related topics of interest

- Craniosynostosis
- Ear reconstruction
- Facial reanimation
- Tissue fillers

Hypospadias

The incidence of hypospadias is 1 in 300 live Caucasian births. The abnormally proximal urethral meatus is found in the ventral aspect of the penis or less commonly, the scrotum. There has been an increasing incidence in recent years that may be partly accounted for by increased awareness and surveillance. Other features include

- Dorsal hooded prepuce with ventral deficiency
- Chordee is a fibrous band that may cause a curvature either at rest or during erection. The exact aetiology is poorly understood (may occur without hypospadias). A curved penis is a normal stage during embryogenesis and thus in some cases may represent an interruption of development. It may be classified as mild (most common), moderate or severe. It tends to be more pronounced and involve deeper tissues in the more proximal forms of hypospadias
  - It can be assessed intraoperatively with an artificial erection test (Horton's test: Performed with a tourniquet applied and sterile saline injected into the corpora)
  - Paraurethral sinuses, urethral valves and flattened glans (which may be spatulated)

Approximately 10% of patients also have inguinal hernias or undescended testes. Patients with hypospadias and one non-palpable testis are usually referred for karyotyping (intersex especially mixed gonadal dysgenesis) and for exclusion of congenital adrenal hyperplasia (genetically female) by measuring 17-hydroxyprogesterone. Apart from the cosmetic issues, there may be functional problems.

- Unable to micturate standing up
- Reduced fertility
  - Severe chordee may make penetration painful or difficult
  - Deposition of semen in the female reproductive tract may be hindered

There is a 10% risk with hypospadias in first-degree relatives. Identical twins are not always both affected, lending credence to environmental influences. Implicated environmental factors include xeno-oestrogens (DDT) and phyto-oestrogens (in soya beans). As urethral development is under DHT control (peripheral conversion from testosterone), reductions in androgens, their receptors or 5-α-reductase, or an increase in exogenous oestrogens may be important. IVF babies are at 5x higher risk and may be related to maternal progesterone levels. The risk is also increased in mothers having oestrogen therapy during pregnancy.

The urethral folds close over the urethral groove and plate to form the penile urethra at 12 weeks. A week later, the glanular urethra is canalised to form the external urethral meatus.

Hypospadias are classified according to the position of the meatus after chordee correction, often making it more proximal than initially apparent. The subcoronal ectopic meatal position is the single most common location.

- Distal, middle or proximal
  - Distal (50%): Glanular, coronal or subcoronal
  - Middle (30%): Distal penile, mid-shaft or proximal penile
  - Proximal (20%): Penoscrotal, scrotal or perineal

Assessment

Counselling is an important part of the management. Reassure parents that it is not their fault and was not preventable. It can be treated successfully in most cases. Important aspects of the physical examination include

- Assessing penis size (almost normal in simple hypospadias)
- Verifying testicular descent
- Observing urine flow (if possible)

The presence of hernia should be specifically excluded. The incidence of upper urinary tract anomalies in uncomplicated non-syndromic hypospadias is not significantly greater than the general population (0.4%)

and routine investigation is not indicated in the absence of anorectal anomalies.

Surgery

Surgery aims to provide the patient with a normal-looking penis with normal sexual function, normally positioned urethral meatus and a normal urinary stream. It is important that circumcision is not performed before surgery.

Timing

Previously, surgery was delayed until the patient was aged 3 years or older. The larger penis size facilitated easier surgery and patients were perceived to demonstrate better comprehension and cooperation. Preoperative testosterone to increase the penis size prior to surgery can be used (Snodgrass), but not universally adopted.

- Current practice aims to perform surgery between 6–18 months for one-stage surgery or slightly later for two-stage surgery. The child remains amnesic to the procedure and is still in nappies, making postoperative care simpler. The aim is operate when technically feasible, but before the patient is aware of the difference. Fitness for surgery is the primary limiting factor (general anaesthesia after 6 months of age)
- Surgery at 2–3 years of age is generally avoided due to a perceived increase in psychological adjustment problems

Techniques

Over 200 named procedures have been described, all of which may fall into one or more of the following categories:

- Single-stage vs. two-stage techniques
- Pedicled flaps vs. grafts
- Tubularised versus onlay grafts

Consequently, there are many different protocols/preferences.

- Meatal advancement and glanuloplasty incorporated (MAGPI) for glanular hypospadias, with Bulbar Elongation and Anastomotic Meatoplasty (BEAM) for slightly more proximal problems

- Flip flap/ Mathieu or Snodgrass/ Tubularised incised plate (TIP) for most distal types
- Vascularised preputial flap or Bracka two-stage reserved for more proximal types

The most widely adopted procedure worldwide is the Snodgrass TIP repair, due to its simplicity and reproducibility.

Other general points:

Surgery is performed under GA, often in combination with a caudal block that anaesthetises skin, mucosa, lessens bladder neck spasm and allows a lighter GA to be given with fewer opiates. However, it produces a partial erection, which a penile ring block and dorsal penile block do not. After infiltration with 0.5% lignocaine and 1:200,000 adrenaline, the penis is degloved in the plane between the Buck's fascia and Dartos' fascia.

- Orthoplasty for chordee: Correction can be obtained in increasing degrees by degloving, dissection of the spongiosum, 'fairy cuts' in the Buck's fascia, supplementation with Nesbitt stitches (plication of the tunica albuginea), resection and transection of the fibrotic tethering urethral plate and conversion to a 2-stage procedure with grafting of the defect at the first stage
- The urethra is repaired where possible using the urethral plate. If insufficient, the urethra may be reconstructed with other tissue (flap or graft)
- Foreskin repair is possible, unless substantial portions of it have been used in the repair. This is also technique dependent

Single-stage techniques

The urethra is reconstructed with vascularised tissue as onlay (incomplete tube that is completed by the urethral plate) or inlay tube grafts (complete tube). The additional tissue that is needed can be transposed

- As a reflected flap, such as the Mathieu flip-flap
- As an islanded preputial flap: Duckett onlay or inlay flaps

Hypospadias in the middle

portions   These can be treated by Snodgrass/TIP, Mathieu **(Figure 10)** and onlay techniques.

Mathieu ('flip flap') 1932   This is most suited for distal hypospadias:

- A wider proximal flap is raised and flipped over to meet a strip of glans mucosa that is not raised or undermined. The flap is as long as required to cover the meatus to tip, with a width of 7.5 mm tapering to 5.5 mm at the glans and sutured with running subcutaneous 7-0 PDS under loupe magnification
- Glans wings are brought around the tube distally, while the proximal part is covered with a pedicled flap of redraped penile skin from the dorsum
- A urethral stent is used in older boys, while a catheter is used for younger patients in nappies. The penis is dressed with a clear occlusive dressing

Snodgrass (1994)   The Snodgrass or TIP technique is simple and versatile. A width of mucosa between the urethral opening and its desired position is isolated and then tubularised after a mid-line relaxing incision (this reepithelialises spontaneously). If there is insufficient tissue, an interpositional graft ('Snodgraft') can be used at the relaxing incision site, to allow 1 stage tubularisation. Caution is needed to avoid tightness with the distal sutures. Strategies to reduce the fistula rate include

- Two layer closure: A running subcutaneous suture and interrupted Lembert inverting sutures. It is important to preserve the more vascularised periurethral tissue (reduce undermining to preserve vascularity) for suturing
- Dartos flap (split in mid-line to avoid torsion or distally based turnover) over this as second waterproofing layer, avoids overlapping sutures lines, which decreases the rate of fistula formation

Onlay techniques   A pedicled preputial flap 9-10 mm wide and as long as the meatus to tip distance is raised and inset into the urethral defect with running full thickness sutures on one side, and subcutaneous sutures on the other, advancing the base of the flap. A pedicled flap is used to cover the anastomosis.

Posterior/ proximal hypospadias   These can be treated with Duckett (transverse preputial), onlay and the two-staged Bracka repairs.

Transverse islanded preputial (Duckett)   After excision of fibrotic tissue, a 15 mm wide transverse preputial pedicled flap is raised and tubularised over 6F catheter using running subcutaneous suture and inverting Lembert sutures as a second layer.

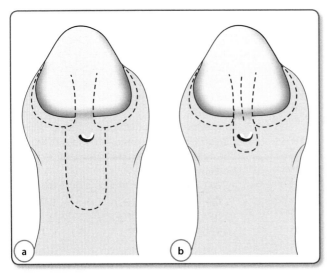

Figure 10 Common methods of hypospadias repair. In the flip-flap repair (a), a distally based flap of skin is used to complete the urethra whilst in the Snodgrass repair (b) the urethral plate is incised to allow tubularisation.

This is tunnelled (excisional to avoid stenosis) to the meatus or placed in a deep glans split and wrapped.

- Suture one end of the tube to the meatus after fixing to the corpus cavernosa for anchorage. The vertical suture line should face tissue
- A 'V' meatus for oblique closure. The proximal anastomosis should be spatulated and covered with subcutaneous tissue or a tunica vaginalis flap

Two-stage techniques: Bracka (modified Cloutier)

The Bracka technique is a workhorse technique for more proximal forms of hypospadias and revisional surgery.

- The first stage is performed at the age of 1. The shaft is degloved and the dorsal skin split and wrapped around the shaft and sutured together ventrally. The glans is split longitudinally to the meatus, the chordee released and the defect covered with an inner preputial skin graft (alternatives see below) secured with a tie-over dressing. This is removed on the 5th postoperative day under sedation and EMLA
  - Bladder mucosa tends to shrink, thus it is common to harvest 10% more. Revision may be needed for protruding mucosa
  - Buccal mucosa can be harvested at a 1:1 ratio as it contracts less and is relatively stiff due to the thick epithelium
- The second stage is performed 6 months later, when the 15 mm width of skin is tubed with minimal undermining over a catheter in two layers with waterproofing, and the skin brought back together as an uncircumcised penis. A catheter is kept for 6 days with co-amoxiclav cover (prophylactic trimethoprim is given for the first stage)

There are obvious disadvantages of having to undergo two operations, including the extra cost and the additional anaesthetic. Controversy exists with regard to the amount of psychological trauma sustained. Proponents argue that it is the final appearance of the genitalia that has a greater impact than the number of operations. Two-stage operations can provide good cosmesis with a slit-like meatus that is less likely to stricture by avoiding a circumferential anastomosis. The operation is technically simple (compared to one-stage), reliable (3% fistula rate) and suitable for revision surgery. It is of particular use in cases with severe chordee.

Advancement techniques These are suited for carefully selected patients with distal defects that were often ignored in the past because of lesser functional problems. Older repair techniques, such as Dennis Brown, Byars and Thiersch Duplay may leave a retrusive meatus that can be corrected.

- MAGPI (Duckett) is suitable for glanular hypospadias only. Subcoronal hypospadias are better treated with other techniques. A longitudinal incision is made distal to the abnormal meatus and closed transversely to provide some advancement. The glans tissue is then closed over the advanced meatus in two layers. The fish mouth deformity can be a complication of the MAGPI
- BEAM: Dissecting a length of penile urethra free advances the meatus. An advancement of up to 5 cm in adults and 2.5 cm in children can be obtained this way, through a tunnel or split glans. Ventral curvature may result from overzealous stretching

Postoperative care

The use of stents or catheters is variable, although urinary diversion for 2–6 days with a silicone catheter is a common practice.

- The original Mathieu operation was performed without stents
- Traditionally after a TIP repair, a catheter is left in for 7–14 days but some studies have shown that early removal of the catheter does not affect the final results or increase the risk of complications

As long as a watertight urethroplasty is performed without overlying suture lines, catheter drainage and urinary diversion may not be necessary in most cases of distal

Table 29 Complications encountered in treating hypospadias	
Early	**Late**
• **Erections,** particularly in young adults, can disrupt the surgery and are suppressed by commencing cyproterone acetate 10 days before surgery with or without desipramine daily.	• Splaying may indicate stenosis (at neourethra and meatus). 15% require further surgery, usually VY advancement flaps.
• **Wound infection** and dehiscence are less common with the routine use of prophylactic antibiotics. It is difficult to resuture dehiscent wounds and it is more common to leave them to heal and then repair any fistulae 6 months later.	• **Fistulas:** The overall rate is 15% (higher in revisions). Most appear early (90% within a week) due to obstruction, haematoma or infection. They rarely close spontaneously. It is common practice to wait 6 months and to exclude distal obstruction before repair. Late fistulae are usually due to turbulent flow.
• **Bladder spasm** from the catheter may be treated with oxybutinin.	• Recurrent urinary tract infections can occur, especially if hairy skin was used to graft the urethra
	• **Strictures**
	• **Glans dehiscence:** Common but to a degree that is infrequently recognised.

repair. Suprapubic drainage (with risk of bladder neck spasm) is usually regarded as being over-the-top. Overall, there has been a move away from stents as well as long-term (1–2 weeks) catheters after hypospadias repair. Hypospadias surgery can often be performed as a day case.

There is a tendency for oedema that may cause sutures to cut through (albeit rarely). Studies have failed to show any difference in the repair result with the different dressings.

The area is inspected at around the second/third postoperative day.

Complications

The complications commonly encountered during treatment of hypospadias are shown in **Table 29**. Most complications such as haematoma, skin loss and wound infections are easily managed.

Further reading

González R, Ludwikowski BM. Importance of urinary flow studies after hypospadias repair: a systematic review. Int J Urol 2011; 18:757–61.

Keloids and hypertrophic scarring

Dermal injury triggers a cascade that results in the deposition of a vascular collagen matrix that manifests as a red, raised scar as it accumulates. As the matrix matures and remodels, the scar becomes flatter and paler over approximately 9 months (longer in children), although remodelling continues beyond this time point. Scar scales (**Table 30**) offer useful methods of describing and recording scar appearance during their evolution.

Problematic scars fall into two main categories:

- Hypertrophic scars follow a similar but protracted course to normal scars, and have a tendency to involute. The hypertrophy remains within the confines of the initial wound
- Keloids (from 'cheloide' after the Greek 'chele' for a crab claw) typically appear after a variable delay, after an initial and apparently normal healing process. They have a tendency to spread beyond the initial wound into previously normal adjacent skin

These problematic scars follow a variety of injuries, but display the following associations:

- Site predilection:
  - High risk: Ears, deltoid, pre-sternal areas and upper arms
  - Low risk: Palms, soles, eyelids, and genitalia
- High wound tension and scars that cross skin tension lines or joints
- Wound infection
- Relationship with wound infection/wound tension during closure

These associations may be stronger in hypertrophic scars compared with keloids.

Differences between hypertrophic/keloid scars and normal scars

Both hypertrophic scarring and keloids are more vascular and have thicker epidermal layers than normal scars when compared histologically. In addition, the matrix contains more type III collagen and has collagen nodules that are not found in mature normal scars.

Differences between keloids and hypertrophic scars

Keloids and hypertrophic scars differ in their clinical characteristics and response to treatment. Although the literature on the subject is plentiful, most are flawed.

- Very few published studies are of sound methodology. The lack of randomisation and lack adequate follow-up are the most common shortcomings
- Many studies do not properly distinguish between keloids and hypertrophic scars

The history is focussed on determining the stage of scar evolution. Keloids and hypertrophic scars can look very similar, histological differences can be subtle and equivocal and both types of scarring may coexist in a single scar. These factors may account for the confusion in the published literature. See **Table 31** for a comparison of keloids and hypertrophic scars, as commonly accepted, given the limitations described above.

Table 30	The Vancouver scar scale		
Vascularity	**Score**	**Pigment**	**Score**
Normal	0	Normal	0
Pink	1	Hypopigmented	1
Red	2	Mixed	2
Purple	3	Hyperpigmented	3
Pliability	**Score**	**Height**	**Score**
Normal	0	Flat	0
Supple	1	< 2 mm	1
Yielding	2	2–5 mm	2
Firm	3	> 5 mm	3
Ropes	4		
Contracture	5		

Table 31 Comparison of hypertrophic scars and keloids		
	Hypertrophic scar	**Keloid**
Onset	Early, within weeks to months.	May be delayed up to several years.
History	Tends to regress with time.	Tends to progress with time.
Extent	Stays within the boundaries of the original wound. Enlargement tends to be expansile (when excised, the defect is smaller than the scar).	Extends beyond the boundaries of the original wound. Enlargement tends to be contractile (when excised, the defect is larger than the scar).
Microscopy	Wavy, loose bundles of collagen with many fibroblasts. Lesions have nodules comprising cells and collagen (seen less in keloids). Compared to normal scars, • Collagen synthesis is 3x higher • Collagenase activity is 4x higher	Disorganised, sparse bundles of large irregular collagen fibres with reduced cross-linking. Greater disorganisation and more ground substance than hypertrophic scars. Compared to normal scars, • Collagen synthesis is 20x higher • Collagenase activity is 14x higher • More type III collagen

Keloids

The overall risk of having a keloid scar is estimated at 5–15%, but accurate and reliable figures are not available. Keloids are more common in darker skin types and there may be genetic susceptibility, as demonstrated by keloid diatheses in some families. It has also been theorised to be an immune reaction to sebum or a type of inclusion cyst (ear keloids). Overall, the causative mechanisms are poorly understood. They may be related to:

• Reduced apoptosis and increased proliferation of fibroblasts
• Role of TGF-β (subtypes 1 and 2 are increased) and IGF-1 in the formation of keloids

While spontaneous keloids have been described in the sternal region, the majority follow a seemingly trivial skin injury such as acne or an ear piercing. Adolescents tend to scar worse than other age groups, possibly reflecting the different inflammatory and cytokine profiles. There is evidence to suggest that the rate of keloid formation following ear piercings is lower if performed before the age of 11.

Treatment

There is a range of treatments used for both scarring types, although underlying mechanisms of action have not been fully elucidated. Proper comparison and applicability to either keloid or hypertrophic scarring or both is difficult as many studies fail to properly and consistently distinguish between them. Furthermore, there is a general lack of standardised treatment regimes. As hypertrophic scarring tends to regress spontaneously, it can be difficult to judge whether or not a treatment has been successful or that there has simply been natural regression of the lesion.

Pressure

Pressure may work through local tissue hypoxia and ischaemia. The exact mechanism of action is unknown but pressure may limit collagen synthesis by limiting nutrient delivery and allow realignment of bundles. Older scars tend to respond poorly and it is more useful in hypertrophic scars.

Pressure garments have been used since the 1970s and have a large body of evidence supporting its use. They can be fitted as soon as the wounds are healed, and should be used continuously until the wound is mature. The optimally effective pressures remain elusive, but it is commonly believed that the compression pressure should be higher than capillary pressure (25 mmHg).

Compliance can be a problem, with only 41% of patients reported to be fully compliant. This is attributed to a variety of factors that include lack of perceived benefit, unattractive appearance (non-beige bright colours may be more acceptable in children) and discomfort (sweaty, rash or pruritus). Complications per se are rare, but pressure (garments) may deform skeletal tissues in young children and cause oedema distally.

Silicone gel

Silicone gel may work by occlusion and hydration of the scar surface, reducing transepidermal water loss that reduces profibrotic cytokine production by the keratinocytes. If used for 24 hours a day for 3 months, the response rate is approximately 65–88%. Self drying silicone gels (Dermatix Ultra) have a greater compliance rate and thus overall efficacy compared to silicone sheets. Some guidelines suggest that silicone should be used to prevent problem scarring in the higher risk patients including Asians.

Steroids

The reported response rate (reduced pain, pruritus, hyperaemia and bulkiness) to intralesional injection varies widely between 30–100%. The mechanism of action is unknown but may involve decreased collagen synthesis, increased collagen degradation or both.

Steroid injections are first line treatment for smaller keloids. Many systematic reviews have been published but provide little useful information on optimal concentration and frequency. Triamcinolone, available in concentrations of 10 mg/ml and 40 mg/ml can be combined with lignocaine to improve (postinjection) comfort. Local side effects include dermal thinning, atrophy, telangiectasia and pigmentary change. Systemic effects, such as endocrine disturbance and osteoporosis are rare. The value of topical steroids is unclear.

Excision

Excision or ablation by surgery, cryotherapy or laser have all been used but have similarly high rates of recurrence (> 50%), although the numbers are low and the follow-up duration too short or unclear. Scar reexcision may be considered for those with specific identifiable causes such as wound infection during healing. Surgery is probably best combined with other modalities such as steroids, pressure or RT to reduce the risk of recurrence.

Lasers

- Vascular lasers such as the pulsed dye laser (PDL) may be effective for relieving itching and redness, particularly in hypertrophic scars (this was discovered by accident when treating port-wine stains (PWS) scarred by previous Argon laser therapy). It may be particularly useful for recent scars (< 1 year), but its efficacy has not been definitively established
- Laser ablation (with CO_2 lasers) may be useful for contour defects in mature scars
- Nd:YAG lasers are reported to have variable effectiveness

Radiotherapy

Radiotherapy inhibits fibroblast proliferation. Although there is no role for radiotherapy alone, an early (24–48 hours) postoperative dose (single 10–14 Gy) reduces the rate of recurrence compared to surgery alone. Malignant complications (thyroid, breast and skin malignancies) have been reported, are extremely rare, but must be considered when treating young patients (thus some defer this treatment until after 21 years of age). Radiotherapy is uncommonly used in the UK for this purpose and reserved for severely recalcitrant keloids.

Less commonly used treatments include

- Immune response modifiers: Interferons (γ for hypertrophic scarring, α-2b for keloids) and the immunomodulator, imiquimod. However, the study numbers are small and of low evidence level . Interferons can cause significant side effects and therefore are rarely used to treat scarring
- Chemotherapeutic agents: 5-FU (intralesional and intrawound topical), bleomycin, mitomycin C. Some have combined pharmacological agents with fractional laser

Further reading

Wu XL, Liu W, Cao YL. Clinical study on keloid treatment with intralesional injection of low concentration 5-fluorouracil. Zhonghua Zheng Xing Wai Ke Za Zhi 2006;22:44–46.

Related topic of interest

- Lasers: Principles

Lasers: principles

Lasers have rapidly developed into invaluable therapeutic tools. However, the perception of lasers as a side-effect-free general panacea for skin conditions is prevalent in both patients and practitioners alike. Consequently, expectation management is vital, as an understanding of the physics and principles of lasers to permit improved decision-making, better patient counselling, and the safe and effective use of the technology.

Laser (light amplification by stimulated emission of radiation)

When an excited atom spontaneously returns to the resting state, it will emit a photon of a certain wavelength. If this photon hits another atom in the resting state it will raise it to an excited state. However, if this photon hits an atom that is already in an excited state, then two photons are released that are in phase (Einstein's theory of stimulated emission).

A laser system provides:

- An external energy source that increases the proportion of excited atoms held in the laser medium
- An arrangement of mirrors (a fully reflecting mirror at one end and a partially reflecting mirror at the other) that allows the light emitted to be reflected back and forth. This arrangement allows the amplification of light energy

A laser will deliver energy in the form of a collimated, coherent and monochromatic light. These terms mean that the light travels in a single direction, single phase and single wavelength respectively and are in decreasing order of importance to the clinical effect.

When such light impinges on tissue, it will be transmitted, scattered, reflected or absorbed to differing degrees, depending on the relationship between wavelength of the light and absorption characteristics of the tissue. The stratum corneum reflects 4–7% of light, whilst the dermis scatters light. When laser light is absorbed, it is predominantly converted to heat (photothermal interaction), leading to a range of temperature-dependent effects. In other situations, depending on the intensity and duration of energy transfer, the light energy can lead to photomechanical or photochemical interactions.

- Shorter wavelengths have higher energy (have ionising effects)
- Longer wavelengths scatter less and therefore penetrate deeper (simplification)

Basic laser technology constitutes a very precise and controllable source of intense heat. Its suitability for clinical use involves matching these properties to the problem. This is where experience is crucial.

Photothermal effects: The CO_2 laser

The CO_2 laser was one of the first lasers to be used for medical purposes and remains a workhorse due its versatility. Its wavelength of 10,600 nm preferentially targets water in the tissues, where heating leads to destruction. This ranges from denaturation and necrosis to vaporisation, depending on the fluence (energy density in J/cm^2) delivered. If vaporisation is incomplete, the tissues retain the heat and charring results.

Pulsing (see below) reduces charring by increasing vaporisation (which actually cools the skin). A defocused CO_2 laser beam can be used to ablate or vaporise superficial lesions. When focused into a narrow beam, it cuts like a scalpel with excellent haemostasis (except for larger-calibre or high-flow vessels). Equipment costs are high, the process is relatively slow and initial healing may be slower with the concomitant risk of poorer scars compared to the conventional scalpel (arguably dependent on the operator). Methods of creating laser pulses include

- Continuous wave (CW): 100 W
- Shuttered: 100 W, pulses in seconds
- Pulsed: 10 W in microsecond pulses. The higher peak power stacks up and tapers off quickly
- Superpulsed: 2000 W microsecond pulses
- Q switched: 1,000,000 W (gigawatt) in the nano/pico second range with fast electromagnetic switches

Applications of lasers in plastic surgery

If the inherent properties of a particular laser can be matched to the clinical problem, then lasers can be used with good effect in a variety of conditions with relatively few complications and side effects (**Table 32**). A summary of common lasers and their applications is given in **Table 33**.

Melanin and pigmented lesions

Melanin has absorption peaks in the 500–600 ηm range. The highest selectivity is in the red end since there is less absorption from haemoglobin in this area. Similarly the blue-green range is relatively selective for melanin over haemoglobin. Selected naevi can be treated with lasers. With QS lasers, the response is variable and those that tend to respond well have melanocytes located mostly in the superficial reticular dermis. Deeper dermal lesions require longer-wavelength lasers. Dysplastic or atypical naevi should not be treated with laser as it does not permit histological diagnosis or examination of margin clearance.

CO_2 lasers are precise, but non-specific. They cannot be used to destroy pigmented or vascular lesions without causing damage to surrounding and overlying normal tissue, leading to a significant risk of scarring. Problems can potentially occur because it is impossible to limit exactly the amount of damage and where the damage occurs. An element of collateral damage is unavoidable. Lasers are not good for

- Postinflammatory pigmentation
- Melasma
- Warts: Not a first line treatment. PDL (warts being relatively vascular) may be a better treatment than CO_2 ablation (which tends to have variable response)
  - HPV has been found more than 1 cm away from a visible wart, and therefore treatment only lessens the viral burden and does not to eradicate infection Shaving the top off the lesion prior to PDL laser may help penetration
  - Prolonged healing times

Table 32 Clinical conditions effectively treated by laser	
Condition	**Typical laser used**
Skin resurfacing	CO_2, Erbium:YAG
Pigmented lesions	Q-switched ruby, Alexandrite, Nd:YAG
Tattoos	Q-switched ruby, Alexandrite, Nd:YAG
Hair removal	Long-pulse ruby, Alexandrite, diode
Vascular lesions	Pulsed dye laser 585 ηm (changed from 577 ηm for better absorption), CW may be used for large vessel diameter lesions

Table 33 Common lasers and their applications	
Laser	**Application**
Argon (488–514 ηm) continuous	Photocoagulation (eye) Skin [vascular lesions and port wine stain (PWS)]s
Alexandrite (755 ηm)	Tattoos
Excimer (193–351 ηm)	Keratotomy: Very precise high energy source
Holmium (2140 ηm)	ENT, Orthopaedics: can be used in liquids
Nd:YAG (1064 ηm)	Tattoos, other pigments (has deep penetration) Can also be used as a scalpel
Frequency doubled Nd:YAG (532 ηm) Sometimes called KTP because wavelength is changed by passing through KTP	Tattoo, pigment Vascular lesions
Ruby (694 ηm) pulsed red light	Pigment when Q switched
Tunable dye (400–800 ηm) exact wavelength determined by medium	504 ηm kidney stones 585 ηm oxygenated haemoglobin 630 ηm haematoporphyrins (PDL)

- Laser plume found to have viable viral particles, although no evidence of infection of staff occurs

Selectivity of lasers

Several conceptual advances have improved the understanding of lasers and made their clinical application more logical. Selective thermolysis (Anderson) is the targeting of a specific tissue component to be heated and destroyed without damage to neighbouring tissues. This may be met if several criteria are met:

- Wavelength suited to target
- Sufficient energy to destroy target
- Exposure duration is less than or equal to time necessary for cooling of target structures

Central to this, is the concept of the thermal relaxation time (TRT), which is the time for the target to cool to 50% of the maximum temperature rise without conducting heat to the surrounding tissue. Thus, if the rate of heating is greater than the rate of cooling, then the target is selectively heated, leading to its destruction before significant conduction to surrounding tissues, causing selective damage. On the other hand, if the rate of heating is less than the rate of cooling, then both target and surrounding tissue are heated, and the effect is less specific.

Approached slightly differently, assuming that there is instantaneous heating with a laser pulse and TRT is the cooling time after a pulse. If the laser pulse is long (energy spaced out in time), the target can cool during the pulse, analogous to a filling a leaky container that leaks faster than it fills. It is necessary to confine the heat (spatially) by using a short pulse (energy concentrated in a short time) that roughly coincides with the TRT of chromophore. This is analogous to filling the leaky container at a higher rate so that it fills faster than it leaks. The ablation threshold should be attained in or under the TRT. On the other hand, if the pulse is too short, there is violent vaporisation and significant collateral damage results from the explosion.

Chromophores (coloured molecules) in the skin preferentially absorb light of a particular wavelength. Heating can be effectively restricted to the target chromophore if laser light of a suitable wavelength and appropriate pulse duration is chosen. However, perfect selectivity is not possible, as other chromophores will still absorb some of the energy, causing a degree of collateral damage. For example, when targeting haemoglobin (absorbs at 580 ηm) with a PDL, some of the 585 ηm light will also be absorbed by melanin (absorbs between 500–600 ηm), leading to dyspigmentation and by water (leading to non-selective skin damage, pain and erythema). While unwanted effects cannot be completely eliminated, they can be minimised by optimal choice of laser parameters. Most lasers are in or near the visible light spectrum (400–700 ηm), except CO_2.

Fractional thermolysis

This modification creates an array of microscopic treatment zones with a density of 2–3000 per cm^2, arranged in a grid. Small but evenly distributed amounts of skin are treated, with the intervening skin left uninjured. Keratinocytes have a shorter migration path allowing rapid healing of these zones with minimal erythema and downtime, at the expense of a less marked improvement and potentially a greater number of treatment cycles. It has been used to treat many problems including wrinkles, acne scars and photodamage. There is less pain associated with the treatment and topical anaesthetics are usually sufficient. The anaesthetic can be combined with a blue tracing ointment to help control the velocity/repetition rate. Both ablative and non-ablative laser systems have been adapted with this function.

Intense pulsed light

This is noncoherent light with a range of wavelengths (515–1200 ηm), pulse durations (relatively long) and fluencies. The use of IPL developed from the prior use of infrared light for treatment of tattoos and vascular lesions. The machines are essentially high-intensity flash lamps with cut-off filters narrowing the output to a range that covers the melanin/haemoglobin spectrum. Its popularity is partly due to

- Relatively low incidence of side effects apart from slight erythema for up to 48 hours
- No anaesthetic is usually required as discomfort is limited to a mild burning sensation
- Can be combined with cooling (usually with a gel)

Proper parameter selection is important, as with increasing power, transient purpura, blistering, crusting and pigmentary changes can occur. The main indications for IPL are

- Hair removal (though the exact mechanism of action is unclear)
- PDL resistant PWS (the vessels are deeper and bigger)
- Deeper vascular malformations resistant to laser

IPL can also be used as second line treatments for:

- Pigmented lesions including postinflammatory pigmentation
- Rejuvenation: Non-ablative subsurfacing due possibly to heat denaturisation of collagen with subsequent increased synthesis
- Fine wrinkles
- Facial telangiectasia: PDL is better. Other alternatives include diathermy or using sclerosants
- Leg telangiectasia: These are > 0.1 mm in diameter, have thicker walls and are deeper compared to facial vessels. Sclerotherapy is still the gold standard. Lasers are an alternative for the needle phobic and in those with allergies

Further reading

Wattankrai P, Mornchan R, Eimpunth S, et al. Low-fluence Q-switched neodymium-doped yttrium aluminum garnet (1064 ηm) laser for the treatment of facial melasma in Asians. Dermatol Surg 2010; 36:76–87.

Related topics of interest

- Hair removal
- Skin resurfacing
- Tattoo removal
- Vascular anomalies

Leeches and maggots

Leeches

The common medical leech (*Hirudo medicinalis*) is one of more than 700 species of annelids. The term 'leech' is derived from '*laece*', an ancient word for physician. The caudal end of the leech is larger than the anterior, and bears the sucker used to attach itself. The more mobile cranial end is characterised by the distinctive 'Mercedes Benz' jaws. Its saliva contains many active substances that include:

- Hirudin is an anticoagulant. It is the most potent natural thrombin inhibitor acting directly on the common final coagulative pathway. This anticoagulative effect is sustained for > 1.6 cm radius from the bite. Recombinant hirudin has been exploited as therapeutic anticoagulants in clinical practice (lepirudin)
- Proteases: Hyaluronidase, collagenase and apyrase
- Local anaesthetics: Controversial

Leeches are used mainly to treat venous congestion after flap surgery, such as in replants. This temporises venous drainage needs until neovascularization occurs at about 4-10 days. Venous congestion can often be more deleterious to a flap than arterial occlusion. An LD flap model demonstrated 40% muscle necrosis after 3 hours of venous congestion, while there was no corresponding necrosis for the same period of arterial occlusion.

Medical leeches are bred specifically for use and ordered from the suppliers as needed. They are bred in a warm environment (24°C) and are hermaphrodites. After hatching and receiving a blood meal, they are then stored in a dark and cold environment (< 15°C) for up to a year in chlorine-free water with 0.5 g of hirudo salt per litre. The solution is changed every 3 days and kept in a covered container to prevent escape.

Using leeches

The use of leeches is contraindicated if there is arterial insufficiency or if the patient is immunosuppressed.

- Select the smallest leech, as it is usually the hungriest
- Leeches can be handled with forceps or the tip of an empty syringe to place it over the intended site. Allow the larger end to attach for support and then direct the head to precise site
- Warmth will attract the leech and stimulate serotonin release from its pharynx causing feeding behaviour. The leech may also be stimulated by sodium, arginine and blood on the surface (skin pinprick can be used to facilitate this)
- The leech can be kept in place by a stack of gauze with the centres cut out, and is usually covered up with a plastic cup. The leech will remain attached until they have ingested a full meal (consumes 5 ml of blood over 20–60 minutes) and may increase in weight up to eight times. This phase of active bleeding is followed by a passive phase, where slow oozing of 50–100 ml of blood occurs over the next 24–48 hours. The bite can be gently rubbed to encourage further bleeding
- The used leech is killed by immersion in 70% alcohol for 5 minutes and must then be disposed as hazardous waste. Leeches can be recycled for use in the same patient by inducing leech regurgitation. Covering it with salt or strong saline does this. It tends to be a hit-and-miss exercise as it can kill it. The maximum number of cycles is unpredictable, as is the relative efficacy of the recycled leech

Complications

- Infection by *Aeromonas hydrophilia*. This is a facultative gram-negative rod that lives as a commensal in the foregut of the leech where it prevents blood putrefaction and aids digestion. The reported infection rate is as high as 20%. It is usually treated with third generation cephalosporins such as ceftriaxone. There are isolated reports of infection by other microorganisms. Antibiotic prophylaxis with either co-amoxiclav or ciprofloxacin is recommended with leech therapy
- Excessive blood loss

Maggots

The larvae of a small number of fly species are used therapeutically to induce benign myiasis. Benign myiasis is the consumption of non-viable tissue, in contrast to malignant myiasis, which is the consumption of viable tissue. Although the larvae do not consume live tissue, the enzymes may cause irritation and erythema. The maggots used in the UK are the sterile larvae of the greenbottle fly. These flies are dipteran (single pair of functional wings) and can reach an average size of 8 mm when fully grown.

Maggots were been used for wound therapy in the military conflicts of the Napoleonic era, American Civil War and the First World War. Crile that showed superior survival in wounded soldiers who had maggot wound infestation. Maggot therapy was popular in the 1930s but declined in use in the antibiotic era of the late 1940s. They were rediscovered following Sherman's work in the 1980s and can now be prescribed in the UK and used in the community. In the US, maggots are categorised as a prescription-only medical device (not a drug). Maggots are suitable for use in many infected necrotic wounds including pressure sores and diabetic ulcers. Their action seems to come from a complex group of substances and physical actions that cannot be substituted for by any single chemical.

- Necrophagous feeding on dead tissue by extracorporeal digestion through chymotrypsin-like enzymes. The maggots have tiny hooks for locomotion and attachment, and may possibly help to disrupt the surface for better enzyme penetration
- Antimicrobial: Maggots directly consume wound bacteria. The increasing exudates may have an irrigation effect and the alkalinisation of wound fluid may be directly antimicrobial. Larval secretions (proteus in gut) and possibly phenylacetic acid and phenylacetaldehyde are purported to have antimicrobial actions as well
- Promote healing: Maggots promote fibroblast growth at 10% of EGF *in vitro*

- May reduce pain (by reducing infection/inflammation) and odours (from volatile amines in wounds)

The cost effectiveness of maggot wound therapy, compared to other methods is good. It has been shown in one study to heal 90% of MRSA infected wounds after 4–6 days or after 1–2 applications of maggots.

- Five to six maggots may be used for small wounds such as the fingertip, while hundreds are appropriate for larger wounds
- Hydrocolloid dressings applied to the wound edge can be used to protect the normal skin and to act as a base for adhesives
- The maggots are applied and covered by a fine mesh. A moist pad is placed on top to prevent drying out, although they are less vulnerable after 24 hours. They can be difficult to contain. Maggots take 10–14 days to pupate, a process that requires a dry place, and therefore maggots will try to leave a moist wound area
- The maggots are removed 1–3 days later and disposed of

Antibiotics or X-rays do not affect the survival of maggots in the wound. Some topical dressings such as hydrogels may have negative effect possibly due partly to the polypropylene glycol content (used to stop drying out and as antimicrobial). Excess wound fluid may drown maggots and dilute their secretions, reducing their effectiveness.

Complications

Overall patient acceptance is high. There are few contraindications to their use, although caution is warranted in wounds potentially connected with body cavities or near major vessels.

- Discomfort (of variable intensity) is the most common complaint particularly in ischaemic limbs and often begins on the 2nd or 3rd day. It may be due to the alkaline secretions and stops immediately with removal of the maggots
- Many patients report a tingling sensation that is tolerable

- There may be irritation of normal skin causing excoriation similar to a superficial burn. Ammonia toxicity is theoretically possible in major infestations

- Infections are rare when sterile maggots are used. There may occasionally be a fever that is transient and of unknown cause
- Bleeding is rare and usually minor

Further reading

Dumville JC, et al. Larval therapy for leg ulcers (VenUS II): randomised controlled trial. Br Med J 2009; 338:b773.

Related topics of interest

- Leg ulcers
- Microsurgery

Leg ulcers

An ulcer is an epithelial skin breach with variable involvement of the deeper structures. Its causes are diverse. In developed countries, venous disease is the most frequent cause. Chronic ulcers warrant biopsy to exclude malignancy (Marjolin's ulcer). Assessment is vital to guide management.

History and examination

- Ulcer characteristics: Particularly, edge and base
- Exclude malignancy: Examine the regional lymph nodes
- Surrounding skin and circulation of the limb
- Sensation (diabetic neuropathy is suggested by a glove-and-stocking distribution)

Investigations

- Biopsy: Long-standing lesions
- Wound swabs may be useful, but colonisation is common and antibiotics are generally unnecessary unless there is evidence of clinical infection
- Ankle brachial index (ABI): An ABI of < 0.8 suggests arterial disease, whereas an ABI of < 0.5 should prompt referral to vascular surgeons
- X-rays may be indicated to exclude osteomyelitis

Venous ulcers

In developed countries, 70–90% of leg ulcers are due to venous disease, of which 10% also have an arterial component. Venous ulcers are typically painless and found in the gaiter area, particularly over the medial malleolus. A gaiter is a protective piece of cloth or leather that covers the area from instep to ankle.

Venous hypertension is often caused by valvular dysfunction, which is usually secondary to previous thrombophlebitis. Prolonged tissue hypertension leads to extravasation of a pro-inflammatory protein-rich exudate into the tissues and formation of perivascular fibrin cuff. This results in scarring (lipodermatosclerosis) and hyperpigmentation (haemosiderin deposition). Duplex scanning is the non-invasive investigation of choice, although superficial reflux is often the only finding. For those with suspected arterial disease, angiography may be indicated.

Management

Treatment of an ulcer is cause dependent. Venous ulcers are generally treated non-surgically with elevation, compression and dressings. Most will heal if the venous hypertension is controlled. However, there is a high recurrence rate (40%).

- Ulcers can be washed with tap water. Debride necrotic material adequately
- While the dressing choices are numerous, there is little evidence to show that any of them give better outcomes than a simple non-adherent dressing. However, the use of hydrocolloid or foam dressings may be associated with less pain
- Avoid topical antibiotics (often become sensitisers). Systemic antibiotics are reserved for spreading cellulitis or preoperative prophylaxis prior to grafting
- Graduated, multilayer, high-compression bandaging aims to provide 40 mmHg of sustained compression at the ankle to reduce capillary transudate. It is kept intact for up to a week (if ABI > 0.8). 70% will heal within months
- Vacuum wound closure may be useful in some cases

There are regional differences in practice.

- In the UK, there is a preference for four-layer bandaging
- In the US, the Unna boot (made of zinc oxide and calamine impregnated bandages wrapped from toes to just below knee that then harden and are wrapped by elastic bandage) is popular. It facilitates ambulation and return to work. The boot needs to be changed once every 1 or 2 weeks and has to be kept dry in the intervening periods

- In mainland Europe, short-stretch bandaging is often used

There is no evidence of significant difference between these practices. If an ulcer fails to heal after 12 weeks of standard treatment, this should prompt further assessment to rule out other causes such as vasculitis, infection, autoimmune disease, sickle cell disease or a tumour.

Surgery

Surgery is generally reserved for cases where conservative treatment has failed or if pain is a prominent symptom and is poorly controlled. Skin grafts offer rapid healing to allow simpler and cheaper compression therapy with graduated stockings. Free flaps are not a commonly used option as they involve major surgery, but may be particularly useful for complex ulcers as they import additional vascularity to the wound bed.

Postoperatively, continued pressure gradient dressings and avoidance of standing for long periods of time is important for long-term success. Simple excision of the ulcer and reconstruction without addressing the underlying cause will almost inevitably result in recurrence (>50%). Procedures such as subfascial ligation of perforators, stripping or valvuloplasty for reflux disease, may be indicated. Superficial system surgery does not accelerate healing but does reduce recurrence. The role of perforator surgery with or without superficial vein surgery is less clear. The ESCHAR trial demonstrated no difference in healing between multilayer compression alone and compression with surgery. However, recurrence was halved in the latter group.

Table 34 shows the appearance, distribution and recommended treatments for the different types of ulcers.

Diabetic ulcers

Diabetic ulcers affect 15% of diabetic patients.
- One third are neuropathic and ischaemic

Table 34 Appearance and treatment of different kinds of ulcers				
Cause	Appearance	Surrounding skin	Typical distribution	Treatment
Venous There is often a history of DVT	Shallow ulcer with flat or slightly swollen borders. Fibrin/slough over a raw weeping base. **Painless** unless infected	Itchy, swollen, eczema, pigmented, lipodermatosclerosis, atrophie blanche. Aching and swelling at the end of the day that is improved by elevation. Capillary refill in <3 sec	Gaiter area especially medial malleolus	Compression: most will heal particularly if venous hypertension is controlled. HBO if available Pentoxifylline has not been shown to provide significant benefit in randomised trials
Arterial Claudication is often a prominent symptom.	Dry, deep punched-out and well circumscribed Base is pale and may be covered with necrotic eschar and sparse granulation tissue. Pain is worse with elevation and at night	Cold, shiny and atrophic (less hair). Pulse is weak. Capillary refill in >4–5 sec Little oedema present	Sides and toes, and dorsum of foot	Revascularisation is required to aid ulcer healing. Veins are preferred over prosthetic grafts due to the risk of infection; amputation may be required. Cilostazol, a type II PDE inhibitor, improves claudication but is not yet a recommended treatment for ulcers
Neuropathic DM, alcoholism, leprosy, tabes dorsalis and spina bifida	Painless. Looks similar to arterial ulcers but variable in depth	Surrounded by callus, may have sinuses. Paraesthesia with repeated trauma causes ulceration	Commonly, but not exclusively, at pressure points eg sole of foot under metatarsal heads and heel	In the absence of ischaemia, 90% heal without surgery. Control infection. Becaplermin gel (recombinant PDGF) is an adjunct for diabetic ulcers that may shorten healing time but has no effect on recurrences (FDA 1997)

- One third is purely neuropathic (especially mid-foot ulcers)
- One fourth is purely ischaemic (dry and painful). Major vessel disease must be ruled out (and treated). Normal pedal pulses do not represent normal perfusion, as vessel calcification can give anomalous results. Similarly, vessel calcification and also elevate pressures making the ABI unreliable. Toe pressures of > 60 mmHg may be a more useful criterion, as vessel calcification tends to be limited to larger arteries. Although the microcirculation is structurally intact, it is affected by stiffened erythrocytes, increased blood viscosity and oxygen affinity of glycosylated haemoglobin. There is also thickened capillary basement membrane

The aetiology of diabetic ulcers is often mixed, but most have neuropathic component. This is due to decreased circulation to nerves and alteration of endoneural flow, causing variable degrees of pain and discomfort, typically in a glove and stocking distribution.

- Somatic neuropathy: Protective sensation is lost
- Autonomic dysfunction leads to opening up of AV shunts (reduced skin flow) and dry skin that may crack and become infected
- Motor dysfunction leads to intrinsic contracture and claw toes

Management

- Offloading and avoid mechanical stress: Boots with windows
- Check for bony involvement and osteomyelitis by probing. X-rays (signs are late), nuclear scan and MRI (sensitivity and specificity 80–90%) may be used. Biopsy if suspicious
- Debridement and dressings: Surgery, wet-to-dry, Versajet, maggots. Repeated inspections and further debridement may be needed
- Manage infections: The infection risk is increased due to impaired phagocytosis and B cell function, in addition to ischaemia. Superficial infections are usually due to *Staphylococcus/ Streptococcus,* while deep infections are

usually polymicrobial and may have anaerobic contribution (Meleney's synergistic gangrene)
- Microangiopathic disease does not play a significant role in diabetic ulcers and thus patients may benefit from vascular reconstruction (endovascular, bypass and free flap as salvage). The mortality associated with revascularisation is approximately 1% but 50% of patients need a second procedure within 3 months. The current management consensus is for aggressive conservative management to postpone amputation for as long as possible because
- one third of stumps fail to heal and require a more proximal amputation
- one half have the contralateral limb amputated within 5 years
- The 5-year survival is 40% after the first amputation

HBOT has been shown to reduce amputation rates in patients with diabetic ulceration and is covered by Medicare (US), if ulceration has been unresponsive to 30 days of standard treatment.

Miscellaneous ulcer disease

Hydroxyurea is an antineoplastic agent used particularly in haematological malignancies that can cause painful leg ulcers, typically around the malleoli. The ulcer is refractory to local care and the drug discontinuation is required for ulcer to heal. The ulcers usually occur only after prolonged use, but its appearance after 2 weeks of treatment has been described. The mechanism is unknown but may be partly related to the primary disease.

Vasculitic ulcers and pyoderma gangrenosum (PG) are uncommon and difficult to treat. PG is a necrotising cutaneous vasculitis that may be associated with rheumatoid arthritis, inflammatory bowel disease or carcinoma, but no cause is found in at least 20% cases. The diagnosis is clinical (ulcer with purple undermined border, skin abscesses) as histological findings are non-specific. Treatment may require anti-inflammatory or immunosuppressive medication (steroids, azathioprine and cyclosporine) as well as local wound care. Those associated with inflammatory bowel disease may respond to control of their disease. Surgery is contraindicated as it may exacerbate the disease. New foci may form at skin graft donor sites.

Further reading

Klode J, Nelson EA, Hutchinson J, et al. Impact of multi-layered compression bandages on sub-bandage interface pressure: a model. Phlebology 2011; 75:83.

Related topics of interest

- Hyperbaric oxygen therapy
- Leeches and maggots
- Pressure sores
- Squamous cell carcinoma
- Vacuum wound closure

Lip cancer and reconstruction

More than 95% of lip cancers are SCCs that most commonly affect the lower lip (> 90%), particularly the mucocutaneous junction of the middle third. Less than 1% of cases involve the commissures. SCCs of the lip can be considered as part of the oral cavity or as a skin cancer. The lip is more susceptible to the effects of ultraviolet light due to the lack of a keratinised layer. Certain lesions such as leukoplakia and erythroplakia (high risk) are premalignant. Typical patients are elderly males.

- Squamous cell carcinoma: Lower lip, upper eyelid
- Basal cell carcinoma: Upper lip, lower eyelid

Multifactorial risk factors have been identified (The 6 'S's)

- Sunlight: Higher incidence in farmers and those working outdoors
- Smoking: Both from heat and the chemicals
- Spirits
- Spices: Betel nut chewing
- Sharp teeth
- Syphilis: < 2%. There is also an association with tongue cancer (classically tip) but there is no definite evidence of a causative role

The overall mortality rate is quoted at 10%. Most cases are detected early due to the obvious site and the slow growth characteristics. Survival is reduced to 50% in advanced lesions with lymphadenopathy. Increased pain or touch sensitivity may suggest perineural invasion particularly in the edentulous. There is a 5% risk of recurrence and a 5% chance of a second lip primary.

TNM staging

Note that the American Journal of Critical Care (AJCC) recognises lip as a part of the oral cavity and includes only the portion from vermilion border to the part that is in contact with opposite lip. It is staged as seen in **Table 35**.

Investigations

- Panendoscopy is part of the work-up: There is a 14% risk of a second primary in the larynx or oesophagus, with one third found at diagnosis or within 1 year
- Imaging
- CXR for synchronous lung primaries (smokers)
- Screening for mandible involvement

Treatment

Small lesions can be excised under LA. The upper lip is suitably anaesthetised with an infraorbital block. This can be done through an extraoral (just lateral to the alar base) or intraoral (above canine) route. A finger is placed on the infraorbital rim to gauge the position and the foramen is found 1 cm below this in the midpupillary line facing inferiorly. The lower lip can be anaesthetised with bilateral mental blocks (nerves can be seen through lower lip mucosa just lateral to canines) but will also require supplemental anaesthesia for the part below the labiomental fold. Attention to oral hygiene is important to reduce complications after surgery, radiotherapy or chemotherapy.

Table 35 TNM staging of the lip						
T1	< 2 cm	N1	< 3 cm	Stage I	T1
T2	> 2 cm < 4 cm	N2	3–6 cm	Stage II	T2
T3	> 4 cm	N3	> 6 cm	Stage III	T3 or N1
T4	> 4 cm and invasion of local structures			Stage IV	T4 or N2 or M1

- Stage I and II: Excisional surgery with 1 cm margins or radiotherapy. The success of local control is the same
- Stage III or IV: Excisional surgery with or without adjuvant radiotherapy

Radiotherapy is useful for positive margins (particularly if re-excision is not possible), lesions with perineural invasion or in the presence of positive nodes. Chemotherapy is not useful for lip cancer.

Neck disease

The lower lip drains to the ipsilateral submental and submandibular nodes, while the central part drains bilaterally. The upper lip drains to parotid, preauricular, facial and submandibular nodes. The incidence of nodal disease is primarily related to diameter of the primary lip lesion and its degree of differentiation. The rate of occult metastasis for lesions < 4 cm (< Stage II) is < 5%.

- Palpable nodes (10%) even though often inflammatory, warrant radical ND. It may also be worth performing a contralateral node sampling
- Clinically negative
  - Stage I and II: Expectant treatment. Salvage surgery (15%) has the same survival rate as elective ND
  - Stage III and IV: Node sampling is recommended

Reconstruction

Preservation of oral competence with maximal aesthetics is the priority. Good functional results depend on the following components:

1. Restoration of muscle continuity
2. Preservation of sensation
3. Maximisation of the aperture

The white roll should be marked preoperatively before LA is injected, but sutures should not be placed through it, as it may cause it to blend in and lose definition. If muscle is not repaired, the scar droop will mirror the muscle droop.

Lower lip reconstruction

The lower lip acts against gravity and is responsible for the oral seal. It retains the salivary pool and resting tone is required to prevent dribbling. If possible, intact sensory and motor function should be maintained. The reconstructive options are outlined in (Table 36).

Defects one third to two thirds

Such defects are reconstructed with local flaps using lip tissue.

- Advancement: These will narrow the commissure. E.g. Gillies and Karapandzic (modification of Gillies that preserves pedicle)
- Rotation: These alter the muscle fibre orientation and require vermilion reconstruction. E.g. McGregor, Nakajima (maintains pedicle)

With the exception of the Abbé flap, most named flaps were originally designed for the lower lip (where most pathology occurs) but can be applied, with modifications, to upper lip defects. The vermilion can be

Table 36 Options for lip reconstruction	
Less than 1/3 (more in elderly)	Direct closure after a V-shaped, shield-shaped, wedge or splayed W-shaped incision, designed to avoid violating the mentolabial crease.
1/3 to 2/3	Local flaps • Commissure: Estlander, Karapandzic • Lateral: Abbé, Karapandzic • Central: Abbé, Karapandzic, Johanson's step (up to 50%)
2/3 to total	• Gillies fan flap, McGregor flap • Webster modification of the Bernard-Burrow
Total	Pedicled or Free flap

restored by buccal advancement, but the movement of bulky and redder mucosa may cause feminisation of appearance and facial hairs may be pulled inwards towards mouth. Alternatives for vermilion reconstruction include tongue flap (two-staged, dividing pedicle after 2 weeks), whereas small defects can be closed with horizontal advancement (A-T/O-T). Tattooing of the lip margin is an alternative.

The Abbé flap produces good results for central or near central defects. It is a transoral cross-lip flap and is designed with its width half as wide as the defect (2 cm limit), with the pedicle on one side. It is based on the inferior labial artery (which runs under the orbicularis muscle, on the lingual side at the level of the vermilion border). A cuff of soft tissue is preserved around the artery to provide venous drainage. The patient has a liquid/soft diet through a wide straw whilst awaiting the second stage 2–3 weeks later. The bridge is divided with a Z-plasty at the donor site to avoid potential notching.

- As the flap is denervated, there may be reduced oral competence. Some sphincteric function returns within a year (60–70%). Sensory recovery may take 2 years and returns in the following order of pain, touch and temperature, and sweating. The transposed segment may trapdoor and move oddly
- It is a good method for reconstructing the philtrum or can be used in combination with bilateral perialar crescentic advancement for wider central upper lip defects. It can also be used for more lateral defects by altering the pedicle position, aiming to leave the largest opening possible for feeding. Bilateral flaps can be used for larger defects

The Estlander flap is a better choice for lateral defects especially those involving commissure. It is similar in principle to the Abbé flap but can be designed as a single stage procedure. Lip tissue is rotated around edge of mouth, which may flatten or round out the commissural angle. This deformity is accentuated when the mouth is open and may be repaired with a commissuroplasty. The flap needs to be designed to be half

as wide but slightly (1–2 mm) longer than the defect. Although the sphincter is reconstructed, the transferred muscle is denervated due to the full thickness incisions severing the nerves. In the presence of an intact commissure, a two-staged procedure, similar to the Abbé, should be used to preserve it.

The McGregor Modification of the Gillies fan flap is used to reconstruct lateral defects, with sphincter repair and mucosal advancement. The flap is raised laterally from base of the defect up to nasolabial fold with a backcut. The medial edge of the flap (which is the lateral edge of the lip defect) is rotated up to become the upper margin of the lip (and thus needs to be covered by a lip advancement). The original Gillies flap was a medial translation instead of a rotational advancement and was thus more distorting. One of the aims of the McGregor is to remove the vermilion tissue with malignant potential. The Nakajima modification (of the McGregor-Gillies flap) preserves the vessels (like the Karapandzic). There is less microstomia compared to the Estlander flap (and Karapandzic) as it recruits a larger amount of tissue. However, the orbicularis oris orientation is changed, and as the flap is denervated, there is limited return of sensation and motor function.

The Karapandzic flap is suitable for central and subtotal defects of lower lip (and can be modified for upper lip defects). It uses upper lip and cheek tissue, which is rotated in as bilateral advancement rotation flaps. The width of the flap is equivalent to the height of the lower lip defect. The incisions around the flap are taken through the skin and subcutaneous tissue whilst preserving the neurovascular bundles by careful blunt dissection. The end of the flaps (1–2 cm) are cut full thickness and approximated to restore muscle continuity. Small Burrows triangles may be excised inferiorly on the chin. Major problems include microstomia (therefore should be limited to defects < two thirds of the lip), commissural distortion and extensive scarring (therefore better in older patients).

The Johanson step technique is used to

reconstruct defects of up to two thirds. It was subsequently modified by Blomgren to preserve the commissure, and a further modification by Grimm for the curved steps. It is in essence, a lip and chin advancement that is more commonly used in Europe. Recently, Taiwanese surgeons have modified it further by altering the composition of each step.

- First step: Full thickness
- Second step: Skin to split muscle
- Third step: Dermis only

Defects greater than two thirds

Few good options exist for reconstruction of wide defects. Surgery often results in a tight inverted lower lip that disappears under the upper lip. Objective evidence of muscle function in reconstructed lips is rarely observed, and in most instances the flap serves as a static sling. They thus serve as a platform for the upper lip to move against. Likewise, sensate reconstruction is emphasised but prospective comparative studies have found no differences in functional outcome. Neurotisation from adjacent tissues may occur if there is sufficient muscle in the flap.

The Bernard-Burrow method of reconstructing subtotal lower lip defects recruits more cheek skin and hence less microstomia compared to the Karapandzic, but at the cost of greater scarring and poor lower lip sensation. Horizontal incisions from commissure to melolabial groove, and long full thickness triangles (Burrows triangles to aid advancement) at the melolabial groove are excised. The lower lip lesion itself is excised as a long V. This allows medial advancement of lower lip/chin tissue.

Webster modified the full thickness triangles to partial thickness (skin and subcutaneous tissue) perialar crescents that are more laterally placed, at the nasolabial fold. The lesion is excised as a trapezium with inferior partial thickness wings. The reconstructed lip is made deliberately tight to act as a static dam to reduce incontinence, although drooling can still be significant. In addition, there is significant scarring especially at the commissures and normal

skin is sacrificed. However, it is achieves good aesthetic results for defects of up to 75% and should not be applied to larger defects, except in patients with substantial cheek laxity. Total lower lip reconstruction usually requires flaps:

- Pedicled: E.g. Deltopectoral or pectoralis major, generally give poor results due to the large bulk and non-functionality
- Free: E.g. Radial forearm with a palmaris longus sling (medial cutaneous nerve of forearm), gracilis, ALT with fascia lata and vastus lateralis (may also be innervated)

Skin taken from outside the head and neck will usually result in a colour mismatch. Functional recovery is usually limited.

Nasolabial flaps are an alternative and can be raised as musculocutaneous flaps (often bulky) or cutaneous flaps based on their very rich subdermal plexus. Bilateral inferiorly based flaps can be used for total defects of lower lip. There are many variations, such as the Von Brun technique or Fuijmori gate flaps (larger triangular flaps rotated on inner corner and the pedicle dissected out, with the ends staggered). These flaps sacrifice less tissue than the Bernard Burrows technique for total lower lip reconstruction. However, the latter gives a better cosmetic result for subtotal defects.

Reconstruction with innervated (motor and sensory) composite (skin, muscle and mucosa) flaps based on depressor and levator anguli oris have also been described.

Upper lip

Reconstruction of the upper lip is more complex, due to presence of the philtrum and the two adjacent lateral subunits. These components must be considered separately in the reconstruction (**Table 37**) and combination procedures are common.

Defects of the philtrum only can be reconstructed with an Abbé flap. Lateral defects (**Table 37**) can be closed directly if <25%, but will distort the upper lip pulling it over to one side. Perialar excision and advancement is thus preferable (can close defects up to 40% this way). FTSG may be an alternative.

Table 37 Options for lower lip reconstruction		
Lateral defects only	< one third	Primary closure
	> one third	Unilateral perialar crescentic flap
Combined lateral and philtrum	Entire lateral lip	Commissure involved: reversed Estlander Commissure not involved: Abbé
	one third–two third	Reverse Karapanzic, Abbé with perialar Advancement (Websters combination)
	> two thirds	Reverse bilateral Gillies or Karapandzic
	Total upper lip	Free or pedicled flap Bilateral Gillies and Abbé Von Brun Bernard Burrows

Further reading

Hanasono M, Langstein HN. Extended Karapandzic
    flaps for near-total and total lower lip defects.
    Plast Reconstr Surg 2011; 127:119–205.

Related topics of interest

- Anterolateral thigh flap
- Neck dissection
- Radial forearm flap
- Squamous cell carcinoma

Liposuction

Illouz, who used blunt cannulae to remove fat under suction, first used the term liposuction. This was an advance over early lipectomies that used unmodified uterine currettes to remove fat, similar to a D&C. The term liposculpture has sometimes been used synonymously, although it was originally used to describe the aspiration and subsequent reinjection of fat.

Liposuction is one of the commonest cosmetic procedures performed and is generally used to reduce focal deposits of adipose tissue that are unresponsive to diet or exercise. It should not be regarded as a method of weight loss or treatment for morbid obesity. Good skin tone is preferable as liposuction relies on tissue elasticity to compensate for the newly 'created' excess skin. The metabolic benefits of liposuction are unclear and controversial (increased HDL, reduction in serum lipids but no changes in glucose or insulin).

Other indications include:

- As an adjunct in abdominoplasty, breast reduction (Hall-Findlay) and treatment of gynaecomastia and lymphoedema
- Harvesting of fat for injection
- Lipomas or pockets of localised fat: Abnormal fat distributions caused by HIV protease inhibitors, Madelung's disease (multiple symmetrical lipomatosis, with deposits of unencapsulated adipose tissue)
- Axillary hyperhidrosis or bromidrosis
- Secondary thinning of flaps

Patient satisfaction tends to be low for the leg, medial thigh and the abdomen in male patients who tend to have more intra-abdominal and subfascial fat. True cellulite will not be addressed by liposuction, which in fact may make it worse.

Subcutaneous fat is divided into superficial and deep compartments:

- The superficial layer (Camper) has a densely packed fibrous stroma with septae. These tethering fibres underlie the formation of cellulite in women. This layer is best kept intact to avoid irregularities of the skin surface
- The deeper layer (Gallaudet) is less compact with sparse septae. The fat is of a deeper orange or yellow colour, and is of variable depth that is dependent on body site. It is thus primarily responsible for shape of the body contour and is the target layer for liposuction. Neurovascular bundles are protected by the stroma, and are relatively safe from damage. Over the dilatable parts of the trunk, fascial condensations form between the deep and superficial layers and are often called Scarpa's fascia

Adipocyte numbers are fixed after adolescence (numbers are genetically determined), but the remaining cells can increase in size (hypertrophy not hyperplasia). Twin studies have shown that there is a significant genetic and gender influence on fat distribution.

Principle of liposuction

The general principle of liposuction is to create a series of tunnels and spaces by evacuation of the intervening fat in the deep layer, that subsequently collapse down. The zones of adherence described by Rohrich, where the skin tightly adheres to the underlying fascia, are areas to avoid, as liposuction is likely to cause contour irregularities. These are:

- Lateral gluteal depression
- Gluteal crease
- Distal posterior thigh
- Medial mid-thigh
- Inferior lateral iliotibial tract

Liposuction at a more superficial level carries a greater risk of skin damage and irregularities, but can induce skin retraction and tightening, which may be desirable. Superficial layer liposuction of the axilla is sometimes used to treat hyperhidrosis.

Types of liposuction

Liposuction techniques can be classified according to the type of suction used and the amount of fluid infiltrated.

Pretunnelling is the process of passing a narrow cannula through the fat layer without suction, to create a pseudoplane that demarcates the most superficial level of the intended treatment. It may make liposuction safer. By comparison, cross tunnelling is to tunnel with suction in approximately perpendicular directions/planes to allow more uniform fat removal with a reduced risk of contour abnormalities.

Types of suction

Vacuum-assisted liposuction is standard liposuction. A vacuum (of approximately 1 atm) sucks fat into the openings of a cannula, while the back and forth motion of the cannula detaches this fat. A suction pump is more efficient for large volumes, but can be performed manually with an attached syringe. The latter is cheap, quiet, less traumatic and is the preferred method, if the fat is to be subsequently re-injected elsewhere.

Ultrasound-assisted liposuction uses a cannula with a 20 kHz mechanical tip vibrator that induces fat fragmentation, which is then aspirated by suction. The cannula must be kept at least 1 cm deep to the skin and moved constantly to prevent skin burns (protective port sleeves are recommended and require longer skin incisions). Although the technique does not necessarily give better results, the effort required is decreased substantially. It is slightly more time consuming due to the extra liquefying step. UAL preserves more fibro-connective tissue with less disruption of blood vessels and nerves, and greater skin contraction. At higher settings, it can disrupt and remove the dense fibrotic parenchyma found in the buttocks, male back, gynaecomastia or secondary procedures.

- VASER (vibration amplification of sound energy at resonance) is a newer variant that uses small solid probes with grooves near the end that increase fragmentation and redistributes some of the energy proximal to the tip. It is a pulsed machine (on for less than half the time) and these combination of factors claim to reduce thermal injury. It has been recently established that VASER does not liquefy fat, but instead separates cells into a fine suspension that can be reinjected

Power-assisted devices use an electrical or pneumatic motor to move the cannula tip back and forth rapidly by 2–4 mm. It may be advantageous for large volume liposuction, particularly those involving fibrous or scarred fat (revisions) with less surgeon fatigue. It is noisy.

Laser-assisted liposuction requires an 'emulsification' step with a laser for about 12 minutes prior to suction. The lipocytes are deflated but membranes remain unruptured after the initial step. Like the UAL, skin tightening can be achieved. External ultrasound (without suction) has also been used but have been shown to be of little demonstrable benefit (no better than massage) at causing cellular disruption. Jet-assisted liposuction uses fluid infiltration to loosen fat prior to suction.

Fluid infiltration

Prior to the development of tumescent and superwet techniques, liposuction was a procedure with a significant amount of blood loss (up to 40% of aspirate). Tumescent and superwet infiltration techniques have made liposuction much safer by reducing blood loss and have also been used as a delivery method for large area local anaesthesia. Wet and dry techniques are of historical interest only (**Table 38**).

- Only 1–3% of aspirate is blood due to the vasoconstrictive effect of the infiltrate. Approximately 20% of infiltrate is aspirated
- There is no need for a general anaesthetic for smaller procedures and analgesia up to 24 hours postoperatively is possible. Even when 35 mg/kg of lignocaine is used (Klein), maximum plasma levels at 11–15 hours only reach half of toxic levels (5–6 µg/ml, seizures occur at levels > 10 µg/ml). The absorption of lignocaine is slower due to the vasoconstriction, the low vascularity of fat and the low concentration of lignocaine used
- Early signs of toxicity are subjective: Circumoral numbness, light-headedness, drowsiness

Table 38 Comparison of tissue infiltration techniques for liposuction		
Technique	**Infiltrate**	**Blood loss**
Dry	None Effect of aspiration is more obvious but no longer in common use.	May have significant blood loss, up to 40% of aspirate (average 25%). Needs GA
Wet	Infiltration of 200–400 ml fluid (mixture of saline, adrenaline, lignocaine, bicarbonate) per average area suctioned	Blood loss around 20–25% of aspirate, reduced further to 15% by addition of adrenaline (Hettler 1983)
Superwet	One mm of infiltrate per mm of aspirate, using saline, adrenaline and lignocaine (added later)	Reduces blood to less than 2–4 ml/L of aspirate
Tumescent	Infiltrate to skin turgor (2–3 ml/ml aspirate) • 1 L of saline/lactated ringers • 1 ml of 1:1000 adrenaline (giving 1 in 10^6) • 50 ml of 1% lignocaine • Bicarbonate (variable) Many variations, but few studies to determine which is best.	Less blood loss, 1–2 ml/L of aspirate Vasoconstriction begins at 10 min but is more effective after 20 min, and lasts for 6–10 hours. Allows liposuction to be performed under LA with or without sedation.

- In anaesthetised patients, the first signs may be cardiac
- Adding fluid allows a smoother mechanical action. Superwet techniques involve smaller volumes than the tumescent techniques and thus have relatively fewer problems with fluid overload (and less time spent on infiltration), but the lower dose of adrenaline translates to slightly greater blood loss. While clearly superior to dry or wet liposuction, the advantages of tumescent over superwet liposuction (and vice versa) are unclear. In practice, modern liposuction tends to be somewhere between the two
- Typically, a long 3 mm blunt multiple hole infiltration cannula is used (fluids should be warmed) and the endpoint (for tumescence) is firm turgor with blanching and a fountain sign (pressure causes a jet of infiltrate out from the infiltration site). A *peau d'orange* appearance is a sign that the fluid is being infiltrated too superficially. Some areas have lighter and looser fat, such as the abdomen and hold more tumescent fluid, while the denser regions of the back fill more quickly

Preoperative considerations

Patients should be in good health, usually ASA I/II. Preoperative photography and thorough documentation including recording the aspirated volumes are important as some patients gain weight after the procedure.

- Liposuction is generally contraindicated in those with disorders of coagulation and severe systemic disease. Medications that affect coagulation, including herbal remedies, should be stopped 2 weeks prior
- Medications that are metabolised by hepatic cytochrome p450 such as cimetidine, erythromycin and β-blockers may potentially increase lignocaine toxicity

Procedure

Prophylactic antibiotics are commonly used, although infections are rare. The patient is best marked upright, with concentric circles to mark the contours. Access sites are best planned in advance, hidden in inconspicuous sites but permitting access to the areas required. The sizes of incision sites tend to be inversely related to the number used, whilst using multiple sites for cross tunnelling reduces the risk of localised depressions.

- Stop regularly to assess results and feather the edges. Fanning is desirable and the process begins superficially first and then proceeds to deeper layers. The procedure is stopped when the desired appearance is achieved, satisfactory pinch testing (1–3 cm), when blood appears in the tubing or when there is a gritty feel to the process. Undercorrection is preferable to overcorrection

Postoperative

- Incision sites are left open and covered with absorbent pads. Patients should be warned of copious leakage for up to 48 hours. Furnishings may require protection
- Keep the patient warm and comfortable. Patients can go home as soon as they feel well enough although larger scale procedures may warrant an overnight stay
- Immediate postoperative pressure garments (17–21 mmHg, particularly for the lower limb) are used to decrease bruising, avoid unevenness and improve skin retraction. The use of pressure garments varies, but is usually worn until drainage through the incision sites stop. Gentle support is advisable for subsequent period (usually 6 weeks) to reduce seroma formation, but excessive compression at this stage may actually promote oedema by blocking lymphatic drainage
- On average, patients should expect to have 1 week off from work after large volume liposuction under GA

The definition of large volume liposuction is arbitrary, but the American Society of Aesthetic Plastic Surgeons strongly recommends a maximum limit of 5 L per session. There is an average 4-unit haemoglobin drop with 8 L liposuction and there may be an increased risk of TED. It may be safer to stage liposuction procedures. Other measures include:

- Avoid volume overload: Administration of one quarter of the volume over 5 L aspirated is recommended
- Reduce lignocaine dosage
- Monitor vital signs especially urinary output

Complications of liposuction

Complications increase with higher volume injections, higher volumes of fat aspiration, simultaneous procedures (10% average), inadequate monitoring and poor patient selection. Some make the distinction of undesired sequelae (irregularities, hypoaesthesia that improves after 3–6 months, oedema, bruising and discolouration) that are expected to a certain extent.

- A 0.1–0.5% major complication rate is quoted in the literature. There have been isolated reports of deaths from PE, fat embolism and necrotising fasciitis
  - Full DVT/PE prophylaxis according to local protocols
  - Some studies show that all patients with a sizeable liposuction procedure (> 900 ml) have fat particles in their blood. However, this asymptomatic form rarely translates, as the incidence of an overt fat embolism syndrome (tachypnoea, tachycardia, petechiae with severe hypoxaemia leading to death) remains extremely rare
- Fluid overload: The need for (additional) fluid delivery is controversial. The exact resuscitation formula is less important than good record keeping, good monitoring (catheter) and communication with the anaesthetist. In general, fluid replacement is not necessary for small volume aspirations (< 1–1.5 L with the tumescent technique). When aspirating more than 2 L, fluid replacement and an overnight stay is prudent but not mandatory. With larger volume (> 4–5 L) aspirations, meticulous fluid balance takes on greater importance
- Other complications such as lignocaine toxicity and visceral injury are rare. Less serious problems include:
  - Damage to neurovascular structures causing haemorrhage, bruising (lasting 2–3 weeks, may be reduced with postoperative compression), paraesthesia, skin trauma and hyperpigmentation. Patients should be aware that a certain degree of neuropraxia is to be expected
  - Contour irregularity: Wait for at least 6 months to allow swelling and changes in skin elasticity to settle before revising. Irregularities can be more common with larger cannulae and with subdermal suctioning
  - Seromas: May be more common with UAL

Further reading

Wells JH, Hurvitz KA. An evidence-based approach to liposuction. Plast Reconstr Surg 2011; 127:949–54.

Related topics of interest

- Abdominoplasty
- Gynaecomastia
- Hidradenitis suppurativa and hyperhidrosis
- Local anaesthetics
- Lymphoedema

Local anaesthetics

Current commonly used anaesthetics include:

- Lignocaine (lidocaine) was developed in Sweden in the 1940s and is a good anaesthetic. It is often combined with adrenaline (epinephrine) to prolong its effect
  - Adrenaline: Reduces local blood flow thus reduces the systemic absorption of lignocaine. This prolongs its action, reduces the dose of LA required and reduces the risk of toxicity, and thus permits a larger dose to be used. The time for onset of vasoconstriction is 5–7 minutes (note that maximal vasoconstriction occurs at 20 minutes, Lalonde 2013) depending on the concentration used. Concentrations of 0.8–1 in 10^6 are sufficient with 1 in 200,000 perfectly adequate for most clinical situations. No additional benefit is seen when the concentration is increased beyond 0.8–1 in 10^5
  - Adrenaline is safe for use with local flaps (studies have not shown increased failure rates, except in delayed flaps). Although traditionally dogma recommends its avoidance in fingers, toes, penis, nose and ears, actual use is fairly common and safe. Thomson dispels the myths of adrenaline use in the finger (PRS 2007)
  - There is a risk of arrhythmias with adrenaline and its use is contraindicated in phaeochromocytoma, severe hypertension, hyperthyroidism, severe peripheral vascular disease and Raynaud's disease
- Bupivacaine is longer-acting than lignocaine (can be combined), but its slow onset of action limits its wider use. It also has a higher risk of toxicity. A direct effect on Purkinje fibres can promote re-entry rhythms and negative inotropy. It is contraindicated for use in Biers blocks, as it has been associated with several deaths even at low concentrations. Levobupivacaine is the isolated S(-)-isomer

of bupivacaine that has lower cardiotoxicity. Ropivacaine is another S(-)-isomer and has less cardiac toxicity and more specificity for sensory neurones over motor but also less potent

- Prilocaine has a duration of action and potency similar to that of lignocaine, but it is less toxic. It is generally considered to be one of the safest LAs, and is therefore recommended for intravenous regional anaesthesia, and is a constituent of EMLA. However, it can cause methaemoglobinaemia in susceptible individuals. This is a rare complication that causes cyanosis, tachypnoea, dyspnoea and death (treat with IV methylene blue)
- Amethocaine is a potentially toxic ester that is only used topically in ophthalmic drops and as Ametop for cannulation sites in children. It is cheaper, quicker acting (30 min) and longer lasting than EMLA. Its vasodilatory property may facilitate IV cannulation particularly in children (even in premature babies)

Action of local anaesthetics

Lignocaine causes reversible blockade of voltage-gated sodium channels by binding to a site on the inside of the axon. It affects C pain fibres first as these are thin and unmyelinated (and subsequently cold, heat, light touch and deep pressure).

LAs are generally weak bases and equilibrium exists between the non-ionised and ionised (charged) forms. Only the non-ionised form can cross lipid membranes, but it is the charged form that is active and binds to the target (inside axon). With a higher H+ (lower pH), more of the cation form is present, resulting in less penetration. Lignocaine is about 25% diffusible at body pH. At abscesses or in areas of inflammation where the pH is lower (typically 5–6), the amount of the diffusible form is reduced substantially and its efficacy is poorer. Solutions with adrenaline are often buffered to a lower pH and hence the block is similarly less efficacious. Lipid solubility influences potency and the speed of onset, which is most related to the pKa. The lower the pKa the better the absorption into the nerve, while a higher pKa provides for a better block. The closer the pKa is to the local pH, the more the non-ionised lipid-soluble form, and the more rapid the onset.

Types of local anaesthetics

Examples of LAs and their metabolism are described in **Table 39**.

For amides, true allergy should be distinguished from toxicity. Most reports of allergy to lignocaine are probably due to inadvertent intravascular injection or due to overdosage. Allergies while rare are likely from the preservative agent rather than the anaesthetic itself. Preservative-free preparations are available that may reduce this risk.

Toxicity

Avoiding toxicity/overdosing require knowledge of the maximal doses, which are related to body weight, with adjustments in the presence of liver and renal disease. Toxicity may be potentiated in pregnancy or at the extremes of age. It is particularly important to calculate doses precisely for children. Under most circumstances, peak levels of LA occur after 10–25 minutes, although absorption is dependent on many factors such as the vascularity of tissues, dosage and concentration. Once absorbed, the LA will move to organs with higher perfusion, and thus the cardiovascular and central nervous systems will be the most affected. The commonest cause of toxicity is inadvertent intravascular injection. Lignocaine is a type Ib antiarrhythmic (and is a common treatment for ventricular tachycardias) but can cause arrhythmias itself.

- Early signs (3–6 µg/ml) of toxicity include circumoral numbness, light-headedness, tinnitus and a metallic taste. These may be missed if the patient is sedated/anaesthetised. Cardiac effects such as negative inotropy, negative chronotropy and arrhythmias may be particularly resistant to treatment. Initially there may be tachycardia (probably due to CNS excitation), but with more severe toxicity there is bradycardia, hypotension and asystole
- Intermediate signs include anxiety and tremors. CNS toxicity is a combination of direct effects and hypoxia. First, there is a depressant effect allowing loss of cortical control of lower centres leading to excitation (twitch and convulsions), whilst higher levels cause depression (coma and respiratory depression, late signs)
- CNS toxicity tends to occur before cardiovascular toxicity and is easier to manage

Care is largely supportive with standard resuscitative protocols. Benzodiazepines are useful for seizures. Bradycardia is usually temporary but may need pacing, if persistent (typically resistant to treatment). Intravenous intralipid has been recently used successfully for local anaesthetic toxicity. These are liposomes that attempt to reduce plasma levels of the local anaesthetic by providing a fat-soluble medium for it to partition into.

Lignocaine is an LA with moderate potency and duration (similar to Prilocaine),

Table 39 Metabolism of local anaesthetics		
Types	**Examples**	**Metabolism**
Esters	Amethocaine, benzocaine, cocaine	Metabolised rapidly by plasma pseudocholinesterases thus short acting; except cocaine, which is metabolised by liver (slower). Structurally related to para-aminobenzoic acid (PABA) and can cause allergy in one third of patients, although most cases are minor with temporary itch or rash. Higher pKa (8.5–8.9).
Amides	Lignocaine, prilocaine	Metabolised by liver at a slower rate. Lower risk of allergy but may trigger malignant hyperthermia Excretion in urine (less than 10%) pKa closer to body pH (7.6–8.1)

Table 40 Characteristics of lignocaine and bupivacaine			
Local anaesthetic	Onset	Maximum dose (adrenaline)	Duration (adrenaline)
Lignocaine	Rapid – less than 4 min depending on concentration	3.5–4.5 mg/kg (7 mg/kg)	1–2 h (2–4 h)
Bupivacaine	2–10 min	2.5 mg/kg (3 mg/kg)	4 h (8 h)

whilst bupivacaine has high potency and long duration. Their respective times until onset, the maximum doses and the durations of action are given in **Table 40**.

- 1% = 10 mg/ml, therefore one can give 4 × 50 = 200 mg or 20 ml of 1% plain lignocaine in a patient with a 50 kg body weight
  - Lignocaine will still work at 0.25% (or lower), but onset will be delayed
- Adrenaline will still work at concentrations of 1 in 1,000,000 but will take longer. In practical terms, no more than 1 in 200,000 is needed. The addition of adrenaline increases the maximal doses of lignocaine that can be used but has less of an effect on bupivacaine. As a general guideline, do not inject more than 20 ml of 1 in 200,000 adrenaline in 10 min

Potential problems using local anaesthetics

- The area injected does not become numb: This may be an error of technique, but in rare cases this may also represent anomalous anatomy. True resistance to LAs is rare, but has been occasionally reported. Commercially prepared lignocaine with adrenaline is stable only when kept refrigerated. Prolonged exposure to room temperature reduces its efficacy substantially
- Severe pain: A shooting pain may occur if the needle impinges directly on the nerve. Withdraw the needle and discontinue injection in that location. There may be prolonged numbness lasting weeks to months, but usually no permanent damage results
- Prolonged pain/numbness/paraesthesia: This may be due to direct injury to nerves, which is a particular risk when infiltrating after partial/previous block.

In addition, there is individual variation in the susceptibility to the drug or it may have been inadvertently injected under the periosteum, forming a reservoir
- Ischaemia with pain and blanching may be due to inadvertent intra-arterial injection of LA with or without adrenaline (or Epipens). The half-life of adrenaline is 2 min (although the vasoconstrictive effect is longer lasting) and usually no permanent damage results. Aspirating prior to injection may reduce the risk
- Signs of ischaemia (rare, 3%) and can be treated with phentolamine (either infiltration or intra-arterial), but can take up to 1–2 hours to reverse blanching. It may be repeated as needed
- Tachycardia: Injection of vasoconstrictor into the circulation may quicken the pulse or cause arrhythmias, but this usually passes within a minute

Reducing the pain of injection

- Warm the anaesthetic
- Use a needle of the smallest calibre possible and minimise the number of times you need to enter the skin. Try to inject sequentially so that you inject through partially anaesthetised skin
- Inject slowly
- Avoid inflamed areas. Efficacy is reduced and there is an increased risk of infection
- Part of the burning sensation is due to the low pH (4–5) caused by the preservatives. Buffering the solution with 0.1 ml of 1.26% bicarbonate per ml of LA will reduce this and also speed up the onset of action. Due to the need to add bicarbonate manually, it is relatively inconvenient and is susceptible to error

Mixing LAs may improve profiles, such as combining a fast, short-acting agent with a slow, long-acting agent. A typical example is a lignocaine-bupivacaine mix.

Topical anaesthetics

EMLA (eutectic mixture of local anaesthetics – 2.5% prilocaine and 2.5% lignocaine) is often used to anaesthetise the skin of cannulation sites, especially in children, but unfortunately does not reduce apprehension (eutectic means that it is a mixture with a melting point lower than either constituent alone). The speed of action varies by site depending on blood flow. The effect is evident after 15 minutes on the face, but may take up to 60 minutes in other areas. Roughly 1 mm depth is anaesthetised per 30 minutes, up to a maximum of 5 mm at 120 minutes (90 min with 30 min wait) and the anaesthesia lasts 3–4 hours. It has an unwanted vasoconstrictor effect (skin blanches) as it potentially makes cannulation more difficult. This effect lasts for 30–90 minutes and is followed by vasodilatation after 180 minutes. Due to the prilocaine content, there is a risk of methaemoglobinaemia in sensitive patients and is therefore not recommended for use in the very young and infants.

For maximum effect, it needs to be applied generously and covered with an occlusive dressing such as Tegaderm. Some cream should be visible at the end of the administration period as an indicator of sufficient quantities used. Treated zones are usually obvious (blanching) but it is wise to mark out the treated area, if used for procedures such as harvesting of a SSG. Alternatives include:

- Ametop (4% amethocaine): Works within 30 min. Price restricts its use to children
- ELA-Max 4 (4% lignocaine)
- ELA-Max 5 (5% lignocaine) delivered as liposomes, faster onset and longer duration

Further reading

Wolfe JW, Butterworth JF. Local anesthetic systemic toxicity: an update on mechanisms and treatment. Curr Opin in Anaesthesiol, 2011; 24:561–66.

Related topics of interest

- Liposuction
- Suturing

Local flaps and flap classification

Skin has a rich blood supply in excess of its metabolic needs (related to thermoregulation and metabolism) that is organised into several plexi:

- The subcutaneous plexus at level of superficial fascia
- The subdermal plexus that provides the main supply to the skin with arterioles and is sensitive to thermoregulation
- The subepidermal plexus is mainly nutritive and thermoregulatory. It comprises vessels with very little muscle in their walls

This rich redundant blood supply provides the basis for flaps.

A local flap is simply a flap that uses tissue adjacent to the defect. Numerous classifications exist, a commonly used one categorises flaps by composition, contiguity and movement.

- Random pattern: Vascularity is dependent on the (random) subdermal plexus and not on known vessel. Such flaps have a recommended maximum width to length ratio that is site-dependant: Leg = 1:1, Face up to 1:6. The length is limited by the perfusion pressure (must be above critical closing pressure of the arterioles), and widening of the flap only works up to a point as a wider flap base will only recruit more vessels at the same pressure
- Axial pattern: Recognised blood supply from direct artery (running within or close to fascia/subcutaneous tissue) or from perforators from branches of a deeper axial vessel running either in a septum or through muscle

The concept of angiosomes (the 3D block of tissue supplied by a particular artery, Taylor) is useful. An angiosome represents the safe mass of tissue that can be transferred on that supplying vessel, often together with the adjacent angiosome (dynamic territory). Adjacent cutaneous arteries are connected by true anastomoses (no change in calibre) or choke vessels (reduced calibre with more smooth muscle).

Delay is the surgical interruption of part of the blood supply of a flap at a stage before its transfer, with aim of improving survival of the flap. A period of 7–14 days is sufficient and the adequacy of perfusion can be checked with IV fluorescein and a Wood's lamp. The exact mechanism(s) are not fully understood, but include:

- Opening of choke vessels between angiosomes
- Increased axiality of vessels
- Sympathectomy with vasodilatation
- Improved tolerance to ischaemia
- Hyperadrenergic (vasoconstrictive) state after surgery diminished

Local flaps can be classified according to mode of movement of the flap into the defect:

- Advancement: Flap slides forwards without rotation or lateral movement. It relies on skin elasticity and may be facilitated by small Burrows triangles or pantographic expansion by widening the base and incurving the incision. Some so-called advancement flaps, such as cheek flaps have an element of rotation. The greater the angle moved, the shorter the flap effectively becomes
- Transposition: Flap moves laterally on a pivot point and carried over intervening normal skin. It differs from rotation flaps in that the flaps are usually square/ rectangular and their axis is mostly linear. The distance from end of flap from the pivot point should be longer than distance to edge of the defect
- Rotation: These flaps are usually semicircular and move around a pivot near the defect through an arc of rotation. A backcut (in or out, to change the tension vector) or Burrow's triangle may be needed to facilitate movement but the benefit is often modest
  - Many flaps combine transposition and rotation and may best be called pivot flaps

- As shortening occurs, the greater the angle the flap is rotated, the flap should be designed with a wider arc than apparently necessary to compensate for this
- Others:
  - Interpolation: The flap moves laterally into a defect that is not immediately adjacent. There is a bridge of tissue in between (also called islanded)
  - Crane principle (Millard): A flap is moved onto an ungraftable defect bed and then returned to the donor site after 3 weeks, leaving a graftable defect bed

Specific flaps

The Limberg or rhomboid flap aims to close a defect that is an equilateral parallelogram with angles of 60° and 120°. Four flaps can be designed around the defect. The Dufourmentel is a variant on this with different angles and a shift in the axis of flap, along a line that bisects the short diagonal and the continuation of long side. Flaps should be designed to have a final donor scar parallel to RTSL and to utilise areas of skin excess.

- The reading man flap is an alternative to the Limberg flap that results in less distortion, a shorter scar and less sacrifice of tissue. It is most suited for a circular defect (alternatives include double V-Y advancements, double transposition flaps and skin grafts). The long central limb from the tangent is perpendicular to an RSTL and 150% of the defect diameter, a second limb runs from the end of this line at 60° to touch the opposite/parallel tangent, and a third limb from the beginning of the first limb at 45°. The flap and defect will close as a tight '5' or 'S' scar. There are two flaps (thus sometimes called unequal Z-plasties) in the reading man, versus only the one in a Limberg flap
- Bilobed flap (modified by Zitelli): The double transposition flaps lie at 45° and 90° to the defect respectively. They are of decreasing size but increasing length. This flap is useful for certain areas, such as the nose and axilla

The Z-plasty is the transposition of two adjacent triangular flaps that can be used to:

- Increase length: Angles are important to optimise the length gained
- Change scar direction: Final scar orientation is more important than any length gain, hence angles are of lesser concern

Z-plasties gain vertical length at the expense of transverse laxity. Classically, the flaps have equal sides and angles of 60° that provide a theoretical 75% gain in length. They can be designed with angles of 30° to 90°, which increases length gain as the angle is increased, but at the expense of increased tension and increasingly difficult inset. The tension in 90-90 Z-plasty is ten times that of a 30-30 Z-plasty, although the former can be divided into two flaps, two 45-45 Z-plasties), reducing tension somewhat. The central limb changes direction to become perpendicular to the original direction, and should be planned to be parallel to an RTSL, where possible. For scar revisions, there is less freedom to choose the direction, and additional incisions will roughly double the length of scars.

- Z-plasties can also be used for lengthening scars (releasing contracture) and to treat trapdoor scars ('U' or circular)
- Multiple Z-plasties
  - Serial flaps: Length gain is additive but the tension affects neighbouring flaps, thus reducing gain by about 75%. The double-opposing Z-plasty (125% gain) is an example of flaps in series, whilst a four flap Z-plasty is a parallel arrangement with 100% gain
  - The five-flap plasty or jumping man flap incorporates a V-Y advancement giving an additional 50% scar lengthening over a double opposing Z-plasty alone (125%)

The W-plasty was first described by Borges and consists of multiple small triangles that need to be matched up on the other side (use a template for one side and shift it for the other side) for interdigitation. The edge is undermined slightly. The new scar lines will fall close to or near RTSLs by chance only. In addition, there is no lengthening effect and the small flaps may heal unevenly. The triangles must be small to minimise excision of normal tissue, and to not make the scar look worse.

The basic keystone flaps (Behan) can be used for closure of an elliptical defect by a neighbouring islanded flap of a keystone shape (see **Figure 11**). It is of the same width but its length is determined by intersection of the lines. The edges are released with blunt dissection with no undermining below the flap. The deep fascia may be divided, only if necessary. Bilateral keystone flaps can be used to close larger defects. Behan describes the 'red dot sign' that occurs at suture points, where arterial blood oozes onto the surface of flap (but not the other side). There may be a vascular flare, and there are claims of a sympathectomy-type effect that has not been proven.

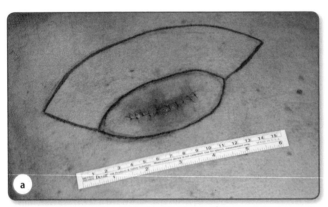

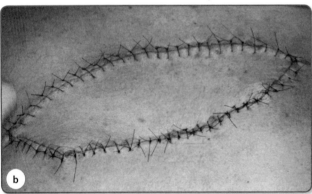

Figure 11 Use of the keystone flap to close the defect (a), following wider local excision of a melanoma scar on the back (b). The flap is mobilised by blunt dissection around the cut border and the ends are closed in a VY manner.

Further reading

Seyhan T, Caglar B. 'Reading man flap' design for reconstruction of circular infraorbital and malar skin defects. Dermatol Surg 2008; 34:1536–43.

Related topic of interest

- Burns reconstruction

Lower limb trauma and leg reconstruction

Lower limb trauma

Important considerations in trauma involving long bone fractures include:

- Severity of injury: High or low energy.
- Bone injury
- Soft tissue injury
- Skin injury

Infection at the fracture site is of major concern, whether open or closed. Repeated debridement of necrotic tissues may be required and may lead to significant defects of:

- Bone
  - Small bone gap < 3 cm: Bone grafts taken from the iliac crest may be sufficient (taking about 9 months to heal) if vascularity is good. It may be delayed for 6–12 weeks until soft tissue cover is complete. Temporary gentamicin impregnated MMA spacers may be used in the meantime
  - Moderate bone gap (4–8 cm): The limb may first be shortened by apposing the bone ends and then gradually distracted with an Ilizarov frame over 18 months (see 'Hypoplastic facial conditions'). Excessive shortening may kink vessels
    - Bone transport is an alternative where the fragments are held at length. Osteotomies are made in the cortex elsewhere and the segment distracted to meet the other fracture end. Normal distraction is preferable when the soft tissue is also deficient, although the use of free flaps to cover a bone transport has been described
  - Massive losses > 8 cm require vascularised bone, such as the fibula flap. It hypertrophies but is still weaker than the tibia, with an average success rate of 88% and weight bearing resumed at 15 months (double barrelling may be better). Bone transport may work for defects up to 12 cm
- Skin and soft tissue

Delayed closure/secondary healing and skin grafts are good alternatives when bone is not exposed. However the paucity of tissue in the pretibial area prohibits the primary closure of many open fractures. Exposed fractures require rigid fixation and vascularised coverage.

Scoring systems

Several scoring systems exist for the grading of injuries, and can be useful for assessment, documentation and for comparisons. Generally, they evaluate the vascularity, bone, soft tissue and nerves. An ideal scoring system should be able to predict which injuries are suitable for reconstruction and those that have a better outcome with amputation. None of the scoring systems do this reliably.

MESS (mangled extremity severity score)

- Skeletal soft tissue injury (1–4)
- Limb ischaemia (1–3, doubled if ischaemia is present for more than 6 hours)
- Shock (0–2)
- Age (0–2)

Byrd/Cierny

I. Low energy, oblique fracture, < 2 cm clean wound
II. Moderate energy, comminuted fracture, > 2 cm wound, moderate contusion with viable muscle
III. High energy, significant comminution or bone defect, skin loss or devitalised muscle
IV. III with crush, degloving and arterial injury

Gustillo and Anderson

Gustillo and Anderson scoring system is given in **Table 41.**

Reconstruction is required for Gustillo IIIB/C injuries. Francel reviewed IIIB patients who had limb salvage versus below knee amputation (BKA) and found that the former group had a lower return to work rate by

Table 41	Gustilllo and Anderson classification of open tibial fractures (subdivision of III by Gustillo in 1984) is frequently used but has its limitations
I	Wound less than 1 cm, clean.
II	Longer than 1 cm but without extensive soft tissue damage.
IIIA	Adequate soft tissue coverage despite damage in the form of lacerations or flaps. High energy trauma (irrespective of wound size).
IIIB	Extensive soft tissue injury with periosteal stripping and bone exposure requiring coverage. Usually grossly contaminated.
IIIC	Arterial injury requiring repair.

42 months, took longer to reach full weight bearing, with higher hospital costs. However with longer follow-up, patients with salvaged limbs are more likely to return to work with some taking more than 10 years after the injury. In short, salvage is a long complicated process and both patients and surgeons need to be aware of this.

IIIC injuries may be successfully salvaged with vascular repair in selected cases with a late amputation rate of only 7%. However, salvage may not be the optimal option.

Amputation

Salvaged limbs may function very poorly; require prolonged rehabilitation and eventual amputation. Patient morale is very poor if late amputation is eventually required after failed reconstruction, and represents the worst of both worlds. Making a correct early decision is important, but so is allowing sufficient time for the patient and family to accept the situation.

- BKA greatly reduces the work of walking compared to AKA (25% increase vs. 65% increase over no amputation), and the quality of life is significantly better. Midfoot amputations (Symes) have little functional advantage over BKA. The ideal length is at least 6 cm of tibia below the tubercle. In practice, as much as soft tissue possible is preserved for cover. In selected cases, a (free) flap may be used to cover the stump

Management of open tibial fractures

Open tibial fractures are a severe injury and a team approach is recommended. In the UK, there are well-established guidelines (Table 42) agreed between orthopaedic surgeons and plastic surgeons with a common aim of salvaging a limb that will be more functional than an amputation, if appropriate.

History: Delineate the level of energy transfer as it determines the severity of damage. High-energy trauma is indicated by:

- History: RTA, fall from height.
- X-ray features: Multiple or widely displaced fragments, air in tissues and segmental fractures of more than one fracture in same limb.

Other important considerations include:

- Crush, entrapment and ischaemia
- Contamination
- Closed degloving: Tissues have a 'boggy' feel or looseness
- Compartment syndrome is not uncommon (9%), even in open fractures, as some compartments may remain closed and the syndrome localised (see 'Compartment syndrome'). The main feature is pain out of proportion to the injury
  - With an unconscious patient, objective monitoring is needed, either in the form of serial pressure measurements or continuous methods. All compartments should be measured
  - If in doubt, treat actively with decompression (see 'Acute Burns')

The emphasis is on speedy treatment and in most cases, aiming for soft tissue coverage of fixed bones by day 5. The infection risk should be minimised by avoiding unnecessary wound exposure. The use of photos taken at first examination should eliminate the need for repeated examination. Antibiotics are

Table 42 Typical protocol for management of open tibial fractures	
Day 0	Combined orthopaedic and plastic surgery consultant assessment or communication with management plan. • Wound debridement and fracture stabilisation • Compartment monitoring
Day 2	Second look • Further debridement, as needed • Soft tissue cover, if possible
Day 4	Third look, if required Soft tissue cover

paramount and anti-tetanus therapy should be given as appropriate.

First procedure

Obviously dead or contaminated tissue is removed meticulously in a zone-by-zone fashion, with view to re-explore within 48 hours to ensure that the debridement has been sufficient.

- Lavage with at least 6 L of crystalloid is common. High-pressure pulse lavage is not recommended. There is little evidence for lavage with antiseptic/antibiotic solutions
- Skin should be trimmed back to viable bleeding dermis. With avulsions, tissue may initially appear viable and subsequently thrombose. Fluorescein and Wood's lamp may help in cases of doubt. Nonviable skin may be salvaged as graft but only on the day of injury
- Muscle: Signs such as colour and contractility can be unreliable. The threshold for reinspection needs to be low and serial débridements may be necessary. Muscle loss is not an absolute contraindication for salvage/ reconstruction (ankle fusions can great simplify muscle needs)
- Bone: All loose and free-floating fragments are removed. It is easier to reconstruct a defect than to manage the consequences of inadequate excision, such as non-union and infection. Bone repair is performed prior to vascular reconstruction
- Fracture stabilisation:
- External fixation: Pins positioned with caution to avoid compromising skin flaps or access to vessels
- Interlocking medullary nail: Reamed pins allow better bone healing and are stronger, but disrupt endosteal blood supply

- Plating: Preserve periosteum and adherent soft tissues

Stabilisation should be definitive and metalwork should be covered immediately with good soft tissue. Thus intramedullary nails and plates are unsuitable options if serial debridement is still anticipated. For bone gaps, see above.

- Nerves should be repaired where possible, but the prognosis is relatively poor due in part to the long distances involved. Sensation is important. Reconstruction with sensory loss to the plantar foot from tibial nerve injury is not an absolute contraindication. Many can still ambulate on this limb, as long as they remain aware of the potential problems

Soft tissue closure (Table 43)

- Skin grafts require vascular recipient beds and take poorly on infected beds
- Local flaps: Although technically simple, planning is of paramount importance. They can be rather unattractive with dog-ears, long scars and require skin grafts for the donor. In general, large FC or muscle flaps need to be raised to cover relatively small defects
  - Fasciocutaneous flaps can be raised on either side of the calf, usually proximally based. FC flaps are bigger, more versatile and of better quality compared to local muscle flaps
    - All three major vessels in the lower leg give off perforators, but ones from the PTA tend to be more reliable and predictable. Using a single sturdy perforator facilitates rotation for propeller flaps. The PTA perforators are located at a distance of 5, 10 and 15 cm from the medial

Table 43 Options for soft tissue cover of leg/tibia	
Proximal 1/3 of tibia	Proximally based medial or lateral fasciocutaneous flap Medial or lateral head of gastrocnemius: The use of the medial prevents potential injury to peroneal nerve, is bulkier and longer (lateral limited mainly to small lateral defects)
Middle 1/3	Proximal/distally based medial or lateral fasciocutaneous flap Proximally based soleus Flexor digitorum longus, extensor hallucis longus: Small defects only Free flap
Lower 1/3	Free flaps are first choice Local distally-based posterior tibial perforator flaps (limited reach) Cross leg flap

MM to tibial tuberosity

malleolus, along a line between it and the tibial tuberosity

- Muscle: Reliable and useful to cover bare bone and combat deep infection. The commonest choice is gastrocnemius (plus skin graft) for knee and proximal third tibia (and very small defects in the middle third)
- Free flaps are mainly used to cover large and distal defects. They also bring in new blood supply. End-to-side anastomoses allow distal run off whilst other options include a 'T' anastomosis or flow-through flaps to simultaneously reconstruct short vascular gaps. Preoperative angiograms are generally not necessary if the distal pulses are normal
- Cross leg flaps are rarely used and still need a vascular bed to sustain the flap before division after 2–3 weeks. They should be regarded as a last option in young patients. Immobilisation for the requisite 2–3 weeks may cause contractures or DVTs

Lower third leg

The tibia has a subcutaneous border that is easily exposed. The lack of local skin laxity and muscles make reconstruction of the lower third of leg particularly difficult. Free flaps are the workhorse method here, but local flap options exist.

- Early leg flaps were raised in subcutaneous plane and were thus dependent on the subdermal plexus and had strict length-width ratio restrictions. The subsequent FC flaps, such as Ponten's superflap, are perforator-supplied, allowing longer, larger flaps with better survival
- Reverse flow FC flaps based on the posterior tibial, peroneal and anterior tibial as well as reverse flow sural artery may be raised to cover heel and foot dorsum but venous congestion is a risk
- Skin-sparing distally-based lateral adipofascial flaps have also been described
- Cross leg flaps

Further reading

El-Sabbagh AH. Skin perforator flaps: an algorithm for leg reconstruction. J Reconstr Microsurg 2011; 27(9):511-23.

Related topic of interest

- Acute burns
- Compartment syndrome
- Hypoplastic facial conditions
- Vacuum wound closure

Lymphoedema

Lymphoedema is the abnormal collection of protein-rich fluid in the interstitium causing swelling that is limited to tissues superficial to deep fascia. It is caused by a reduced efficiency of lymph clearance due to an underlying lymphatic problem that may be congenital (primary) or acquired (secondary).

There is on average, a 7 mmHg pressure gradient driving fluid from the blood vessels into the tissues. The lymphatic system returns proteins and fluid that have accumulated in the interstitial space to the venous system, with 100% of the total body albumin recirculated every 48 hours. The lymphatic transport capacity has an inbuilt resilience factor (flow can increase to 10 times resting levels) and symptoms will not appear until this resilience factor has been nullified. During this latent period, the smooth muscle cells become fibroblast-like, the vessels become dilated with a fibrinoid cuff and the lymph nodes harden with fibrosis.

- Stage I: Early decompensation where lymphatic load exceeds capacity and protein rich fluid accumulates. This is potentially reversible and elevation helps
- Stage II: Brief compensation as all lymphatics open up. Eventual flow reversal leads to reaccumulation
- Stage III: Increase in cells within tissues
- Stage IV: Brawny non-pitting oedema from fibrovascular proliferation

The presence of protein-rich fluid in the interstitium triggers a vicious cycle making the disease progressive (also known as 'protein-poisoning of tissues').

- The disruption of the oncotic pressure gradient promotes further accumulation of protein-rich fluid that is prone to infection. Phagocytic efficiency is reduced
- The protein promotes inflammation and fibroblast activation leading to fibrosis and oedema, which causes hypoxia and further fibrosis. Macrophage numbers increase up to 30 times and contribute to a chronic infection-like state, with cytokines further promoting fibrosis and angiogenesis

- When the condition becomes chronic, the typical skin changes are: dryness, hyperkeratosis, papillomatosis (thickened warty texture), lymphangiomas and cracks/fissures (which increase infection risk)
  - Oedema on the back of the foot and toes is a useful sign. The Kaposi-Stemmer sign is the inability to pinch the skin on base of second toe. This distinguishes lymphoedema from lipoedema
  - Flow between watershed areas via superficial dermal system, giving rise to a *peau d'orange* appearance
- Lymphangiosarcoma: Malignant transformation is a significant risk (10%) after 10 years of disease. It occurs in 0.5% of those with chronic lymphoedema after mastectomy (Stewart–Treves syndrome). The prognosis is poor and may require amputation, with an average survival of 19 months.

Differential diagnosis

- Oedema: Due to generalised states, such as salt retention and fluid excess. This is commonly due to renal or cardiac causes or low protein states (nephrotic syndrome, malnutrition or cirrhosis) that generally cause pitting oedema
  - Early lymphoedema may pit, but subsequent fibrosis abolishes this
  - Elevation improves simple oedema quicker than lymphoedema
  - There are fewer skin changes such as thickening and ulceration in oedema
- Obesity
- Lipoedema: This poorly understood condition, also termed lipohyperplasia dolorosa, occurs almost exclusively in females beginning at puberty. There is symmetric maldistribution of adipose tissue, particularly in the extremities from abdomen to ankle (sparing feet, Kaposi-Stemmer negative). The texture is rubbery and non-pitting rather than hard, with pain (including pins and needles) and easy

bruising due to increased blood vessel fragility. Lymphoscintigraphy is normal as the condition is not caused by malformed or dysfunctional lymphatics. Many patients are labelled as obese
- Venous oedema is due to deep venous disease
- Miscellaneous, such as Parkes–Weber, Klippel–Trenaunay, gigantism and AVF

Lymphoedema is generally classified by cause, but this has little practical significance in terms of treatment. An alternative classification is based on lymphangiographic appearance.
- Acquired: Distal or proximal obliterative (more severe)
- Congenital: Hyperplasia (usually bilateral, below knee and associated with other tissue abnormalities), megalymphatic (usually unilateral affecting whole limb), aplasia or hypoplasia (more likely to be familial)

It has been suggested that lymphoedema patients (primary and secondary) are a subset with pre-existing abnormal lymphatics, but that the secondary/acquired groups have a milder problem that predisposes them to only develop swelling when triggered by a serious event. This may explain why the condition does not universally affect those who have axillary surgery/radiotherapy.

Primary lymphoedema

Primary lymphoedema is less common (15%) and generally shows slower progression. No precipitating cause is found and is thus a diagnosis by exclusion. Patients are often female (2:1 overall). It is either isolated or inherited and can be further sub classified according to timing. Note that the inappropriate use of eponyms has confused things somewhat. The terms *congenita, praecox* and *tarda* refer to the time of appearance and encompasses numerous different diseases.
- Congenital (10%): Involves the lower limb most frequently and one third of cases are bilateral. Milroy's disease is a subset of primary lymphoedema showing familial inheritance but incomplete penetrance.

It is inherited in an autosomal dominant manner and a defect in a tyrosine kinase receptor VEFGR3 (FLT4 gene, required for lymphatic development) on chromosome 5q has been described. It is one of the rarest causes of lymphoedema and thought to be due to lymphatic aplasia. The swelling is present at birth and is usually limited to below the knee and tends to be non-progressive but may be complicated by recurrent infections. The term Milroy's has been applied inappropriately to various forms of primary lymphoedema. Milroy described the condition in 1892, in a missionary and his mother
- Praecox (80%): Sometimes called Meige's lymphoedema (but is better regarded as a subset of praecox) and is disproportionately common in females (10:1) with an autosomal dominant pattern of inheritance. The swelling usually begins at puberty but can occur from age of 14–35 years. The lymphatics are hypoplastic in most cases. It is particularly severe below the waist, affecting the dorsum of the foot first. Dr Henri Meige was a French physician who described a hereditary form of lymphoedema in 1891
  - Lymphoedema distichiasis: There is a mutation in the FOXC2 gene on chromosome 16q and is associated with pubertal onset lower limb oedema that is preceded by double row of eyelashes. The extra set is usually soft and pale, located in the Meibomian gland openings and may cause irritation. Vessels tend to be hyperplastic and may be associated with clefts, heart defects, ptosis and vertebral anomalies
- Tarda (10%) is a less common variant with later onset, typically after 35 years of age. Vessels are hyperplastic, tortuous and abnormal

Secondary lymphoedema

Secondary lymphoedema is more common.
- Malignancy: Primary lymphatic neoplasm, secondary metastasis blocking nodes and lymphatics, or external compression may cause this. Cancer rarely presents with

lymphoedema, unless very advanced (except for prostatic carcinoma). Breast cancer surgery is the most common cause in the developed world with an 8% patient prevalence. The onset may be delayed by up to a year. Mastectomy-related lymphoedema may become less common with more sentinel node biopsies

- Radiation and surgery, particularly of lymph nodes, are important iatrogenic causes. It may also follow burns or burns surgery, and occasionally follows varicose vein stripping
- Infection with Wucheria bancrofti leading to fibrosis is the most common cause worldwide and may lead to massive enlargement, commonly called elephantiasis. Tuberculosis may also cause lymphoedema

Investigation

Investigation often yields little information on the cause of the lymphoedema. Other causes should be excluded.

- Lymphoscintigraphy: Intradermal or subcutaneous Technetium-labelled antimony is preferentially taken up by the lymphatics. This investigation is useful to define anatomy, patency and dynamics, and is the current standard investigation for lymphoedema. A gamma camera is used to visualise nodal uptake after a specific post-injection interval. Lymphoedema is distinguished from oedema by the presence of dermal backflow. This presence of tracer outside the main lymph routes, such as the skin, combined with poor transit indicates hypoplasia. It cannot distinguish between primary or secondary lymphoedema
- Lymphangiography was a standard investigation but it has been largely replaced by less invasive techniques (see above). A blue dye is injected into the first web space to reveal the lymphatics that are subsequently injected with radio-opaque dye, e.g. lipiodol. It is tedious, time-consuming and poses a risk to the patient (including exacerbation of the condition by inducing further fibrosis and valve damage) with little actionable information obtained
  - Interstitial lymphangiography relies on the uptake of interstitial contrast by the lymphatics without direct cannulation
- CT/MRI provides little extra information above that obtained with lymphoscintigraphy. It can confirm the diagnosis by demonstrating the classic honeycomb pattern with normal subfascial tissues, differentiating it from oedema and fat or a post-thrombotic limb with a thickened muscle compartment. It may be useful to rule out malignancy in selected cases
- Doppler ultrasound can assess lymphatic and venous flow, and is primarily used to exclude DVT

Management

Treat any treatable identifiable causes, e.g. diethylcarbamazine for early-stage filariasis (in later stages, when the worms die, they will still block the lymphatics). In essence, lymphoedema requires long term, life-long medical/non-surgical management with good patient understanding and compliance.

Conservative

These measures (elevation, hygiene/antibiotics, massage and compression) are more effective when started early in the disease progression.

- Avoid standing for long periods of time
- Meticulous skin care to eradicate/prevent infection, especially of fungi
- Drug treatment
  - Antibiotics should be used to treat infections aggressively to minimise fibrosis. Long-term use of antibiotics such as penicillins and cephalosporins for streptococcal prophylaxis, in particular, may be required in recurrent cases. Topical antibiotics/antifungals are often needed for the feet
  - Diuretics are generally contraindicated. Although there may be a minor initial improvement, the effect is usually transient and is counter-productive in the long run. This is because the loss

of interstitial fluid increases protein concentration in the tissues and may lead to more fibrosis. In fact, oedema that improves significantly with diuretics is unlikely to be lymphoedema

- Benzopyrene (a class of drug originally used in patients with vascular disease, e.g. coumarin and troxerutin) can induce phagocytosis by binding to interstitial proteins, thus allowing fragmentation of proteins into particles that can be cleared. Clinical results have been mixed. Daflon (a bioflavonoid) has been shown to be more effective than placebo but poor quality data prevents its recommendation
- Heat treatment may soften up the tissues and may induce macrophage activation
- Low-level laser therapy is an FDA-approved for treatment of lymphoedema

Physiotherapy

- Complex/ comprehensive decongestive therapy (CPT or active physiological drainage) is the application of skin care, massage, compression bandages and exercises in stages:
  - Inpatient (or intensive outpatient) decongestive phase: Good hygiene and skin care measures are enforced. Manual lymph drainage (MLD) performed aims to encourage lymph flow from the swelling towards healthy channels, by first emptying proximal areas on the trunk. Compressive bandaging and exercise follow this. The compression opposes filtration pressure and provides a counterforce to muscle contraction during exercises
  - Outpatient: Lifelong use of support stockings, compression garments and a regular exercise regime is required maintenance therapy, with 54% maintaining volume reduction at 3 years
- There are many different protocols based on similar principles of compression (manual or pneumatic), exercise and pressure garments. Proximal emptying manoeuvres (MLD) must precede pneumatic compression, otherwise scrotal oedema may result

Surgical

The role of the surgeon in lymphoedema is difficult to define. It is a condition without a cure, lymphatic function cannot be permanently restored/improved and surgery is symptomatic and temporary. Recurrence is common. Thus surgery is not the first option, and is used in only 10% of patients when conservative treatment fails. It is conventional to describe procedures as either physiological or excisional, but there is considerable overlap. Although there are other aspects to the disease, patients are often most concerned about the appearance, and many surgical treatments may worsen this. The evidence for many physiological treatments is limited to series of case studies, representing low levels of evidence.

The feet are particularly difficult to treat with verrucous changes, and oedema of skin grafts is common. Preoperative preparation with at least 72 hours of skin care and elevation should be performed. Postoperative elevation and splintage is also important. The results for postmastectomy patients tend to be less predictable and less successful overall.

- Physiological procedures aim to recreate working lymphatic channels. Results are variable and the long-term effects unclear and largely unproven. Patients often report subjective success/relief, even if there has been no objective reduction
  - Lymphangioplasty: A variety of materials including silk sutures (historical interest only, Handley 1908), Teflon or rubber tubes have been implanted into the subcutaneous tissue in an effort to create drainage channels. It can be complicated by infection and extrusion, and long-term results are poor (average 13 months benefit, although patients perceive a benefit for longer)
  - Bridging techniques
  - Thompson dermal flap (see below)
  - Pedicled omental transfer: In practice, the denuded mucosa of the omentum tends to be quickly surrounded by fibrosis rather than lymphatics and the long-term results are poor, with risk of donor site hernia development

- – Enteromesenteric flap: A flap of ileum denuded of mucosa is used to cover transected lymph nodes below the level of obstruction
- – Anastomoses (supposedly more effective before further lymphatic damage)
- – Lymphovenous shunts (lymph node to vein or lymphatic to vein). May work better for early disease, particularly for genital lymphoedema but less so in hypoplastic type disease. Nodovenous shunts often work in the short-term, but the swelling invariably rebounds
- – Lympholymphatic anastomosis (vein grafts) may be useful in cases where the disease is localised to a short segment, e.g. genitalia, but is ineffective in those with hyperplastic disease
- – Lymphaticovenular anastomosis (LVA): This involves supermicrosurgery. Multiple anastomoses can be performed under LA and thus potentially low morbidity, but expertise is not widely available
- Excisional
  - – Charles procedure (1912): Excision of lymphoedema tissue (almost all except foot and ankle tendons) and coverage with split skin grafts (occasionally FTSGs, from excised skin where suitable) is usually reserved for extensive cases with unhealthy skin, particularly ulceration. The results are aesthetically poor, the skin unstable and prone to changes such as hyperkeratinisation. It is rarely used. Thick leathery skin that does not mobilise well is better suited to this procedure than a Homans procedure
  - – Homans procedure (after Sistrunk) is the most popular surgical technique for lymphoedema and may represent the best surgical compromise. This is a staged excision of subcutaneous tissue and excess skin after 1–1.5 cm thick flaps are raised (thus only suitable if the skin is healthy). The medial side is usually excised with a second operation on the lateral side 3 months later. A variation of this is radical reduction with preservation of perforators that allows thinner flaps (5 mm)
  - – The Thompson buried dermal flap is rarely used. Subcutaneous tissue is excised and a dermal flap is buried into the muscle compartment with the aim of merging the dermal lymphatics with deep lymphatics. The results are generally poor and no definite connections have been demonstrated

Liposuction has been used by a small number of practitioners with some success, although its effects are temporary and requires patients to be meticulous with maintenance therapy with compression postoperatively. Patient selection is critical. There are concerns that it may exacerbate fibrosis but modalities such as Vaser or jet-assisted liposuction may be less traumatic. It may have a role as an adjunct to surgery in certain cases.

Further reading

Koshima I, Yamamoto T, Narushima M, et al. Perforator flaps and supermicrosurgery. Clin Plast Surg 2010; 37:683–89.

Related topics of interest

- Liposuction
- Skin grafts

Mandibular fractures

The most common causes of mandibular fractures are RTAs, sports and interpersonal trauma, with alcohol a frequent contributing factor. Consequently, patients show a male predominance (three times).

The condylar area is the most frequently fractured (29%). Other areas include the angle, symphysis and the body of the mandible, while coronoid and ramus fractures are uncommon. These common sites of fractures are areas of structural weakness (**Table 44**).

The mandible forms part of a ring-like system and hence approximately 50% of cases have another fracture on the contralateral side (contre-coup fractures, average 1.5 fractures per fractured mandible) (**Table 45**) and should be specifically excluded.

Favourable or unfavourable

Fracture stability and displacement depends on the fracture geometry and location, which in turn determines the resultant action of attached muscles on the fracture fragments. In an unfavourable fracture, the muscles tend to pull the fragments apart, whilst in a favourable fractures, the fragments are pushed together by muscle action, opposing displacement.

- For favourable fractures in a horizontal plane, the line runs downwards and forwards. The masseter pulls the fragments together
- For those in a vertical plane, the line runs medially, forwards and laterally. The medial pterygoids pull the fragments together

Symphyseal and high condylar fractures tend to be unfavourable due to pull of suprahyoid (including anterior belly of digastric) and lateral pterygoid muscles respectively. With a trend towards early fixation, the significance of this concept is reduced, but it remains a useful way to rationalise the treatment in selected cases.

Assessment

Initial assessment should always follow ATLS guidelines, i.e. ABC:

- Airway: Obstruction may be caused by the backward displacement of fracture fragments (with or without the tongue), reduced consciousness, soft tissue swelling or from excessive bleeding. Such fractures may require urgent distraction and fixation if an airway cannot be inserted
  - Bleeding is most likely to come from the nose or sinuses, particularly after Le Fort fractures. In most cases, they can be managed with nasal packing/balloons but may require IMF/fracture reduction

Table 44 Pre-existing weak areas of the mandible	
Weak area	**Underlying reason**
Condylar	Narrow thin bone of the neck
Angle	Third molar roots
Parasymphysis	Mental foramen and long canine tooth root
Body	Bone is thin due to resorption. This fracture is more common in the elderly, with fractures nearer the angle in the edentulous.

Table 45 Complementary mandible fractures	
Fracture	**Complementary fracture**
Condyle	Contralateral angle
Angle	Contralateral body
Parasymphysis	Contralateral condyle
Symphysis	Bilateral condyles

- Breathing: There may be coexistent chest injuries such as tension pneumothorax or flail chest
- Circulation: Profuse bleeding from mandibular fractures sufficient to cause haemodynamic compromise is unusual. Other sources of bleeding should be sought if this is the case

It is unfortunate that many trauma patients with obvious facial injuries will be rapidly assigned to the plastic surgery service without adequate multisystem evaluation (studies show that significant additional and undetected injuries were found in up to 12–25%). The plastic surgeon must routinely perform a full assessment when receiving a trauma patient for this reason. Associated injuries are common (45%). Concomitant cervical spine fractures are present in 3%. Loose tooth inhalation may occur.

Specific assessment

The signs of a mandibular fracture are local pain or tenderness, swelling and malocclusion.

- Swelling and bruising may mask deformities. Check for symmetry, palpate for crepitus, instability, focal tenderness or step deformities. Examine systematically in either an up-to-down or down-to-up fashion
- Assess excursion and occlusion
  - Assess the degree of mouth opening. Trismus (less than 35 mm opening; normal 40–50 mm adults and less in children) may be due to spasm, swelling or direct trauma to the muscles
  - An open bite is inability to close the gap between the jaws completely and may be anterior or lateral
  - Wear facets are useful clues to occlusal problems. Many patients do not have normal pre-trauma bite
  - Angle classification for occlusion
    - Class I (74%): The mesobuccal cusp (anterolateral of the four cusps) of the upper first molar fits into the buccal groove (the groove between anterior and posterior cusps) of the lower first molar. The upper teeth are slightly posterior

- Class II (24%): Mandibular retrognathia/ overjet/distocclusion
- Class III (1%): Mandibular prognathia/overjet/mesioocclusion
- Intraoral examination: Haematomas are almost always seen in fractures. A significant proportion of mandibular fractures involve the teeth and overlying mucosa. They are thus open fractures and prone to infection. Antibiotic prophylaxis is recommended. In contrast, mandibular fractures are rarely compounded to the skin
  - Avulsed teeth may be reinserted but success depends on timing. Gently clean without damaging the root surface and transport in milk, Hank's balanced saline or buccal vestibule
- Check for paraesthesia in the trigeminal distribution. Facial nerve function may be affected by swelling

Imaging

- The best single plain radiograph is an orthopantomogram (OPG or Panorex). Subcondylar and condylar regions and the ramus are still not as well visualised as the rest of the mandible. It will demonstrate 92% of mandibular fractures, and more likely to miss fractures in the posterior parts
- A mandibular series of plain radiographs is a reasonable alternative if OPG is not available (requires special equipment and a stable patient)
  - Caldwell: PA view with 15° tilt to remove the shadow of the petrous temporal bones from the orbit with a good view of symphysis and angle
  - Oblique view showing ramus, adjacent body and condyles
  - Towne or reverse Towne views preferably: AP with a 30° tilt that provides a submental view, demonstrating the subcondylar region by projecting it below the mastoid. An OPG and a Towne's view is the best combination
- CTs give exact details of fracture location and extent and may be indicated for surgical planning or for confirming diagnosis if clinical suspicion remains high despite equivocal X-rays, especially for

suspected condylar fractures. In practice, CT scans are often used to screen for other injuries including brain/intracranial. MRI examination is rarely indicated except for TMJ disc injuries or to better delineate soft tissue entrapment in the orbit

Treatment

- Patients should be nursed head up to reduce swelling
- Antiseptic mouthwash and oral antibiotics if the fracture is open
- Prompt surgical management is most important in the prevention of infection

Conservative treatment may be appropriate in selected cases:

- Children, especially with greenstick fractures
- Subcondylar fractures, especially if undisplaced
- Favourable undisplaced fractures with normal occlusion and minimal trismus

Patients who are treated non-surgically should be followed up after 1–2 weeks to check occlusion and healing (reduced pain and mobility, X-rays may not show evidence of healing at this stage but will demonstrate displacement). Proper physiotherapy is important, particularly for subcondylar and condylar fractures. However, with the exception of the above, the general trend is towards operative repair where possible, usually with IMF or ORIF.

Intermaxillary fixation (IMF)

This term is explained by the fact that the mandible was once known as the inferior maxilla. Wires and arch bars are used to fix the mandible to the maxilla after occlusion is restored. Alternatively, elastics may be used. IMF is a non-rigid form of fixation and is thus ineffective for severe bony displacement. The rate of non-union is higher than with miniplates. Closed treatment with IMF is suitable for most condyle, coronoid and ramus fractures.

- It is a significant undertaking for the patient: Oral hygiene must be meticulous. There are potential airway problems and the patient may find it difficult to maintain weight through oral feeding. Wire cutters should accompany the patient and early signs of nausea should be treated actively
- It is generally not recommended for those with poor compliance. The edentulous may be treated with circum-mandibular and zygomatic wiring
- IMF must remain in place for 4–6 weeks if used alone, followed by 2 weeks of training elastics. The trend is for early controlled mobilisation that can often be started in three weeks, particularly for subcondylar fractures, allowing oral cleansing and exercise to decrease stiffness

Open reduction and internal fixation

Open reduction and internal fixation (ORIF) is usually the treatment of choice as it allows direct visualisation of the fracture, precise reduction, and early mobilisation, avoiding TMJ stiffness. IMF is used to fix the occlusion first to provide a stable base. This alone often reduces the fracture, and can be removed after plating is complete. ORIF is recommended for displaced, unstable fractures, particularly those of the angle to symphyseal area (**Table 46**).

Truly rigid fixation (as espoused by the Association for Osteosynthesis/Association for the Study of Internal Fixation (AO/ASIF) School, and more popular in the US) to produce primary bone healing under absolute stability can be achieved by:

- Interfragmentary compression plates (inclines built into screw holes): An inferior border 2.4 mm (or thicker) bicortical plate to counter compression whilst a superior plate (monocortical or an arch bar) counters traction. Complications of infection and malocclusion are more common than with miniplates
- The reconstruction plates lock screws to the plate rather than compressing bone to it
- Lag screws (two) can be used for oblique fractures of the parasymphyseal or symphyseal region, but fracture must be precisely reduced first. It is an exacting technique and not for the occasional operator

Table 46 Characteristics of different sites of mandibular fracture	
Angle	Associated with the highest complication rate and optimal management is somewhat controversial. **Undisplaced:** ORIF by intraoral approach or Risdon (submandibular) approach. Incise two fingerbreadths below angle, elevate flap above plane of submandibular gland to access mandible. This provides a better view of the inferior border but puts the facial nerve at risk (5%). **Displaced:** ORIF and IMF
Coronoid	Generally requires no treatment except for a brief period of IMF (1–2 weeks to allow union) and soft diet
Body	Either open or closed if favourable configuration, but use of IMF alone requires good dentition and may cause displacement, although it can be combined with inferior border plate. ORIF is most the stable, allows early mobilisation, and is thus the preferred option
Symphysis	Isolated (para)symphyseal fractures have tendency for lingual rotation of upper border, hence two plates are preferred. With unilateral subcondylar fractures, plate symphysis only. With bilateral condylar fractures, plate symphysis and subcondylar fracture if low enough, via the Risdon approach

Non-compressive titanium miniplates with 2 mm unicortical screws are more commonly used (in Europe and Australasia). They are simpler, quicker to use and cheaper. Miniplates are semi-rigid which is sufficient for healing of the facial bones, including the mandible. However, it should be used with caution in those unlikely to be compliant. In practice, successful fixation is more dependent on operator technique and bone quality than the plating system per se.

- Champy developed the principle of adaptive osteosynthesis. This is achieved by placing a tension band plate with unicortical screws along Champy's line of ideal osteosynthesis. This stabilises fractures sufficiently (e.g. oblique ridge in angle fractures) to achieve healing while avoiding disadvantages of rigid fixation. If the fracture line lies anterior to the mental foramen then two plates are required, otherwise one plate is sufficient. Champy's line represents the interface or the line of zero force, located in between the superior zone of tension and inferior zone of compression at the angle, generated from muscular action
  - Many actually use a dual miniplate technique (superior and inferior) for the angle and still call it Champy

The major complication rate with miniplates is low, whilst minor complications such as screw/plate failure (fracture/extrusion) are higher.

External fixation is seldom used and reserved for selected situations such as compound or comminuted fractures in the edentulous elderly patient, bone loss, osteomyelitis and massive soft tissue injury.

The timing of surgery depends on several factors:

- Most cases are not urgent unless there is airway compromise or excessive uncontrollable bleeding. Surgery within 48 hours reduces the rate of infection, but there is otherwise little demonstrable difference in clinical results if surgery is delayed for up to 1 week. Two weeks is probably the practical upper limit for primary surgery, bearing in mind the young heal at a faster rate
- Late secondary surgery often requires osteotomy and may be difficult due to soft tissue contraction and rounded bone ends that are more likely to be unstable

Edentulous patients

The risk of complications increase with the degree of mandibular atrophy, especially if < 10 mm in height. There is little cancellous bone and a reduced healing potential. The most common site for fractures in this group is in the body. Stable fractures can be treated conservatively (soft diet) whilst those with minimal displacement can be managed with closed reduction with splints and dentures. For open treatment, circumferential/circum-mandibular wiring is the technique of choice. With this, a wire is passed through a spinal needle or passing needle, from inferior edge of mandible upwards lateral/anterior to the bone. The other end is passed through the same hole medial/lateral to the bone, seesawing to cut through the soft tissue. The wire is then passed back to front through a drill hole in the denture and twisted tight. Bone grafts may be required (primary or secondary).

Paediatric considerations

The incidence of facial fractures in children is low due to parental protection and their anatomy (small face, small stronger sinuses). Treat fractures early but conservatively.

- More likely to be green stick
- They will become fixed in one week
- Avoid iatrogenic damage to tooth buds and causing growth disturbance (which is uncommon except in those under 3 years of age)

If ORIF is required (body, angle, displaced), microplates and wires are favoured over conventional miniplates. Condylar fractures are often treated conservatively with soft diet and analgesia (25%), IMF (50%), ORIF with wires or splints (12.5% each), and early mobilisation (at 7–10 days).

Complications of fixation

A quarter of complications occur with fractures of the angle. Other risk factors for complications include fractures with teeth in the line, comminuted fractures, edentulous patients, those presenting late and those with poor oral hygiene. The removal of teeth in the fracture line is not always necessary with exceptions being comminuted fractures, damaged tooth, gross decay, periodontal disease or non-functional tooth (absent opposing tooth). A tooth can be retained if it is otherwise healthy, and as long as one accepts the increased risk of complications, such as plate removal.

- Infection (6%) is the most common complication and may lead to non-union, delayed union (3%) and pseudoarthrosis. Good rigid fixation is the best protection against infection

- Nerve injury (2–8%), particularly of the inferior alveolar nerve
- Ankylosis is most probably related to excessive immobilisation
- Plate removal is performed most commonly for infection, exposure or discomfort

Condylar fractures

Condylar fractures can be classified as extracapsular, subcondylar, or intracapsular (head). Most are low (with reference to sigmoid notch'). High fractures are more likely to be comminuted and associated with dislocation. Unilateral fractures commonly present with contralateral open bite and deviation on mouth opening, while bilateral fractures may present with premature posterior contact and anterior open bite. The lateral pterygoid tends to cause anterior and medial displacement of the condylar head. Intra-articular fractures (with haemorrhage) have a greater risk of ankylosis. Physiotherapy is important whether or not the patient has surgery.

Treatment of condylar fractures presents a particular problem. Surgical access is often difficult with risks to the facial nerve and TMJ. A patient with a condylar fracture and reasonable jaw opening without pain and malocclusion can often be treated without open surgery. Unilateral fractures treated with ORIF allow earlier mobilisation but long-term results (3 years) show no difference compared to close reduction. In general,

- Closed treatment results in good movement but poor alignment. There may be shortened ramus height and deviation on jaw opening to affected side due to the reduced pterygoid effect on a shortened condyle. Despite this, it is still an acceptable in most cases (> 90% outcome satisfaction). There is room for remodelling in children (< 10–12 years old) but with a risk of growth disturbance if under 3 years old
  - After 2 weeks of IMF (less in children), controlled mobilisation can be considered if the fracture geometry is favourable, along with 2 weeks of elastics to pull the mandible up and forward

- Note that IMF and restoration of occlusion alone does not mean that a displaced condyle will reduce, as room is needed for this to occur
- Open treatment results in good alignment but with a 20% risk of temporary facial nerve weakness (though almost all resolve within 6 months), problem scarring in 7%, pain and stiffness with risk of ankylosis (and risk of condylar head devascularisation)
  - Bilateral condylar fractures are often candidates for surgery, particularly if shortened or with an open bite
  - Low subcondylar fractures are also candidates for surgery as they are reasonably accessible
  - In multiple fractures that involve the condyle and another part of the mandible, the condyle is usually treated by a closed method such as IMF, while the other is fixed by ORIF
- Approaches: Risdon, post ramus (especially for low subcondylar, below sigmoid notch) and pre auricular (for high fractures, also known as a trans-parotid approach). Endoscopic access may reduce scarring and facial nerve injury, though the learning curve is steep

A comparison of open and closed treatment (2002) found no functional difference. Appearance and occlusion were generally acceptable in both groups. The closed treatment group had fewer surgical complications, but more problems with late malocclusion, such as anterior open bite, TMJ dysfunction, asymmetry and chin deviation with mouth opening. There has thus been a recent trend away from conservative treatment, although some say that a trial of IMF before ORIF may be reasonable. The absolute indications for ORIF as described by Zide (1983 and modified in 1989) are:

- Dislocation into middle cranial fossa or EAM
- Lateral extracapsular displacement
- Inability to maintain occlusion with conservative treatment
- Open joint with foreign body or gross contamination

In practice, the relative indications for surgery depend on the preference of the individual surgeons and additional considerations include:

- Bilateral fractures in those with no dentition for splintage (or other situations where splinting is not possible or when adequate physiotherapy not available)
- Severe shortening, angulation or lateral displacement of more than 30° with severe malocclusion
- Patient has panfacial fractures that require open fixation anyway
- A rule of thumb often used is that if the fragment is large enough to fit two screws then one should operate. Placing only one screw leads to hinge motion

Further reading

van den Bergh B, van Es C, Forouzanfar T. Analysis of mandibular fractures. J Craniofac Surg 2011; 22:1631–34.

Mastopexy

The breasts undergo typical changes with age (Table 47), with loss of volume and projection causing ptosis.

Regnault classification of breast ptosis (1973)

I.   NAC above/up to 1 cm below IMF, above inferior convexity/pole
II. NAC 1–3 cm below IMF but above most prominent part of breast, anterior to the breast mound
III. NAC > 3 cm below IMF, also below breast mound with nipple pointing downwards

This traditional classification has many limitations, as does not take account of skin laxity, breast mass, nor distinguish between nipple and glandular ptosis. Other related terms:

- Pseudoptosis describes a dropped lower pole with increased NAC-IMF distance. The breast is bottomed out but the NAC still remains above the IMF
- Glandular ptosis: Excessive inferior displacement of breast volume below the IMF
- Tubular breasts with high IMFs are technically ptotic by Regnault definition, but are due to superior IMF displacement instead of inferior nipple displacement

Management

Most current techniques have similarities to breast reduction surgery and thus represent one end of the spectrum consisting of minimal glandular resection with parenchymal reconfiguration, reliable nipple repositioning and minimal scars. The skin alone should not be used to retain the mastopexied breast.

Skin incision pattern

Periareolar (donut) mastopexies have been popular as the scar lies in the perimeter of the areolar, but the effects are not long-lasting and tend to create a flat, poorly projecting breast.

- Simple periareolar for minimal ptosis with good skin quality: Remodel parenchyma via incision and close with a permanent purse-string suture
- The Benelli (1990) procedure involves de-epithelialisation of a concentric egg-shaped region around the areola that is kept on a wide superior dermoparenchymal pedicle. The lower breast flap is undermined, split and then criss-crossed by tacking it to the chest wall. The NAC is closed with a non-absorbable purse-string suture
- Periareolar with vertical ellipse: Enables more tailoring than a periareolar approach alone and is suitable for moderate ptosis with good skin quality
- Periareolar with vertical ellipse and short horizontal: Similar to Wise and is suited for moderate ptosis with poor skin quality. Augmentation may be required
- Wise pattern: Allows very predictable results but at the expense of extensive scarring, and the undermining involved may increase the risk of skin complications. Inferior pedicle techniques tend to lower the IMF whilst superior or medial pedicle techniques tend to lift the IMF

Table 47 Age related changes of the female breast	
Young breast	Firm texture with fuller nipple that projects upwards Inferior hemisphere from nipple to IMF is rounded Superior hemisphere has subtle convex slope
Older breast	Glandular involution – Increased fat content, tissue is less firm and softer Gravitational pull with loss of elasticity of skin and ligaments Inferior hemisphere ptotic with inferior drift Superior hemisphere striae
Postmenopausal	Atrophic breast

Projection

Projection can be maximised most consistently by coning the parenchyma. Other options include stacking (Graf Biggs: An inferior dermoglandular pedicle is passed under a 3 cm muscle loop at the inferolateral edge of the pectoralis major, then tacked to fascia), flip-flap (lower glandular tissue is folded under the upper pole and sutured to the muscle fascia about the level of the second rib) and dermal cloak (a 2–3 cm periareolar dermal layer used to shape the breast and fix it to the muscle fascia).

Implants are more likely to be needed in those with relatively poor skin quality and deficient parenchyma particularly in the upper pole. Subcutaneous implants alone tend to produce a relatively poor and very round shape. Submuscular placement may allow the native breast to droops over the implant, producing a 'double bubble' deformity, as well as superior migration. Thus, most cases usually require a mastopexy and augmentation preferably in two-stages (usually augmenting before mastopexy, but can be done either way). One-stage procedures are possible, but the conflicting tissue principles to achieve mastopexy (envelope reduction) vs. augmentation (envelope expansion) raise the risk of complications.

A subglandular implant will fill the skin envelope better and is often preferred.

For submuscular placement, the lower pole is opened up at the IMF, and then repaired after implant inset. The muscle edge can be fixed to the IMF with various techniques such as sutures/mesh, autologous abdominal dermis or acellular dermal matrix (that vascularises/incorporates).

Postoperative

There are inherent problems with mastopexies:

- The effects will only be temporary but the scars are permanent. Cooper's ligaments are not reconstructed but their role is 'substituted' by the skin, which will stretch with time. Glandular rearrangement techniques produce longer-lasting results
- Any manoeuvre designed to enhance upper pole fullness will be compromised by the volume loss inherent to the condition. Rearrangement of the parenchyma will result in a smaller breast that may necessitate use of implant
- The most common side effect after mastopexy is widening of the areola. Non-absorbable periareolar purse string sutures or reducing the areola as part of the procedure have been used to combat this with varying success

Further reading

Rinker B, Veneracion M, Walsh CP. Breast ptosis: causes and cure. Ann Plast Surg 2010; 64:579–84.

Related topic of interest

- Breast reduction

Maxillary fractures

The maxilla is the keystone of the face, and can be viewed as being composed of a series of buttresses or pillars. Reconstruction of these buttresses is the key aim of surgery for maxillary fractures. There are three vertical buttresses (thicker portions of bone) on each side that maintain the relationship between cranial base and mandible, including occlusion. They can be conceptually visualised as legs of a three-legged stool.

- Nasomaxillary/nasofrontal
- Zygomaticomaxillary/lateral orbital margin
- Pterygomaxillary

The horizontal buttresses are:

- Supraorbital ridge
- Zygomatic
- Inferior orbital rim
- Palate
- Mandible

Maxillary fractures are classified according to Le Fort patterns. Fractures involving both sides are not necessarily symmetrical. Le Fort II or III fractures are usually comminuted to a degree. Isolated Le Fort IIIs are rare as usually there is a zygomatic fracture on one side and a Le Fort II and I on the other side. Note that 10% of patients with a maxillary fracture will have a concomitant cervical spine injury.

Le Fort patterns

I. A horizontal fracture line that lies above the floor of nose, through piriform fossa, lower third of septum and pterygoid plates
II. A pyramidal fracture line in an inverted-V, with the apex at the nasal bridge that continues down to the orbit and lateral two thirds of the rim, close or through the infraorbital foramen and extending to lateral wall of maxillary antrum. This is the most common
III. Craniofacial dysjunction. The midface is detached from the skull base due to a fracture line through the orbits and parallel to the cranial base. Least common

Diagnosis

The diagnosis is made on clinical examination and imaging. Symptoms include swelling, bleeding, pain and malocclusion. The telltale sign is mobility of the maxillary segment, which it is often found retruded and tilted. The assessment should be systematic either top to bottom or bottom to top, incorporating a bird's eye view.

- Palpate orbital rims
- Check eyes
- Nose/palate/teeth

Imaging

X-rays may show the fractures and sinus opacification with fluid levels. For suspected trauma to the maxilla and orbits, the standard series is:

- Occipitomental (OM): Orbitomeatal plane is 45° (chin on plate, beam from posterior). The horizontal beam goes through the nasal spines and projects the top of petrous temporal, below floor of the maxillary sinus
  - Visualises the maxillary sinuses +/– fluid level, orbits and zygomatic arches
- Occipitomental 30 (OM 30): Orbitomeatal plane is 45° (chin on plate beam from posterior) and the beam is 30° down from above the occiput
  - Visualises the anterior aspect of facial bones and zygomatic arches while the maxillary sinuses and orbits are less well demonstrated
- Lateral facial bones (coned lateral of facial bones): Orbitomeatal plane is parallel to film, interpupillary at 90°. The beam passes through centre of maxillary sinus
  - Visualises the anterior wall, posterior wall and floor of maxillary sinus, sphenoid sinus and postnasal space

The name of view is named after the position of head, with the baseline being the orbitomeatal line running from EAM to lateral canthus and the interpupillary line. The degree (if any) refers to the angulation of the X-ray tube relative to this line.

Treatment

The aim is to re-establish the mid-facial height, width and projection and to restore normal occlusion. It is conventional to work from the stable to the unstable, and to reduce and stabilise the buttresses. It is important to expose all fracture sites for a proper assessment.

- Le Fort I: First, an IMF is placed, and then the two central sets of pillars are plated via upper oral sulcus incision
- Le Fort II: After IMF, the orbital fracture line is identified through coronal (for higher level nasofrontal fractures) and subconjunctival/subciliary incisions. Bone grafts may be required for bone gaps > 5 mm and to repair the orbit. There may also be naso-orbitoethmoid (NOE) fractures that need treatment (open reduction). Arch bars are left in place, even if semi-rigid fixation has been performed. The patient is allowed a soft diet and occlusion is monitored regularly with problems corrected by fine tuning with either elastics or rewiring, using the arch bars as anchors
- Le Fort III (usually with concomitant level I or II fractures): A coronal incision is usually required. The zygomatic arch is fixed, followed by the ZF sutures. NOE fractures may need treatment. Soft tissues should be suspended to fixed points

Le Fort types osteotomies

- Type I (most common) osteotomies are performed horizontally, in between the infraorbital foramen and roots of canines (at least 4 mm above), above the nasal floor. It lies slightly above the level of classical Le Fort I fractures and there is additional separation of septum from vomer and pterygoid plate from maxillary tuberosity, allowing completion fracture of the bone by finger pressure with protection of the palatine vessels. The segment can be moved by lengthening with bone grafts, retruded, advanced or segmented. This is often used as part of orthognathic surgery to repair malocclusion in combination with sagittal split osteotomies of the mandible
- Type II is less common
- Type III can be used to advance the mid-face in craniosynostosis. It will enlarge the orbital cavities

Further reading

Yu J, Dinsmore R, Mar P, et al. Pediatric maxillary fractures, J Craniofac Surg 2011; 22:1247–50.

Related topics of interest

- Orbital fractures
- Zygomatic fractures

Melanoma

Malignant melanomas (MMs) are neoplasms of the epidermal melanocytes that are embryologically derived from neural crest cells. Melanomas tend to affect younger patients compared to BCC and SCCs. The lifetime risk of a Caucasian living in the UK is estimated to at 1 in 80, but this increases 5 times if they emigrate to sunnier climes such as Australia or South Africa. Survival is improving but the increasing incidences result in an increase in absolute mortality numbers (in the UK, the incidence has doubled over 20 years). Although it only constitutes 5% of skin cancers, it is responsible for 50% of skin cancer deaths.

Risk factors

The risk increases with age. Overall, females have a lower risk of developing MM (though it depends on the subtype) and better prognosis. Having a previous melanoma carries a 3–5% risk of second occurrence.

- Ultraviolet light: Sunlight, especially short and intense exposures (as opposed to chronic occupational exposure) resulting in sunburn as a child (before age 10) in the fair-skinned and freckled (Fitzpatrick type I) is a major risk factor. Both UVA and UVB have a role and the relationship is strongest for lentigo maligna melanoma (LMM) and superficial spreading malignant melanoma (SSMM) subtypes
- Xeroderma pigmentosum is a rare sex-linked recessive disorder with faulty DNA repair. The inability to repair UV damage results in increased melanoma rates and many die from metastatic disease
- Giant pigmented naevus (20 cm or 2% body surface area in size or greater, see below). Generally, early excision of these lesions has been recommended but the benefits are not clear-cut
- Dysplastic naevus syndrome is a familial condition (various modes of inheritance) in which those affected have many (> 100) small pigmented naevi (with lymphocytic infiltration) or > 8 mm in size or with atypical ABCD features (see below). These patients should have lifelong screening for melanoma as they have up to a 50 times increased risk (depending on number of atypical moles and family history). Prophylactic removal is not useful as the majority of melanomas arise de novo. The moles are a marker for increased risk but are not usually precursors in themselves
- Familial melanoma occurs in a small number of cases with evidence of autosomal dominant inheritance

Common acquired naevi appear at ages 4–8 years old, and numbers increase up to adolescence. Other types of naevi include:

- Halo naevus: A pigmented naevus with a pale zone (due to an intense inflammatory infiltrate). It is benign but must be differentiated from melanoma
- Spitz naevus: A small pink to dark brown raised naevus with variable pigmentation found in children. They are almost always benign they can histologically appear aggressive with MM the main differential diagnosis. The latter has been labelled an atypical Spitz naevus. The pathology community argues that the atypical Spitz is a different condition and that all Spitz naevi are benign
- Dysplastic naevus (or 'atypical mole'): Dysplasia refers to architectural disorder with some atypical features. These moles appear flat, brown variegated (darker in centre) and variably symmetrical. They are slightly larger than typical moles measuring 6–8 mm in size, with a 'fried egg' architecture and an irregular, indistinct outline. Those with severe atypia may be regarded as premalignant
- Congenital naevus (see below) (**Figure 12**)

Giant congenital melanocytic naevus (GCMN)

Congenital melanocytic naevi (CMN, **Figure 11**) occur in 1% of the Caucasian population and new incidences estimated at 1 in 20,000. Rarely, they can appear after a 1–2 year delay (naevus tardive). The definition of 'giant' is widely accepted as

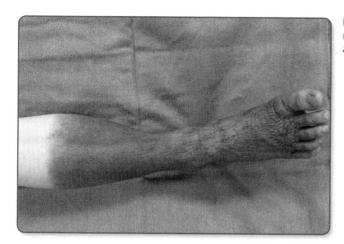

Figure 12 Congenital melanocytic naevus involving the leg in a glove and stocking distribution.

being > 20 cm in the greatest diameter in an adult (or projected to be) or 2% surface area. Naevus dimensions of > 10 cm and > 5 cm are designated medium and small respectively. Satellite naevi are present in 80% of GCMN patients. Affected areas have less subcutaneous tissue and heal poorly in comparison to normal skin. Skin markings/appendages, including hair and piloerector apparatus, (causing goosebumps) are exaggerated. Pigmented cells may extend into fat or muscle layers.

Apart from cosmetic issues, the greatest concern is the potential for malignant change. Early studies estimated this to be up to 40% but more recent systematic studies/reviews place this closer to 3–6%. Most occur in the first decade (50% in first 3 years, 70% by 13 years). The risk is greater in larger lesions with increased numbers of lesions/satellites, or darker/more variegated. The increased risk in small melanocytic naevi is negligible. Melanomas in GCMN tend to arise in the dermis but have also been found in deeper tissues. The risk of extracutaneous (GI, CNS and retroperitoneum) melanomas is 4%. Consequently surgery cannot totally eliminate the risk of MM, rather it aims to reduce the risk by prophylactic reduction of the cell load. Evidence-based protocols are lacking.

Neurocutaneous melanoses (found in one third with one third becoming symptomatic) are more common in those with many satellites (> 20) or midline lesions. Symptoms include raised ICP, hydrocephalus, development delay or space occupying lesion. The development of symptomatic disease is grave as most die within 2–3 years. The management of asymptomatic neurocutaneous remains controversial.

From a cosmetic point of view, any treatment should be able to pass the stare test (i.e. stop a person from staring when they pass the patient on the street). Otherwise, its usefulness is doubtful even if there has been an objective improvement. The choice of reconstructive methods depends in part on the site and there may be limitation of donor sites for reconstruction with massive lesions or satellites. Treatment has to be individualised and includes:

- Dermabrasion: The hair follicles are often deep and there is often pigment seep-back and regrowth of hairs
- Laser, especially QS ruby or long-pulse Alexandrite, has been used but the response is unpredictable (usually a 50–70% reduction) and often leaves a 'polka dot' appearance. The hair removal effect is generally poor. Carbon dioxide laser resurfacing has also been reported
- Skin grafts have been popular in the past but long-term follow-up has usually shown regret and dissatisfaction. The grafted skin is dry, insensate and fragile compared to naevus skin. Contour defects on the limb are more obvious with more proximal

lesions/defects. Skin substitutes, such as Integra, can be used but there are no large studies on their long-term results

- Tissue expanders have the potential for the best cosmesis particularly in those with few satellite naevi

Histological malignant melanoma subtypes

Various histological subtypes exist:

- Superficial spreading MM is the most common subtype in Caucasians (70%). They are flat or slightly raised variegate lesions with a prolonged radial growth phase at the level of the epidermal-dermal junction before vertical growth leads to deeper invasion. They often occur on the legs in females and on the trunk in males (though trunk and upper limb lesions are also increasing in females probably reflecting changes in clothing styles) and arise in pre-existing naevi with a stronger connection to ultraviolet light exposure than other subtypes. It affects males and females equally, although some studies suggest a higher frequency in females
- Nodular MM (NMM) (15–20%): Typically a blue-black nodule that may ulcerate or bleed with minor trauma. They tend to be more aggressive. NMM is more common in males and the association with sunlight is not as strong. Five percent are amelanotic and have a poorer prognosis
- Lentigo MM (5–15%) appears as a brown macular patch with or without a discrete nodule, typically in the sun-exposed areas of an elderly (F>M) patient. It has a prolonged radial growth phase (up to 30 years) and a better prognosis overall. The onset of the vertical growth phase marks the change from lentigo maligna to LMM. It is the least aggressive melanoma subtype and has the strongest association with sun exposure. Due to the vague margins, the recurrence rate is high and close follow-up is generally recommended
  - Lentigo maligna (LM, Hutchinson's freckle) is a precursor lesion (intraepithelial melanoma or in situ disease) and frank dermal invasion

(LMM) develops in 5%. It should not be confused with lentigo simplex/solar lentigo, which develops secondary to actinic damage and is very common with increasing age
  - Optimal treatment is uncertain. The aim is to excise with a clear margin and no further treatment is needed. In some situations close observation or radiotherapy may be appropriate. Cryotherapy is often used while imiquimod is unproven (causes regression in 80% but recurrences may be non-pigmented)
- Acral lentiginous MM is the rarest subtype in Caucasians (2–8%) but is more common in dark-skinned races (29–72% of all melanomas). They can occur on the palms, soles, mucocutaneous junctions or classically under the toe/finger nails (subungual MM). Half of subungual MM involve the hallux and a significant proportion are amelanotic (30% vs. 7% overall). The optimal level of amputation is somewhat controversial
- Rare subtypes are amelanotic and desmoplastic melanomas. Mucosal MMs are also rare (< 2%) and are usually large on presentation. Wide resection margins are not particularly useful. Ocular MM is the most common site of non-cutaneous MM comprising up to 5% of total MMs. Three percent of melanomas present with enlarged nodes in the absence of an identifiable primary

Signs

The suspicious signs of a pigmented skin lesion are listed below and are commonly summarised mnemonically as ABCD (and also EF). Only 10–20% of MM develop from a pre-existing naevus (and these tend to have a better prognosis).

- Asymmetry
- Border irregularity
- Colour: Variegated (i.e. more than two colours), irregular brown–black colouring
- Diameter > 6 mm,   >6mm

Also, Elevation/evolution/enlarging faster than other moles and Funny looking lesions.

A change in the lesion is more predictive than the absolute size. A lesion is unlikely to be a melanoma unless at least one major criterion (**Table 48**) is present.

Prognostic factors

The prognosis of melanoma is related to many factors including:

- Thickness of lesion (most important parameter, **Table 49**): Note that this is a continuous variable, with no natural breakpoints. It is thus not absolute but are based on best-fit data. The Breslow thickness is a better prognostic indicator as it is quantitative, more accurate and easily reproducible between pathologists. However, it tends to underestimate the thickness of ulcerated lesions and can be compromised by previous non-excisional biopsy
- Presence of lymph node metastases (microscopic and macroscopic N1/2 a and b respectively) and in transit/satellite as N2c
- Lesions with ulceration (TXb) and high mitotic rate
- Location: Trunk lesions have a worse prognosis compared to lesions on the limbs (excluding the hands and feet). Mucosal lesions also tend to have a worse prognosis

- Males and elderly patients fare less well for unclear reasons

Investigations

Careful physical examination, including regional nodes and entire skin surface, should be performed.

- Excisional biopsy: A 2 mm margin with subdermal fat is sufficient. Shave, punch or incisional biopsies are not recommended, although the latter may have a role in the assessment of larger lentigines
- For the limbs, a longitudinally orientated ellipse is preferred if the suspicion of melanoma is high. (There is still a chance that primary closure after wide local excision can be achieved. Transverse ellipses will almost invariably require a graft after wide local excision)
- Reconstruction of the defect can be delayed until the final histology is known

Staging

Clinical staging consists of excision of primary lesion and assessment of nodal status.

- Stage I: Localised disease, up to T2a
- Stage II: Localised disease, T2b to T4b
- Stage III: Nodal disease
- Stage IV: Metastatic disease

Table 48 Criteria for diagnosis of melanoma (Mackie)	
Major criteria	**Minor criteria (three or more)**
Change in size (94%), shape (95%) or colour (89%).	Inflammation (51%)
	Bleeding/sensory change (46%)
	Crusting or oozing (31%)
	Diameter > 7 mm

Table 49 Methods for measuring histological thickness of melanoma	
Clark's levels describe the position of melanoma cells in the layers of skin. It is more useful in thin melanomas and melanomas in thin skin, e.g. eyelid.	Breslow thickness maximum distance from the top of zona granulosa to base of tumour (5 year survival).
I: Epidermis or carcinoma-in-situ	Thin: thickness less than 1 mm (95–100%)
II: Papillary dermis	Intermediate:
III: Up to papillary-reticular interface	Thickness of 1.01–2 mm
IV: Reticular dermis	Thickness of 2.01–4 mm
V: Subcutaneous tissue	Thick: greater than 4 mm (37–50%)

The AJCC melanoma staging system was updated in 2009 with several important differences. The important points are:

- Tumour thickness is the predominant factor determining the T-stage. For T1 lesions the mitotic rate (number per mm^2) is taken into account (rather the level of invasion, i.e. Clark's level). The presence of histological ulceration (b vs. a, which can be differentiated from traumatic loss of the surface) is a significant adverse prognostic factor that upstages the tumour

  T1 <1mm
  T2 1.01-2
  T3 2.01-4
  T4 >4mm

  pT1, < 1 mm; pT2, 1.01–2 mm; pT3, 2.01–4 mm; pT4, > 4 mm A microsatellite is defined as a discontinuous nest of tumour cells, > 0.05 mm in size and separated from the main tumour by normal dermis
  - The number of, rather than the size (pre 2002) of lymph nodes is important to the nodal stage. Best fit data from studies led to the following categories: N1 is 1 node,

    N1 = 1
    N2 = 2-3
    N3 = 4

    N2 is 2–3 nodes and N3 is 4 or more, or in transit/satellites together with nodal disease (in transit disease without nodal disease is N2c). Satellite lesions are considered together with in-transit lesions as part of nodal disease (N2) and regarded as intra-lymphatic metastases
    - The tumour load in the nodes (micro vs. macrometastasis) is also taken into account and affects survival. The results of sentinel node biopsies are included. Micrometastases (a) are positive nodes diagnosed after sentinel lymph node biopsy (SLNB) and are of a lower stage than macrometastases (b), which are pathology-confirmed clinically detected nodes
  - Metastasis: Lung metastases are considered separately from other types due to the worse prognosis of other visceral metastases. Currently the number of metastasis is not considered in the AJCC. Raised LDH is significant

    b lung
    c viscera
       or ↑LDH

    - M1a Distant skin and nodes
    - M1b Lung and M1c other viscera or elevated LDH

Staging investigations

In general, thin melanomas need no specific investigation, whereas thicker melanomas should be staged by contrast CT (chest, abdomen and pelvis), USG abdomen, CXR, and liver function tests (LFTs) including two LDH measurements more than 24 hours apart; but the yield is low. Positron emission tomography (PET) is sensitive but has low specificity and is not particularly useful in the work up for the initial surgery.

Imaging

In basic terms, stage III and IV disease has poor prognosis with no known life-prolonging therapies (see below). Defensive medicine should be avoided but imaging in the symptomatic may reveal disease that can be palliated or dealt with on an individual basis.

- US [American Association of Dermatology (AAD) 2011]: No imaging is done in the asymptomatic with localised MM. Investigation is guided by history and examination
- UK [British Association of Dermatologists (BAD) 2010]: Imaging is done only for stage IIIB/C; CT (head, trunk, abdomen and pelvis) or CXR and liver USG though evidence to support role of investigations is not strong (Level IIa, Grade A evidence). For stage IV, additional investigations according to clinical need, e.g. PET/CT before metastasectomy, and LDH
- No routine investigations including blood tests, for asymptomatic stage I/II and IIIA. The pick-up rate of true positives is low whilst the rate of false positives is high (increases patient anxiety and prompts more investigations)

Modalities

- CXR: Has a low yield (approximately 0.1%) in asymptomatic patients with a relatively high false positive rate 4.4%. It does have a role as a preoperative screen in symptomatic patients as well as in the asymptomatic advanced T-stage
- Ultrasound is very operator-dependent with a false positive rate of 6%. It can be used to assess nodes. USG with FNA may allow detection of sentinel nodes and is the best alternative if SLNB is not available. The use of high frequency probes (20 MHz) to differentiate MM from other pigmented

lesions and to provide depth information is still being evaluated

- CT chest/abdomen and pelvis: Although it does provide reasonably good imaging of the chest/hila, it is not a good investigation for small deposits
- MRI: Provides better contrast resolution but less spatial resolution compared to CT and images are multi-planar. T1 weighted scans can detect metastasis with greater sensitivity compared to CT (whole body scanning)
- PET–18FDG: This scan is based on the premise that malignant cells are more metabolically active. The spatial resolution is low (4 mm) and lesions that are small or of low activity will be missed. PET is of little use in early stage disease. It is sensitive but prone to false positives (20%), with an overall accuracy of only 85%. It is most useful for stage III and IV disease and may have a role for assessing distant disease in those with nodal involvement or in the detection of an unknown primary
  - CT/PET: The mapping of PET images onto CT images acquired at the same time (CT can be of a lower resolution and without contrast) improves localisation of isotope uptake. The two modalities are synergistic, and permit a lower contrast load
- Bone scan: This only evaluates the bones, which tend to be involved late. The false positive rate is 4% and is unsuitable for routine staging

Surgery

Secondary surgery: Subsequent excision margins are dictated by the thickness of the melanoma on histological sectioning. There are no firm guidelines regarding the timing of the wider excision but the general consensus is that a delay of a few weeks is not harmful. Wide local excision only affects local recurrence rates and not survival. The deep fascia does not need to be included and skin grafts, for reconstruction, when needed are conventionally taken from other limbs. There are various guidelines available for the margins:

2010 UK guidelines suggest:

- In situ disease: 0.5 cm margin is adequate
- < 1 mm to 1 cm margin
- 1–2 mm to 2 cm margin
- >2–4 mm to 2–3 cm
- >4 mm to 3 cm

AAD guidelines 2011:

- 0–1 mm to 1 cm margin
- 1–2 mm to 1–2 cm margin
- >2 mm to 2 cm margin

Wider margins may be warranted to optimise local control, but do not seem to impact on the overall survival. Overall there is little data to support the usefulness of a wider excision margin (more than 2 cm). The classic studies are the WHO (Milan) and Intergroup studies that showed no difference in survival in 1 vs. 3 cm in melanomas less than 2 mm thick (though slightly more recurrence in narrower margin group) and 2 vs. 4 cm in intermediate-thick (1–4 mm) melanomas respectively. Numerous systematic reviews have shown that there are no benefits of excising 3–5 cm margins over 1–2 cm margins in terms of local recurrence, disease-free survival and overall survival. A 2 cm margin may be preferable to 1 cm and in a RCT in 2004; Thomas showed a marginal significance in terms of decreased local recurrence with 3 cm margins compared to 1 cm margins.

Management of lymph nodes

Sentinel lymph node biopsy

Sentinel lymph node biopsy (SLNB): The rationale is that lymph flows predictably to a sentinel node first and then and only then, on to other nodes. If this node can be detected and sampled, then subsequent treatment can be based on this result. There is a discordance of 40% between the predicted and actual drainage basins that is most marked in head and neck lesions, where 10% drain to contralateral nodes although they do not skip. It is contraindicated in those with palpable nodes as nodes filled with tumour will not take up dye or tracer and give a false negative.

SLNB is not routine but there are compelling reasons to use it in patients with melanomas thicker than 1 mm: It is useful for staging, to identify those likely to benefit from adjuvant treatment, avoids unnecessary lymph node surgery (compared to elective lymph node dissection) and provide the psychological comfort of a negative result. Positive SLNB upstages the patient to stage III, and the 5-year survival decreases from 92% to 67% if positive. There is a low false negative rate of 1–5% but there is a learning curve of 25–50 operations (SLNB with completion lymphadenectomy). It has a lower morbidity than elective lymph node dissection (ELND) though there is still a risk of lymphoedema.

The 2010 BAD guidelines suggest that it can be considered for stage IB and upwards with patients being informed that it has no proven therapeutic value and the risk of procedure and of false negatives. There is no survival benefit with SNLB and the large reputable studies (Morton) are said to be flawed both in calculation of survival advantage and definition of disease-free interval (recurrence in the previously dissected lymph node basin of the SNLB patients is always going to be lower than those in the watch and wait group).

- Preoperative formal lymphoscintigraphy with peritumoural Tc-99m is used to identify the nodal groups likely to drain lymph from the melanoma and may also demonstrate identify in-transit lesions. This is less useful in extremity lesions
- Perioperative injection of blue dye and/or radioisotope (Technetium) labelled colloid. After 20 minutes the 'hot' blue node is found and resected. Waiting longer leads to spilling-over into second echelon nodes
- Formal paraffin sections and immunohistochemistry are preferable as they increase detection. Standard pathology techniques have a 70% detection rate. Sensitivity can be increased with serial sectioning and tyrosinase PCR to preselect nodes for serial section immunohistochemistry (S100, Melan A). Completion node dissection can be performed on the basis of these results, after 2–3 weeks
- The questionable need for completion node dissection is in itself the subject of study due to the finding that some positive SNLB patients without subsequent

completion dissection did not recur. This implies that SNLB itself may be therapeutic but there is no evidence that allows this group to be distinguished yet

Clinically palpable lymph nodes

Clinically palpable lymph nodes are initially investigated with USG+FNA or biopsy, and if found to be positive, then a block dissection is offered. Wound problems and postoperative lymphoedema after nodal surgery are not uncommon (25%). There is some controversy with regards to the extent of en bloc dissections required, especially in the groin; there is no evidence of improved survival but there is a risk of increased morbidity especially oedema (others dispute this). See 'Groin dissection'.

Other treatments

For stage III disease the aim should be to increase the survival or quality of life in these patients with a high risk of metastasis (80%). The Cochrane review in 2004 concluded that there were no adjunctive treatments of proven benefit for melanoma, referring to agents such as interferons, dacarbazine and interleukins, however there have been recent developments since then. Those with elevated LDH in particular, are unlikely to benefit from systemic treatments.

- Interferons (IFN α2b) are licensed for use as an adjunctive treatment, i.e. after surgery. The consensus seems to be that they reduce, relapse and increase disease-free survival with little effect on overall survival
- Dacarbazine (DTIC) was FDA approved for stage IV disease in 1975, and is used as part of a trial where possible
- Interleukin 2 was approved for stage IV disease in 1998 as an immune-boosting therapy with a 2-week high dose course. Side effects are severe and possibly fatal

Newer agents include:

- Ipilimumab (MDX-010 or MDX-101 or Yervoy) is a monoclonal antibody with anti-CTLA-4 activity. Cytotoxic T-lymphocyte antigen CTLA-4 inhibits activated immune cells, thus blocking it may enhance the response against tumours. In 2010, Hodi showed improved survival of 24% after 2 years vs. 14% with other treatments as part of a Phase III trial. This was the first time a treatment was shown to improve overall survival in advanced melanoma. Ipilimumab gained FDA approval as immunotherapy for metastatic melanoma in March 2011

- Vemurafenib (i.e. PLX4032) shrank tumours in advanced melanoma patients with the BRAF V600E gene mutation and improved 6-month survival in a Phase III trial. However, the effect on long term/ overall survival is unclear as tumours can switch to other pathways and become resistant to the drug
- The results of TK (tyrosine kinase) gene mutation inhibitors such as imatinib mesylate are on the horizon

Palliation for multiple metastases:

- Isolated limb perfusion (ILP) is a regional palliative therapy that should be performed by expert teams. ILP with melphalan alone is sufficient for low tumour burden, whereas ILP with TNFa and melphalan, preferably also with IFNα (up to 90% response), is indicated for bulky disease and recurrence and/or resistance to melphalan alone. There is no significant survival benefit but it offers better local control and is a safe and effective treatment for locally advanced and symptomatic extremity melanoma. An alternative is isolated limb infusion, which seems to offer comparable results, but can be done under LA and sedation with fewer side effects
- Other palliative measures includes:
  - Metastasectomy: In-transit lesions should be completely excised (not widely) as first line
  - CO_2 lasers for less bulky disease
  - Palliative node dissections can be considered for uncontrolled disease and lymphatic obstruction but the surgery is difficult and often unrewarding
  - Radiotherapy can be used as primary treatment in lentigo maligna or as palliation for cord compression, brain metastases or in the head and neck region, where extensive resection or

isolated perfusion is not possible. The optimal dosages have not been established
- Amputation is generally reserved for fungating disease or exsanguinating haemorrhage

Prolonged survival has been reported for some patients with regional metastasis. For distant metastasis, a low chance of improved survival is only possible by total metastasectomy with curative intent. Those who do not have surgery have a uniformly poor prognosis with an 8.5-month median survival. The most common cause of death is respiratory failure from lung metastases, followed by brain metastasis and raised ICP.

Follow-up

Local recurrence is most common within 5 cm of the primary within 3–5 years and may represent incomplete excision. The risk of a second primary lesion is 2–8%. With regards to starting a family, patients with low risk lesion are advised to wait longer than patients with high-risk lesions, e.g. 5 years rather than 3 years, to avoid developing metastasis during pregnancy. Oral contraceptives and hormone replacement therapy have no effect. It has been difficult to formulate follow-up guidelines, but in general:

- In situ disease does not require routine follow-up
- With invasive disease the duration can be tailored but the frequency should be every 2–3 months otherwise it is essentially pointless:
  - Stage I and II: 2–3 years (studies show that treatable recurrences after excision of thin melanomas are all detected within 2 years). Note that the UK BAD guidelines permit discharge after 1 year for Stage Ia.
  - Stage III/lymph node disease: Life-long (only 2% of patients relapse after 10 years but usually present with stage III/IV)

Routine blood tests and X-rays are not indicated in the asymptomatic. The most accurate way to detect metastatic disease is through a thorough history.

Further reading

Marsden JR, Newton-Bishop JA, Burrows L, et al. Revised UK guidelines for the management of cutaneous melanoma, Br J Dermatol 2010; 163:238–56.

Related topics of interest

- Tissue expansion
- Ultraviolet light

Microorganisms and antibiotics

The overall infection rate after plastic surgery is 6%, of which > two thirds are diagnosed after discharge from hospital. The detected rate of infection depends on the length of surveillance and a 30-day cut-off is commonly used. Risk factors for surgical infections include:

- Length of surgery: Operations lasting > 2 hours are 3 times more likely to have infective complications than those lasting < 1 hour
- Preoperative level of contamination: Infection risk is 10% if clean, 38% if dirty

Basic definitions

Colonisation must be distinguished from infection. Most cultured isolates represent colonisation rather than true infection.
- Contamination is temporary presence with no bacterial multiplication
- Colonisation is permanent presence with no multiplication
- Infection implies invasion, inflammation and tissue destruction

In simple terms, bacteria can be classified as:

- Gram-positive: These have an outer peptidoglycan cell wall that retains the purple dye (crystal violet). These include *Streptococcus, Staphylococcus, Enterococcus* and *Clostridium*
- Gram-negatives have an additional hydrophilic outer lipopolysaccharide coat. Hydrophobic molecules such as penicillin cannot penetrate without modification. They include *Pseudomonas, Haemophilus* and *Neisseria*
- Anaerobes (both Gram-positive and negative) often caused mixed infections that are typically foul smelling. They affect tissues with low oxygen levels such as damaged tissues and tissues in diabetics. The most common are *Bacteroides* and *Clostridium*

The above are extensively discussed in standard texts. This section aims to provide an overview of the *less* commonly discussed bacteria relevant to plastic surgery.

Acinetobacter baumannii

This is an aerobic Gram-negative coccobacilli that is found in 25% of healthy people. It can survive on surfaces for weeks and thus hand transfer is a common mode of spread. It is particularly common in the hospital environment. *Acinetobacter* displays a preference for 'watery' or 'wet' sites such as oropharynx, respiratory tract and urinary tract, as well as skin, although presence in the gut is uncommon and meningitis is rare except after neurosurgery.

It is usually of low virulence but capable of causing infection, especially in susceptible patients such as the extremely ill and immunocompromised. It is common for it to affect the ICU and trauma patients, including burns. Due to its numerous resistance genes (52), multi-resistant *Acinetobacter* can be particularly difficult to eradicate and on occasion has forced ICU closures to curtail epidemics.

Prevention and treatment
- Supportive care and monitoring and appropriate replacement of lines, and removal of unnecessary invasive devices
- Sensitive usually to meropenem/ imipenem, amikacin, third generation cephalosporins, ciproxin or levofloxacin. Severe infections best treated by combination therapy

Eikenella corrodens

This is a facultative anaerobic Gram-negative bacterium that derives it name from its ability to cause pits in agar. In order to culture the organism, it must be grown under aerobic and anaerobic conditions. It is a normal oral commensal, but may contribute to periodontal disease and is the most frequently isolated organism involved in human bites. It has low pathogenicity on its own, but severe abscess disease may result when co-infected with *Streptococcus* or *Staphylococcus*.

- All strains are susceptible to penicillin, but ampicillin or tetracyclines can also be used. There is a variable sensitivity to cephalosporins

Pasteurella multocida

This small Gram-negative coccobacillus is an upper respiratory commensal. It is often co-infects with multiple aerobic/anaerobic organisms. This polymicrobial tendency dictates that broad-spectrum antibiotics are usually necessary, such as co-amoxiclav. *Pasteurella* is sensitive to most antibiotics except macrolides. It is often a component in cat and dog bites and can cause a rapidly progressive cellulitis with local spread and lymphangitis. Early attention is required. Wounds should be irrigated, adequately debrided and only be sutured if there is a low risk of infection. Erythromycin and clarithromycin, both macrolides, and frequent default choices for the penicillin-allergic patient, are inappropriate substitutes for cat and dog bite injuries.

Pseudomonas aeruginosa

This microorganism is ubiquitous and is frequently isolated as opportunistic infection in hospitalised patients. It is the archetypal opportunistic organism, as it almost never infects normal tissue but can cause multitude of infections when given the chance. It is primarily a nosocomial infection accounting for 10% of all hospital acquired infections, commonly affecting the immunocompromised, diabetics and may cause endocarditis in IV drug addicts.

- Burns and trauma: *Pseudomonas* does not grow on dry intact skin, but grows very well on moist skin or environments (swimmer's ear, athlete's foot). It is extremely tolerant of adverse physical conditions (>42°C) and is a cause of hot-tub folliculitis
- Devices

It is a Gram-negative aerobic rod (although it also displays properties of a facultative anaerobe) with very simple nutritional needs (it can multiply in distilled water) and a high level of resistance (outer member LPS, plasmids, biofilm that is resistant to phagocytosis and protects the bacteria from adverse environmental factors). It is toxigenic (produces an exotoxin A, similar to diphtheria) and invasive (enzymes: lecithinase, collagenase, lipase and haemolysin). Wounds are often black/violet with greenish discharge and a characteristic fruity odour. The name 'aeruginosa' comes from the Latin for 'copper rust'.

- Pyocyanin: Bluish-green pigment produced in more than half of the cases. It is also a toxin interfering with electron transport chain
- Fluorescein: Fluoresces yellow-green under ultraviolet light. It is also known as pyoverdin and pyorubin

Severe infections generally require treatment with combination therapy.

- Aminoglycoside plus broad-spectrum antipseudomonal penicillinase, such as piperacillin (with or without β-lactamase inhibitor tazobactam) or cephalosporin
- Monotherapy in the form of ceftazidime or carbapenem. Ciprofloxacin is being evaluated but is probably not suitable for burn infections where multiple resistances are more common
- Topical SSD is useful in burns (also mafenide)

Antibiotics

In very simple terms, there are:

- Penicillins and modified penicillins that attack the cell wall
- Non-penicillins that tend to have intracellular targets

Penicillins

These penicillins belong to β-lactam group that inhibits bacterial wall synthesis in Gram-positive bacteria by inhibiting cross-linkage between peptidoglycan chains. Overuse has led to development of resistant Gram-positive strains. They have almost no activity against Gram-negatives (hydrophobic molecules cannot penetrate hydrophilic LPS wall) but are very effective against anaerobes.

- Antistaphylococcal penicillins: e.g. cloxacillin, methicillin, nafcillin and oxacillin. Dicloxacillin and flucloxacillin are a narrow spectrum (compared to penicillin) β-lactams that are active against *Staphylococcus* (which produces β-lactamase/penicillinase). They are ineffective against MRSA (methicillin-resistant *Staphylococcus aureus*)

- Aminopenicillins, e.g. ampicillin and amoxicillin (related) are more hydrophilic and thus are more effective against Gram-negatives. Both are broad-spectrum antibiotics. Ampicillin can be used in combination with flucloxacillin (Cofluampicil) for empiric treatment of cellulitis
- Antipseudomonals, e.g. carbenicillin, piperacillin and ticarcillin
- β-lactamase inhibitors include clavulanic acid, sulbactam and tazobactam
- Cephalosporins, monobactams (e.g. aztreonam, often used as a less nephrotoxic alternative to aminoglycosides) and carbapenems (e.g. imipenem, often a last resort to reduce bacterial resistance but with risks of opportunistic fungal infections, fluconazole prophylaxis may be added) have β-lactam rings that are modified to make them more resistant to β-lactamases. Allergic reactions may be related to the common β-lactam ring or the distinguishing R group side chain
  – Each subsequent generation of cephalosporins have increased Gram-negative activity at the expense of decreased Gram-positive activity. Their activity against enteric bacteria is poor

Antibiotics with no similarity to penicillin

- Aminoglycosides bind to ribosomal proteins but require transport into the bacteria via an oxygen dependent pump. They have thus little activity on anaerobes. Their hydrophilicity permits good activity against Gram-negatives. Ototoxicity and renal toxicity are the major side effects. Aminoglycosides are not available in oral preparation
- Quinolones: Interferes with DNA replication (topoisomerase)

Empiric treatment

- Gram-positive: First generation cephalosporin, antistaphylococcal penicillin
- Gram-negative: Gentamicin, second or third generation cephalosporin (like penicillins, these display synergistic activity with gentamicin and are often used together for pseudomonal infections)

- Anaerobes: Penicillin, metronidazole, clindamycin

Penicillin allergy

There is a reported 10% cross reactivity with cephalosporins (share β-lactam ring) but this may be overestimated because:
- Early first generation cephalosporins were contaminated with penicillin
- The β-lactam ring in cephalosporins is rapidly fragmented
- Some patients are purely cephalosporin allergic: 2% of general population, with no history of penicillin allergy, compared to 8% if penicillin allergic from history. Risk factors for true cephalosporin allergy include the following:
  – Positive penicillin skin test (5%)
  – Use of a first generation cephalosporin

Many patients with penicillin allergies are not truly allergic in the strictest sense of the word, as the symptoms reported are not typically Type I hypersensitivity reactions (rapid within 1 hour, involves swelling, urticaria, wheeze/stridor and hypotensive) but are often non-specific problems, such as nausea/vomiting/diarrhoea, non-specific rash and toxic effects. If the history is unconvincing of a Type I reaction to penicillin, cephalosporins may be used with caution. If the history suggests a possible Type I reaction, and the antibiotic is essential, then skin testing (IgE) can be useful (4% of patients with a negative test will have non-lethal reactions to penicillin, although not anaphylaxis). Overall,
- 90% of those claiming a penicillin allergy will be negative on skin testing. They should still avoid penicillins but can use cephalosporins (1–2% rate of sensitivity, which is no greater than general population)
- 10% will have a positive skin test. They should avoid both penicillin and cephalosporins (5–8%)

In addition, according to a review, the risk of cephalosporin cross-reactivity in a penicillin-allergic patient depends on the generation. The first, second and third generations have cross reactivity rates of 0.5%, 0.2% and 0.8% respectively.

In summary, it is 'safe' to administer cephalosporins in those with supposed 'penicillin reactions', as long as the reaction is not a Type I reaction and the penicillin skin test is negative. A literature review and analysis by Campagna (2012) showed that the true cross reactivity (cephalosporin allergy in a penicillin-allergic patient) is 1% overall and is mostly due to using first generation cephalosporins (or those with similar R1 chains) and almost negligible with third generation cephalosporins.

Further reading

Campagna JD, Bond MC, Schabelman E, et al. The use of cephalosporins in penicillin-allergic patients: a literature review, J Emerg Med 2011; 2012;42:612–20

Related topic of interest

- Hand infections

Microsurgery and tissue transfer

In 1902, Carrel developed the triangulation technique for anastomosis of small vessels. Zeiss built the first operating microscope in 1951 and by 1960 Jacobsen and Suarez were using adapted jewellers instruments, reporting 100% patency in anastomosing small vessels (1.5–3.2 mm).

Microsurgical free tissue transfer allows a block of tissue to be moved from one part of the body to another with immediate revascularisation, enabling reconstruction and wound closure where grafts are not a viable option (see below). Free flaps are distinguished from local and pedicled flaps that remain attached to the body and their blood supply during transfer.

The anastomosis of blood vessels, an artery and one or more veins require specialised techniques and instruments, and prolonged anaesthesia. Nevertheless, in experienced hands, microsurgical free tissue transfer has a high rate of success in the region of 95–99%, after an initial learning curve. The technique is particularly useful in the following conditions:

- Surface area requirement to provide stable cover for exposed vital structures, such as complex tibial fractures or large vessels
- Vascularised bone requirement, such as for mandible reconstruction
- Functional tissue requirement, such as muscle for facial reanimation
- Volumetric soft tissue requirement, such as for breast reconstruction or to obliterate cavities

Decision making and planning is as critical to the success of flap microsurgery as surgical technique. The choice of flap should be appropriate to the problem with pre-planned alternatives (lifeboats) in case of failure. Planning ahead is vital to reduce the overall operative time and the ischaemic time of the flap (secondary ischaemic time is ischaemia after surgical reanastomosis, which counts as warm ischaemia, **Table 50**).

- The recipient vessel should be out of zones of injury or irradiation. A hand-held Doppler ultrasound probe may be useful to detect suitable recipient vessels and flap donor vessels
- Performing the anastomosis requires meticulous technique, especially limiting unnecessary manipulation of the vessels. The adventitia is trimmed (circumcised) and the vessel ends are sutured tension-free, using the minimal number of sutures possible without leaks. A neat anastomosis is less likely to have flow problems
- A degree of vessel diameter mismatch is common. Differences of up to 2:1 can be dealt with by:
  - Differential suturing
  - Cutting obliquely and spatulating
  - Dilation

Larger discrepancies have increased risks of turbulent flow and thrombosis, and should be sutured end-to-side instead. Only if this not possible should the larger vessel end be narrowed to match.

- Finding recipient vessels can be a major hurdle in certain situations, such as in the irradiated head and neck. Options include the transverse cervical or thoracoacromial vessels. The external carotid itself can be used with a side clamp and good proximal and distal control. According to Batchelor, any artery with pulsatile flow can support a flap whether anterograde or retrograde. For veins, either the external jugular or cephalic can be turned down and used as a recipient

Table 50 Warm and cold ischaemia times		
	Warm ischaemia	Cold ischaemia (cooling prolongs the tolerance of all tissues)
Skin	4–6 h	12 h
Muscle	< 2 h	Up to 8 h
Bone	< 3 h	Up to 24 h

- Vein grafts may be needed when there is insufficient vessel length. The length of the vein graft does not seem to affect patency per se, but increasing the length increases the risk of thrombosis and kinking. Mark the ends carefully and be particularly wary of twisting

Postoperative management

Regular flap observations are important. The window for rescuing a flap is rather narrow, especially for muscle flaps, which can become compromised very quickly and may also cause systemic upset. Patient should preferably be monitored on a 'flap ward' by experienced staff and where ambient temperatures can be controlled. Clinically, a combination of colour, capillary refill (1–2 seconds), temperature and turgor is used to assess the state of the flap. Careful puncture (avoiding the pedicle!) or scratching with a needle-tip to assess bleeding may be used. Do not rely on muscle contraction as a sign of good perfusion as it can persist for hours after the onset of ischaemia. Similarly, tissue can continue to bleed for several hours after the onset of inflow occlusion. In simple terms, the patient should be kept 'well, warm and wet'.

- Well: Give adequate analgesia to reduce pain and anxiety, which can lead to vasoconstriction. Preoperative oral gabapentin has been shown to reduce postoperative analgesic requirements
- Warm: Keep the flap (and the patient) warm
- Wet: A hyperdynamic circulation (systolic blood pressure > 100 mmHg, without use of vasoconstrictors) is maintained to maximise perfusion through the anastomosis. Intravenous fluid is given to maintain a urine output of about 1 ml/kg/h depending on the cardiac status of the patient
- Elevate flap area where possible to reduce swelling and promote venous drainage

More objective measurements for flap monitoring exist that allow continuous monitoring and potentially earlier detection of a problem. To date, none of these show demonstrable superiority over combined clinical assessment, which remains the gold (practical) standard.

- A flap to core temperature difference of more than 2°C suggests a perfusion problem
- Pulse oximetry may be useful for toe transfers and replanted digits
- Transcutaneous oxygen: Relative changes are more useful than absolute values
- pH monitoring: A pH < 7.3 or a difference of > 0.35 compared to control suggests a problem
- Surface Doppler: May record false-positives by picking up other vessels, and an arterial signal may persist even if the vein is occluded. Implantable probes may overcome some of these problems
- Laser Doppler techniques measure blood flow but only penetrate 1.5 mm. Near-infrared spectroscopy has better penetration
- Intravenous fluorescein and a Wood's lamp: The fluorescein takes 12–18 h to clear and is thus unsuitable for continuous monitoring. The use of minidoses may be better
- Intravenous indocyanine green (ICG) is already widely used in neurosurgery and hepatobiliary surgery

Potential flap problems

A free flap may be compromised by inflow or outflow problems. Anastomotic problems are the most common reason for reexploration, followed by haematoma/bleeding as the second most common. Haematomas may develop and compress the anastomosis, or cause kinking or twisting of the pedicle. Perforator flaps are particularly difficult to salvage.

- Arterial problems: Cool pale flap with sluggish capillary refill
- Venous problems (three times more common): Blue congested flap with brisk refill

Simple measures may be useful:

- Assess and optimise haemodynamics and hydration
- Reposition patient or body parts if needed
- Remove constricting dressings or tight sutures

But if these manoeuvres do not make an appreciable difference rapidly, reexploration is required and has a 75% success rate on average if done promptly.

- Consider applying antispasmodics such as verapamil or papaverine (30 mg/ml). 2% lignocaine as a single agent is ineffective and requires 20% concentrations for effect, or combination with papaverine (Gheradini 1998)
- Check for twisting of the vessels or anastomosis. Check for the presence of thrombosis (either fresh or established clot). Do not milk non-occluding thrombi, as this will only cause more damage. A growing thrombus should be irrigated out by opening up a few sutures. Re-do the anastomosis if necessary
- Fibrinolytics, such as streptokinase, urokinase or TPA may be useful in salvage if a thrombus is found, at the risk of haemorrhage. Anticoagulants or dextran may be used postoperatively
  - Dextran 40 (40 kilo-Daltons) at 25 ml/h for 5 days has been used to reduce platelet function/adhesion, reduce blood viscosity and destabilise platelet thrombi. It is a natural product of the *Leuconostoc mesenteroides* from sucrose. The mechanism of action is unclear but may involve its negative charge. Severe complications, such as acute renal failure, pulmonary/ cerebral oedema have been reported and anaphylaxis occurs very rarely. It is commonly used as a 10% solution, with a bolus of 250 ml followed by an infusion of 25 ml/h, but the evidence base for its use is weak and has fallen out of current favour
  - Heparin is a natural substance that potentiates antithrombin III and causes release of plasminogen activator to initiate fibrinolysis. Clot-bound thrombin may be resistant and

effectively hidden from circulating heparin. Hence heparin alone cannot be used to clear blocked anastomoses
  - Prostaglandin E1 is often used in the postoperative regime in supermicrosurgery with very narrow vessels

No single drug treatment can be recommended based on solid evidence. The surgical technique, pedicle choice and position are much more important. With reexploration, the speed of the response is key.

- Flaps may also be damaged by reperfusion injury. Anaerobic metabolites build up in ischaemic tissue and on re-establishing blood flow, oxygen free radicals are generated, causing calcium influx and cell damage. The no reflow phenomenon describes the situation of no flap perfusion despite a physically patent anastomosis. This has been attributed to platelet aggregation, endothelial injury, intravascular thrombosis and fluid shift into tissues (from failing cellular pumps) with arteriovenous (AV) shunting

Failing flaps

- Leeches are useful for cases of venous congestion. The leech itself removes approximately 10 ml of blood, but the hirudin in its saliva is a selective thrombin inhibitor that will promote another 50 ml of loss through oozing. Prophylaxis against *Aeromonas hydrophila* is required
- Poor man's leech: A small area of flap surface epithelium is removed and allowed to bleed freely. The flow is maintained with topical heparin (400 IU/ml) soaked gauzes that are replaced every 30 minutes and can be used for up to 5–10 days
- Hyperbaric oxygen has been shown to be useful for salvaging failing flaps in some animal studies, but there is little clinical data on its role

Further reading

Chiu TW, Chung WH, Vlantis AC, et al. Monitoring a free anterolateral thigh flap for pharyngeal reconstruction. Surg Prac 2009; 13:77–9.

Related topics of interest

- Breast reconstruction
- Hyperbaric oxygen
- Leeches and maggots

Nasal reconstruction

The external nose is a complex structure in terms of shape and layers, and components.

- Different skin characteristics:
  - Zone I: Upper-third skin is thin and mobile, and FTSGs give reasonable results
  - Zone II: Lower-third skin is thick (almost twice that of Zone I), adherent and sebaceous. Flaps (local/distant) will provide better results than grafts
  - Zone III: Alar skin is also sebaceous
- The skeleton is also divided into thirds: Proximal (nasal bones), middle (upper lateral cartilages) and distal/lobule (alar/lower lateral cartilages)
- There are three layers that need to be considered: Skin, support and lining. If reconstruction of the lining is neglected, deformation and stenosis in the long term result. Support is required early on, as secondary modifications are disappointing once the soft tissue collapses and contracts
- There are nine subunits: Single: dorsum, tip and columella. Paired: Sidewalls, soft triangles and alar. A defect that involves > 50% of a subunit will yield a better cosmetic result if the entire subunit is reconstructed, instead of just the defect. The subunit principle of reconstruction is underlined by observation that eyes are trained to see changes in colour, texture and contour. While the quality of scarring cannot be controlled, the site of scars can be to an extent. Scars can become raised or spread, in which case they reflect a line of light, or they become depressed and cast a linear shadow. Ideal placement of scars along the borders of the nasal subunits provides optimal cosmesis

General observations on nasal reconstruction:

- Colour: Patients who are Fitzpatrick I/II tend to heal well without a pigmented scar, and thus may be acceptable to have scars crossing subunits if there is a good colour and texture match
- Texture: Certain skin textures that are very sebaceous, rosaceous or very tight and smooth, may be better reconstructed using adjacent skin of the same quality, even if subunit principles are not adhered to (e.g. bilobed flaps and dorsal advancement flaps). FTSG are likely to be of a different texture and noticeable unless subunit principles adhered to
- Contour: Hide scars in concavities or points of inflection. Some areas are particularly difficult to reconstruct, such as the alar facial junction that has a gentle sloping concavity, and may be best to preserve it and only replace part of the subunit

Reconstruction is often most straightforward after cancer resection as it does not have the following complexities:

- Trauma may displace adjacent structures
- Burns may affect potential donor sites
- Congenital: Generally hypoplastic structures

Small defects (<0.5 cm)

- Primary closure: Angle oblique to alar margin, if possible
- Secondary healing can be considered around the medial canthus (concavity)
- Zone II
  - Banner flap for up to 1 cm defects (similar to a single lobed bilobed flap)
  - Bilobed flap (Zitelli) for up to 2 cm defects
  - Sliding glabellar flap which is based on infratrochlear artery but will leave scars that cross subunits with blunting of radix and nasofrontal angle
  - Reiger dorsal nasal flap widely based on one side of the nasal dorsum (angular artery) for up to 2 cm defects. The original glabellar extension is not generally used
  - Nasolabial flap (using two or more stages gives the best results) can be pedicled superiorly, inferiorly, tunnelled, islanded or turned over for lining
  - FTSGs

Larger defects >1.5 cm

- Zone I: FTSG particularly postauricular skin that is relatively thin (thinner than preauricular) and vascularises well
- Zone II: Best results are obtained from a multi-staged forehead flap that will require sacrifice of normal tissue and a forehead scar (see below)
  - NLF: Most often superiorly based flaps with the pivot point near infraorbital foramen give the best results (may be islanded but it will not reliably reach the dorsum or tip). As it often contracts significantly or trapdoors, (particularly with islanded flaps or delayed reconstructions) it is a good option for a complete subunit, such as the alar lobule, where the trapdooring may be disguised or contribute to the aesthetic contour
    - Note that nasolabial flaps are not axial as the artery lies below the muscle and is not included with the flap. They are random patterned with a rich vascular territory, and can be pedicled in numerous directions
  - Cheek advancement: The flap is raised at the subdermal level with a large Burrow's triangle along the NLF. It is a good option for side of the nose, particularly in older patients, but suboptimal for the alar region
  - Converse scalping flap: This is fairly mutilating. The whole forehead (including the hairline) based on one superficial temporal artery is used with majority of this large flap simply acting as a carrier for the new nose, which is positioned at the lateral extent of forehead (and arching over superiorly). The flap is raised in the subgaleal plane (except the neo-nasal portion, which is raised in the layer above muscle) and shifted downwards. The neo-nasal donor site defect is grafted (FTSG) while the rest of the flap is returned to its original location after flap division
  - Washio (posterior auricular/temporomastoid flap): This only yields a small amount of thin skin

Forehead flap

Forehead skin is an excellent colour and texture match for the lower nose. Modern forehead flaps are transferred on unilateral paramedian vessels which brings the axis of rotation lower down nearer the defect.

The forehead skin is richly anastomosed and the flap has a rich axial pattern anastomotic plexus centred on the medial canthus that can potentially support the flap even after division of supraorbital, supratrochlear and infratrochlear vessels. Traditionally, the forehead flap has been a two-staged procedure with a 3-week interval. However, this often meant delayed placement of cartilage grafts, which could be difficult in a shrunken soft tissue envelope. Menick proposes a three-stage procedure with an intervening stage for revision and trimming. The flap can be theoretically islanded and transferred in one stage, but the pedicle is bulky and vascularity is at greater risk.

Stage 1

- Cut an exact pattern, using a template from the normal contralateral side. The flap is centred on a line starting just medial to eyebrow, 1.2–1.5 cm wide at the corrugator crease, and includes frontalis muscle at base of flap. It is based on supratrochlear vessels that start off lying just over periosteum inferiorly, which then run with muscle to become almost subdermal at the hairline. Traditionally, the flap has been partially thinned distally at the first stage, but this may diminish the vascularity and the raw subdermal surface is more liable to contract
- Methods of harvesting longer flaps have been described. These include making the flap oblique, horizontal (but elevates/distorts brow), up and down (Gillies). Current choices include extension into the hairline followed by depilation (with lasers), incision of frontalis at 1 cm intervals, taking the base more inferiorly to medial canthal area and/or skeletonizing the pedicle

- Treat the primary defect as priority. Do not compromise by making the flap too small in order to minimise the donor defect, and avoid tissue expansion (the skin tends to thin and retract unpredictably). The forehead can always be closed by other methods. Defects of up to 3–4 cm can be closed primarily after undermining. Gaps with partial closure will eventually heal well with secondary intention, as long as the periosteum is intact to prevent bone drying out. It will continue to contract over 3–4 months, although the time taken for healing may be an issue

Stage 2

- Transect pedicle that is unfurled and inset as inverted-V at medial brow. Forehead flaps are delayed and are thus vascularly robust enough to be completely re-elevated and the layers separated, if required. Quilting sutures can be used to hold the thinned flap to the contoured bed, in particular to define and accentuate the sidewalls and tip

- Further revision as required after 4–6 months after maturation

Lining

It is important to line the flap, otherwise it will tend to distort. Lining can come from folding of the forehead flap, skin grafting (with quilting, good choice in elderly) the undersurface or mobilising intranasal flaps. The latter are capable of supporting primary cartilage grafts. It is difficult to satisfactorily place cartilage primarily in folded flaps because of their bulkiness. Other options for nasal lining include turned over nasal skin, NLF or composite grafts.

- In larger complex defects that require more lining, a thin free flap, such as a FRFF, can used to provide a lining layer, which is then covered with skin grafts on the outer exposed surfaces. At a later stage the skin grafts are removed, the tissues revised and a cartilage framework constructed (usually from costal cartilages) and then covered with a forehead flap

Further reading

Koch CA, Archibald DJ, Friedman O, et al. Glabellar flaps in nasal reconstruction. Fac Plast Surg Clin N Am 2011; 19:113–22.

Related topics of interest

- Facial anatomy
- Local flaps

- Rhinoplasty

Neck dissection

The presence of metastatic neck disease from head and neck cancer halves patient survival. On average, 25% of patients with SCC of the head and neck may have microscopic nodal disease at the time of presentation. This risk increases with posterior cancers and younger patients.

Assessment

Clinical assessment by palpation alone is unreliable and will often miss nodes <2 cm in diameter or those under the sternomastoid. It has a false-negative rate of one third, particularly in those with short fat necks or after radiotherapy, and a comparable false positive rate. Thus a CT/MRI from skull base to sternoclavicular joints is commonly performed in all patients to stage the neck.

- CT can demonstrate features suggesting malignancy, including central necrosis, capsule enhancement and extracapsular spread
- MRI is more sensitive and will demonstrate more nodes (almost all if > 4 mm in diameter), but is less able to differentiate between benign or reactive nodes from malignant nodes. MRI is useful to assess clinically negative necks, due to its high negative predictive value. Positive MRI findings should be assessed further with FNA/surgery
- Ultrasound scan with FNAC has high specificity but low sensitivity of the latter. It is used to clarify equivocality on CT/MRI
- FDG-PET has a role in increasing the accuracy of nodal staging where CT/MRI is equivocal. It is particularly useful for patients who present with lymph nodes with an unknown primary or in cases of suspected recurrence not well demonstrated by CT/MRI. FDG-PET is fluorine-18-fluro-2-deoxy-D-glucose positron emission tomography, and demonstrates increased glycolysis, reflecting high activity, such as in tumour cells. Both false positive and false negatives rates are high. Some tumours are inherently FDG negative, such as chondrosarcoma and adenocarcinoma of salivary glands

Levels of the neck nodes

A significant advance in the discussion/comparison of neck disease and its treatment was the use of consistent nomenclature (Memorial Sloan-Kettering), as described in **Table 51**. The lower the nodal involvement, the worse the prognosis (in very simple terms) with the worst prognosis in IV and V.

Level II–IV nodes occupy the space between the posterior border of sternomastoid and the lateral border of sternohyoid. Perifacial nodes are not included. Some describe level VII nodes in the anterior mediastinum.

Nodal status (from TNM)

- Nx: Not assessable
- N0: No involved nodes
- N1: Single ipsilateral, 3 cm or less
- N2a: Single ipsilateral, > 3 cm, < 6 cm
- N2b: Multiple ipsilateral, < 6 cm
- N2c: Bilateral/contralateral < 6 cm
- N3: Massive > 6 cm

The prognosis is significantly worse if the nodes show fixity, extracapsular spread, perivascular or perineural invasion, or if they occur in the posterior triangle or contralateral neck.

Surgical management

A ND is effectively a block dissection of the regional lymphatic system, with skin flap elevation in the subplatysmal plane.

- Radical ND (RND, Crile 1906) aims to remove the first five nodal levels, from mandible to clavicle, and from lateral sternohyoid to anterior trapezius along with 3 non-lymphatic structures: the accessory nerve, sternomastoid and IJV
- Modified radical ND: As a RND, but sparing one or more of the 3 non-lymphatic structures
- Selective: One or more nodal groups are spared (subtotal)
- Extended ND: As a RND, but with additional lymphatic and non-lymphatic structures included such as the paratracheal, retropharyngeal and mediastinal nodes, and the parotid gland

Node level	Name	Boundaries: clinical and surgical	Comments
I	Submandibular triangle	Between lower mandible border, posterior bellies of digastric muscles and hyoid	IA: Submental triangle—lower lip, FOM, tip of tongue IB: Digastric triangle—rest of oral cavity
II	Upper jugular	From base of skull to hyoid bone or carotid bifurcation	Jugulodigastric node drains oral cavity, face and scalp IIA: Anterior to accessory nerve IIB: Posterior to accessory nerve—dissection may not be necessary if IIa is not involved for tumours of oral cavity, hypopharynx and larynx.
III	Middle jugular	From hyoid/carotid bifurcation to cricothyroid membrane or the omohyoid	
IV	Lower jugular	From the cricothyroid/omohyoid to the clavicle	Contains the thoracic duct on the left. A: Deep to sternal head, higher risk for VI involvement concomitantly B: Deep to clavicular head of sternocleidomastoid muscle, higher risk for V Contains some of the supraclavicular nodes including Virchow
V	Posterior triangle	Posterior border sternomastoid, anterior trapezius and clavicle	A and B according to accessory nerve A: Oropharynx, nasopharynx and skin B: Thyroid Contains cervical plexus and transverse cervical artery
VI	Anterior compartment	Hyoid to suprasternal notch, between lateral borders of sternohyoid	A later addition to the original scheme, includes superior mediastinal nodes

Table 51 Classification of lymph nodes of the neck

The morbidity of a ND is mainly related to the excision of non-lymphatic structures:

- Spinal accessory: Problems include discomfort and reduced abduction, asymmetry of neck outline and drooping shoulder. Symptomatology is variable but older patients tend to be affected more
- Internal jugular vein: Bilateral RND may result in increased facial oedema and intracranial pressure with an increased risk of stroke and blindness. The mortality of bilateral RND is 10–14% compared to 0–3% in unilateral surgery. Generally, it is recommended that bilateral operations should be staged or one IJV should be reconstructed
  - Even when the IJV requires removal, the stump can still be used for (end-to-side) microanastomosis in head and neck reconstruction
- Sternomastoid: Removal of this muscle has the least associated morbidity. The problem is mainly a cosmetic issue, although its preservation offers potential protection for the carotid sheath

Radiotherapy (external beam or brachytherapy) after a ND may be indicated for:

- Positive histology on ND specimens
- Extracapsular spread
- N2 disease (large single node)

Modified radical neck dissection

Modified radical neck dissection (MRND) was designed in an effort to reduce the morbidity by preserving one or more non-lymphatic functional structures when oncologically safe to do so. Bocca originally described this in 1967 (preceded by Suarez in Argentina but reported in Spanish) and its safety was established over the next decade. There is a classification described by Medina (N-M-V):

- Type 1: Accessory nerve preserved

- Type 2: Accessory nerve and sternomastoid muscle preserved
- Type 3: All three (accessory nerve, sternomastoid and IJ vein) preserved

The type of dissection is often decided perioperatively according to the findings. A paring of the specified structures is a viable option if there is no clinical evidence of their infiltration by malignancy. Although it does take more time, MRND is the operation of choice in most cases, except when the extra, perceived safety of RND is specifically indicated (**Table 52**). Outcomes in selected cases are similar, but there are no prospective studies comparing RND and MRND. Studies that do exist suffer from the fact that many preceded the standardised classification of NDs.

Selective neck dissection

From a review of surgical specimens at the Sloan-Kettering hospital, it was found that nodal spread is largely predictable as it follows certain characteristic and consistent patterns. This led to development of selective neck dissection with the aim of clearing levels most likely to be involved and to avoid further unnecessary and additional morbidity, as explained in **Table 53**.

Complications of neck dissection

Intraoperative

- Bradycardia: Due to carotid body stimulation
- Bleeding: Prolongs hospital stay, but shortest in those that return to theatre rather than managed by bedside procedures or observation
- Slippage of ligature on IJV especially at skull base is a very difficult situation to manage. If the stump cannot be identified for ligation, pack for haemostasis, before using either Surgicel or a muscle flap

Table 52 Indications and contraindications for radical neck dissection (RND)

Indications for RND (i.e. MND not good enough)	Contraindications of RND, i.e. futile or not necessary

• High-grade tumours with N2+ neck disease
• **Invasive nodal disease:** extracapsular spread, involving IJV or accessory nerve
• **Recurrent disease**
• **Postradiotherapy,** if the primary is under control.
	• N0 neck
	• Uncontrollable primary
	• Distant metastasis
	• Fixed neck/encased carotid
	  – A balloon occlusion test (risks 1.2% temporary, 0.4% permanent) is advisable if > 270° involvement.
	  – Surgery requiring sacrifice is generally not regarded as potentially curable and even after resection and reconstruction, recurrence and early mortality is high.

Table 53 Classification of selective neck dissection

Selective neck dissection	Levels resected	Indications	Comments
Supraomohyoid	Levels 1, 2 and 3 mandible, to posterior SCM/cervical plexus and omohyoid over IJV	For oral cancer for N0, or TxN1 (less than 3 cm, mobile and in I or II). It can be viewed as essentially being a staging procedure and to gain access.	Spares thoracic duct, accessory nerve, sternomastoid and IJV. Not suitable for tonsillar tumours.
(Antero)lateral	Levels 2, 3 and 4	For laryngeal, oropharynx and hypopharyngeal cancers	Hypo/oropharynx and supraglottic occult metastasis 30%
Anterior	Levels 2, 3, 4 and tracheo-oesophageal nodes	Thyroid	
Posterior/posterolateral	Levels 2, 3, 4 and 5, and occipital triangle (suboccipital and postauricular)	Posterior scalp/neck cancers	

- Breach of the IJV may lead to air embolism (negative intrathoracic pressure sucks air into distal end), possibly leading to a drop in blood pressure, cardiac output and saturation. It is important to control the distal end first. Inform the anaesthetist (to give 100% oxygen and stop nitrous oxide). Positioning in left lateral position may trap air in right atrium for aspiration with a central venous catheter. Prophylactic antibiotics are commonly given, but the evidence is not well established for this practice. The rate of infection after RND is quoted at 10%
- Lymph/chyle leak due to damage of the thoracic duct (left neck, 4% risk) or right lymphatic trunk (less common). It is more common with radical surgery and can be checked for intraoperatively by asking anaesthetist to induce a Valsalva-like manoeuvre (positive airway pressure for 30 seconds or more). If a leak is present, a milky drainage is seen. Triglyceride and chylomicrons levels cannot be used reliably to confirm the diagnosis
  - It can usually be managed conservatively with a low-fat diet (medium chain triglycerides that are absorbed directly into portal system and bypass lymphatics), pressure dressings/suction drainage and head elevation. Electrolytes need to be monitored carefully
  - Total parenteral nutrition can significantly reduce the volume of leakage within 24 hours and can be considered in selected patients
  - High output fistulae (> 600 ml/day) are less likely to respond to conservative treatment. Surgical options include fibrin glue, muscle flaps, sclerosing agents (tetracycline/doxycycline) or mediastinal exploration and ligation of duct more proximally
- Salivary fistula
- Nerve damage causing difficulty in swallowing (glossopharyngeal), shoulder pain and weakness (XI), difficulty in breathing (phrenic: a raised hemidiaphragm is seen on chest radiographs) and tongue weakness

(hypoglossal). Trigger point sensitivity may be due to neuroma formation
- Skin flap necrosis: If this occurs over the great vessels, there is a risk of a carotid blow-out, especially in the radiotherapy patient. Thus, triradiate incisions are at greater risk than apron or MacFee incisions. There is often a minor warning bleed. Semielective treatment involves resection and ligation, with reconstruction in selected patients. Ligation after rupture carries a 50% mortality, compared to 12% with elective ligation (with one-third neurologic deficit)

Skin incisions

Preoperative considerations include the location of adenopathy, type of ND needed, the likelihood of postoperative radiation and the potential for wound healing problems (preoperative radiation, diabetes, vascular disease and previous surgery). There are a significant number of different neck incision lines and the general principles are:

- Skin flaps should be raised in the subplatysmal plane, if feasible and oncologically safe to do so. Scars should be excised for cosmesis, potential harbourage of tumour seeds and because of its poor blood supply. Incisions that cross or join the tracheostomy skin opening risk the formation of fistulae or leakage that is very difficult to manage
- Place incisions along RSTLs with lazy 'S's to reduce the potential for contractures and place junctions at right angles for at least 2 cm to reduce tip necrosis
- Submandibular incisions should be at least 2 cm below the level of mandible (posterior to the facial artery) to avoid damaging the marginal mandibular branch of facial nerve
- Be wary of incisions in the watershed areas of blood supply (mid-neck and in the midline). Y-incisions should not be placed over the carotid artery but at a distance from it (usually posterior) (**Figure 13**)

The archetypal incision was the Hayes Martin (**Figure 13**) with two Y junctions (a larger Y at the submandibular region and a smaller inverted Y at the supraclavicular region)

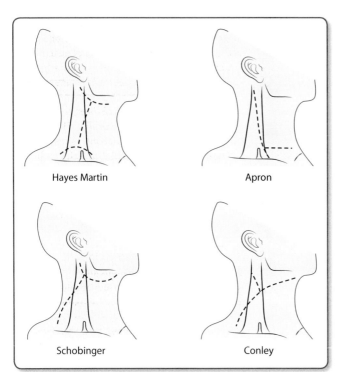

Figure 13 Common types of incision for neck dissections.

that provided good access but had problems with wound breakdown at the three-point junctions and poor cosmesis. The Slaughter modification (1955) eliminated the sharp angles, and improved vascularity. The lower three-point junction was substituted subsequently by a continuation of the long limb, e.g. Kocher, whilst other modifications included shifting of the vertical limb back to avoid the carotid and also to reduce posterior flap dissection, which could be difficult due to lack of a specific plane, e.g. Schobinger.

- Utility Flap: The incision runs from mastoid tip, curving 2 fingerbreadths below the angle of mandible to the midline at the level of the superior border of thyroid cartilage/hyoid bone. It is a useful type of incision with most of visible scar in RSTLs and is convenient for laryngeal tumours, bilateral ND, thyroid surgery and easily combined with parotid incisions. Its disadvantages include the relatively poor exposure posteriorly with a large inferior flap. The apron flap is a modification of the utility flap, which runs from mastoid to symphysis (unilateral) or mastoid to mastoid (bilateral), lying 2–3 fingerbreadths above the sternal notch. It is mainly used for laryngectomies
- Schobinger (1957): The higher horizontal incision allows easier access to oral cavity and the shorter superior flap allows a midline lip splitting extension with less likelihood of tip necrosis
- Conley: The curved vertical limb meets the anterior submandibular incision as a smooth curve (concave anterior) and the posterior submandibular incision meets this at right angles. The main aim is to decrease the risk of scar contracture. There is excellent exposure of the neck, but whilst the superior flap is safe, the lower part is less so. There is a risk here of flap necrosis exposing vessels, making it relatively dangerous for the post-radiotherapy neck. (**Figure 13**)

The MacFee type (**Figure 14**) involves parallel neck incisions with an intervening bipedicled flap at least 7 cm wide. The upper incision lies 2.5 cm below mandible from mastoid

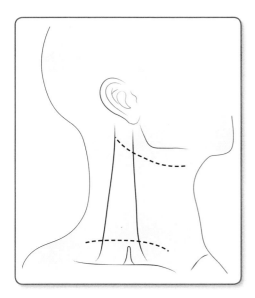

Figure 14 The MacFee type of incision named after William F MacFee (1960) though sometimes spelt in the literature as McFee, is preferred by some surgeons as it avoids some of the drawbacks of three point access methods.

to hyoid and the lower one approximately 3.5 cm above clavicle from anterior trapezius to midline. It is popular is some centres where it may be used almost exclusively but in others, it is usually primarily reserved for irradiated necks and for thyroid cancers in young women. The cosmesis is generally good as the incisions lie in RSTLs. However, the overall cosmetic result after ND is also related to the contour and symmetry rather than the skin scar alone. It is technically more difficult, with the limited exposure making dissection (particularly with bleeding on the undersurface) more tedious. Although blood flow in the neck is predominantly vertical, theoretical vascular problems have not been borne out clinically.

In general, the utility flap and modifications of the Schobinger flaps are preferred for most procedures involving ND alone or with upper aerodigestive tract tumour resections. MacFee type flaps or longer apron flaps are sometimes preferred for cosmetic reasons, if their use does not compromise the resection.

Further reading

Brennan PA, Blythe JN, Herd MK, et al. The contemporary management of chyle leak following cervical thoracic duct damage. Br J Oral Maxillofac Surg 2012;50:197–201

Related topic of interest

- Head and neck cancer principles

Necrotising fasciitis

Necrotising fasciitis (NF) is a rapidly progressive soft tissue infection with widespread fascial necrosis and secondary necrosis of the superficial tissues as a result of vascular occlusion. Bacterial enzymes (haemolysins, hyaluronidase, and streptokinase) and toxins facilitate bacterial spread along fascial planes. The onset of disease is typically insidious and the patient may initially seem deceptively well, with only flu-like symptoms with fevers and chills. However, it progresses very quickly and sudden deterioration can occur. Do not delay surgery. If in doubt, exploratory surgery is indicated.

- Disproportionate extreme pain with few obvious skin abnormalities that changes to anaesthesia with skin changes as the superficial nerves are damaged
- Initial spreading erythema that darkens to purple and grey-duskiness. Multiple areas may coalesce. Swelling with vesicles and blisters may form. Serous-filled bullae are a characteristic feature. Crepitus may be present, especially in diabetics, reflecting gas formation by the organisms involved
- Extreme toxicity and septicaemia develops. The mortality rate is high (25–50%) and is highest in those with sepsis on presentation, delayed debridement, the elderly and those with diabetes mellitus. NF can affect any area. Fournier's gangrene is a subset that is localised to the scrotum/perineum and is typically idiopathic (in the original description) with up to 75% mortality

Although NF may be found in the immunosuppressed (HIV, cancer, diabetes and in transplant patients), half of patients in most literature series were previously fit and well. It can develop after relatively minor trauma, insect bites, surgery (such as drainage of intraperitoneal or perianal/ischiorectal abscesses) or needle puncture.

- Intravenous drugs users are at risk of developing NF from anaerobic *Streptococci*, whereas those with liver disease are susceptible to *Vibrio vulnificus* from raw seafood especially oysters. These patients often have haemorrhagic blisters

NF has become a rather general term to describe soft tissue infections involving the fascia that may have many causes. There are three main types, and distinguishing between them is useful, as the optimal treatment is significantly different in each case. NF may also be classified by the presentation: fulminant (hours), acute (days) and subacute (weeks).

- Type 1—Polymicrobial: This is the most common type, which has a comparatively slower onset and mainly affects the subcutaneous fat and fascia first. There is synergy between anaerobes and facultative aerobic organisms, especially Gram negatives. The organisms proliferate in the hypoxic local tissue that develops after tissue injury, particularly in the unwell (hypoxia reduces neutrophil function that facilitates bacterial growth)
- Type 2—Streptococcal (group A): Streptococcal superantigen is directly toxic in addition to its propensity to induce a massive inflammatory response. The injury may be minor and the overlying skin may look viable despite extensive underlying necrosis. Pure streptococcal infection was described in the classic paper, but most clinical infections involve additional organisms such as *Bacteroides* and *Escherichia coli* with *Streptococci* +/– *Staphylococci* as the initiators. Other organisms may contribute by reducing phagocytic function and interferon secretion. Gas may be present but is not a common feature. This form of NF typically has a worse prognosis and is more rapidly progressive. There is an unexplained association with the use of non-steroidal anti-inflammatory agents such as ibuprofen during zoster infection. The drug may delay or mask symptoms, or may cause direct immunosuppression and renal impairment, but the association itself is controversial
  - Streptococcal toxin shock syndrome (STSS): *Streptococcus pyogenes* exotoxins A and B reduce phagocytosis and cause release of TNF-α, IL-1 and IL-6, leading to systemic response

- Superantigens interact directly with
- T lymphocytes via the $\alpha\beta$ portion of the receptor rather than via pre-processing and presentation. They thus activate up to 20% of the T-cell population rather than 0.01% with regular antigens. T-helper cells then secrete large quantities of cytokines such as TNF, clotting factors and complement, activating inflammation and thrombosis
- Clostridial myonecrosis/gas gangrene can happen after trauma/surgery (*Clostridium perfringens* – Gram-positive spore-forming, gas-producing anaerobes found in soil, GI tract) or spontaneously (*Clostridium septicum*, infection may be associated with colonic carcinoma and leukaemia). Muscle necrosis and toxic symptoms are due to lecithinase (a-toxin causing haemolysis) and θ-toxin. Gas and crepitus is a characteristic feature. Patients are markedly toxic with intense pain and swelling

Investigations ↑WCC

- Blood tests may typically show a raised white cell count and a low plasma sodium level. Formal risk stratification can be performed by assessment of the Laboratory Risk Indicator for Necrotising Fasciitis (LRINEC) score
- The LRINEC score can be used to determine the likelihood of NF presence. It uses six serological measures and a score of 6 or more is highly suspicious for NF
  - CRP (mg/L): > 150 = 4 points
  - WCC ($\times 10^3$/mm^3)
    - < 15 = 0 points
    - 15-25 = 1 point
    - > 25 = 2 points
  - Hb (g/dL)
    - > 13.5 = 0 points
    - 11-13.5 = 1 point
    - < 11 = 2 points
  - Na (mmol/L): <135 = 2 points
  - Creatinine (μmol/L): > 141 = 2 points
  - Glucose (mmol/L): >10 = 1 point

- Wound fluid can be aspirated for urgent Gram staining. The finger test performed via a 2 cm incision is positive if the fascia comes off the subcutaneous layer easily. *[sweep test]* There may also be murky purulent exudate with less bleeding than expected. It is said to be pathognomonic but can be falsely negative when applied incorrectly
- Biopsy is important. It gathers material for culture, Gram staining and histology (necrosis with thrombi in occluded vessels), but it is important to biopsy either the periphery or the deep margin as the central parts may have bacteria that do not actually contribute to the process
  - Bedside (FS) biopsy of necrosis and the leading edge may give a rapid diagnosis at an early stage of disease
  - Rapid streptococcal diagnosis can be obtained by PCR of the spe genes, *[spe genes]* including culture negative cases
- Radiography is generally uninformative unless there is gas. Gas is not specific to *Clostridia*, as it may also be seen in infections of *Bacteroides*, *E. coli*, or *Peptococcus*. The gas composition is a mixture of hydrogen, nitrogen and hydrogen sulphide
- If surgery is indicated, it should not be delayed for imaging. CT may be useful to establish the extent of necrosis and is more sensitive in detecting gas, but is still generally non-specific. Some have pushed MRI as a diagnostic test but the appearances can likewise be non-specific. With MRI (T1 fat white, T2 water white) fascial inflammation or fluid accumulation is demonstrated by low intensity on T1 and high intensity on T2, and fascial necrosis by the lack of gadolinium contrast enhancement. Others believe that there is a use for USG but it will be of limited value with deeper disease. Some literature series showed a sensitivity of 88% and a specificity of 93% with a positive predictive value of 83%, using criteria such as diffuse subcutaneous thickening accompanied by fluid accumulation more than 4 mm in depth along the fascial layer

Treatment

Aggressive resuscitation with fluids and oxygen is required. High-dose antibiotics are administered as guided by the Gram stain results, but empiric treatment (e.g. gentamycin, clindamycin and ampicillin) can be commenced until definitive results are available. Remember that antibiotics only act against the microorganism and have no effect on the toxins (except clindamycin that has antitoxin effects) or microorganisms in dead tissue.

- Aerobes are mostly Gram negatives (ampicillin and gentamicin)
- Anaerobes (metronidazole, clindamycin or a third-generation cephalosporin such as ceftriaxone)
- Streptococcal (penicillin G or clindamycin)
  - Clindamycin may destroy streptococcal superantigen
- Clostridia are sensitive to high doses of penicillin

Immediate aggressive debridement of the necrosis down to viable tissue is important. Muscle is often healthy beneath the necrotic fascia. The wound is dressed and evaluated daily in the operating theatre.

- Intravenous immunoglobins may be used in patients with STSS and work by providing neutralising antibodies and opsonising bacteria, but the evidence is not particularly strong
- Hyperbaric oxygen (20 × 90 minute sessions at 2 atm) may be an option *after* antibiotics and surgery. It may reduce spreading and improve tissue perfusion, but there are no randomised trials confirming its usefulness. It may be most useful as an adjunct to surgery in clostridial disease. However, HBOT chambers are difficult areas to resuscitate in, and are frequently unsuitable for the critically ill

Further reading

Hau V, Ho CO. Necrotizing fasciitis caused by Vibrio vulnificus in the lower limb following exposure to seafood on the hand. Hong Kong Med J 2011; 17:335–37.

Related topic of interest

- Hyperbaric oxygen

Nerve compression and injury

Nerve compression causes conduction block by reduced perfusion in the nerve. With sustained pressures over 60 mmHg, there is complete ischaemia leading to fibrosis, traction, ischaemia or excessive excursion may also contribute to conduction block. The nerve dysfunction disrupts axoplasmic transport and increases susceptibility to damage at a second location (proximally or distally), predisposing to the 'double crush' phenomenon. The main symptom of nerve compression is pain.

- Motor nerves: Weakness and wasting
- Sensory nerves: Numbness/paraesthesia (often intermittent) and pain that radiates distally and proximally (even in pure motor nerves such as the anterior interosseous nerve). Patients are often vague in their descriptions and terms are often used interchangeably/incorrectly, e.g. 'pain' as 'discomfort' or 'numbness'. Similarly, the distribution is not clearly appreciated by the patient in many cases, e.g. the little finger sparing in carpal tunnel syndrome, until the patient is asked to draw it out or pay specific attention to it during the next episode. Provocation tests are part of the examination
- Tinel's sign and tenderness at site of compression

Electrodiagnostic tests can be confirmatory, but normal results should prompt a repeat test if they are disparate with the clinical picture. MRI may be useful if a mass lesion is suspected.

Recovery

Loss of nerve function is the most obvious sign of a complete nerve injury. Clinical signs of nerve regeneration, such as those following repair, are:

- An advancing Tinel's sign
- Increasing muscle power grade (MRC)
- Reappearance of sensory modalities in the following sequence:
  - Moving light touch produces tingling: Semmes–Weinstein monofilament test is sensitive but very tedious to perform
  - Protective sensation to pain and temperature (cold intolerance)
  - Discriminating sensation with some hypersensitivity
  - Two-point discrimination (2pd): Getting two thirds correct is deemed a pass. Dynamic 2pd recovers before static 2pd. 2pd tests are innervation density tests that make them less useful for detecting the gradual decrease in entrapment syndromes, as it can still be in a normal range with a minimal number of functional fibres. By comparison, the Semmes–Weinstein and vibration testing are threshold tests and are thus more useful in this context.
  - Sweating: Once this has returned to normal then no further improvement in 2pd will be seen

General management

The necessity and timing of nerve repair is based on the likelihood of spontaneous recovery. Taking a history aims to elucidate the mechanism of injury but differentiating between a total disruption and a severe stretch can be difficult. The best time for repair is 3–6 weeks after injury, but it is still worthwhile up to 6 months. Indications for exploration (Sunderland) include:

- For diagnosis (especially when symptoms suggest at least a severe stretch)
- Exclude sharp transection by fracture fragment
- Open wounds
- Arrested recovery

Conversely, waiting is worthwhile under the following conditions:

- Likely in-continuity mechanism with good chance of recovery
- Only partial interruption clinically
- Nerve continuity observed
- Steady recovery

Specific nerve compression

Compression or entrapment tends to occur at certain locations rather than being distributed truly randomly. The most commonly affected nerve is the median nerve.

Radial nerve

The radial nerve proper (RNP) and its main branch/continuation, the posterior interosseus nerve (PIN), innervates the extensor compartment muscles of upper limb as well as the overlying skin. It is the largest branch from the brachial plexus and arises from the posterior cord (all posterior divisions of C5–8) to run along the posterior surface of the humerus. It then pierces the lateral intermuscular septum 12 cm from the lateral epicondyle.

- The PIN divides quickly into individual branches after passing through supinator. The order of innervation by the RN/PIN can be useful in determining level of entrapment though variations exist: Brachioradialis (BR), ECRL, ECRB, supinator, EDC, ECU, EDM, APL, EPB, EPL, and EIP last
- The superficial RN runs along with the BR to form a variable number of branches 5 cm from the radial styloid, supplying sensation to the dorsum of radial three and half digits (first web) up to fingernails

Entrapment of radial nerve

The three common syndromes are:

- The radial tunnel at the elbow is 5 cm long and ends at the proximal supinator. Compression may be due to the Leash of Henry (recurrent vessels of radial artery) or tendinous edge of ECRB
- PIN syndrome at the forearm from the arcade of Fröhse (sharp fibrous proximal edge of supinator muscle). This is the classical PIN entrapment syndrome that often spares the supinator innervation
- Wartenberg syndrome at the wrist (relatively rare)

Compression at lateral intermuscular septum is more common than apparent, such as from humeral fractures. Injuries related to the use of tourniquets are uncommon (pneumatic ones are safer than rubber bandages) and seems to be related to direct pressure rather than prolonged ischaemia. Permanent deficits are rare and most resolve within 6 months.

Radial tunnel syndrome Radial tunnel syndrome is predominantly a nocturnal pain syndrome with few sensory/motor deficits. Less commonly, there is some weakness of wrist and finger extension, although this is a secondary sign.

- Pain: In the belly of brachioradialis, 6 cm distal to the lateral epicondyle, that is similar in nature to lateral epicondylitis (thus often incorrectly diagnosed as intractable tennis elbow) but is more distally placed. The pain is worse with resisted supination, such as when using a screwdriver
  - The third/middle finger test: Pain on resisted full extension of middle finger with wrist/elbow extended (to test ECRB) is diagnostic
- NCS/EMG can be unreliable but may help

In general, a 1–3 month trial of conservative therapy is used. Decompression surgery yields good results in 50% of cases, but motor recovery may take 6–18 months.

Posterior interosseus nerve syndrome PIN syndrome can be due to elbow fracture/dislocation, lipoma/ganglia, inflammation or injection/iatrogenic. The pain is similar to above but with more weakness, particularly of wrist and finger extension. Electrical tests often confirm the diagnosis. It is typically treated by decompression if conservative measures are unsuccessful.

Wartenberg syndrome Wartenberg syndrome is often due to external compression, e.g. watches, overuse or following release for de Quervain's disease, causing entrapment of the superficial radial nerve as it emerges from under the BR. This leads to numbness of the entire dorsum of the hand that worsens with pronation (test for 30–60 seconds). Treatment is primarily conservative.

Median nerve

The median nerve arises from contributions from the medial and lateral cords (C5–T1) and does not supply anything above the elbow, although some branches to the pronator teres (PT) arise 4 cm above. The nerve runs downwards within the medial intermuscular septum lateral to the brachial artery until approximately halfway when it crosses medial to the artery and descends into the antecubital fossa, deep to the bicipital aponeurosis. Here, it lies medial to vein and artery and then enters the forearm through PT. It travels down the forearm sandwiched between FDS and FDP until the distal third, when it enters the carpal tunnel between PL and FCR. The carpal tunnel has ten structures—9 tendons and 1 nerve. The median nerve supplies the LOAF (Lumbricals 1 and 2, opponens pollicis, abductor pollicis brevis and flexor pollicis brevis) muscles by its recurrent motor branch whilst the two other divisions supply the fingers.

- The usual order of innervation is: PT, FCR, FDS, PL, anterior interosseus nerve (AION), FDP, and PL
- The palmar cutaneous branches usually arise from the radial side, 4–5 cm proximal to the wrist, and supply the skin of thenar eminence and adjacent palm. It does not travel within the tunnel
- Crossovers with the ulnar nerve are common (Riche-Cannieu anastomosis in 80%)

Entrapment of median nerve

Entrapment commonly occurs at the elbow, wrist and forearm but proximal (pronator and AIO) syndromes are less common than carpal tunnel syndrome (CTS).

Pronator syndrome   Pronator syndrome occurs at the elbow level and is often due to the ligament of Struthers (found in 1% population), from a bony spur, the supracondylar process, lacertus fibrosus, pronator teres belly or proximal edge (arch) of FDS.

- Symptoms include pain in the proximal volar forearm, with a positive Tinel's sign. The weakness and numbness in the radial digits tends to be absent at night and includes the palmar cutaneous nerve. EMG is generally unhelpful and the diagnosis is usually made clinically
- Testing consists of pain with forced pronation of the extended forearm
- It may be confused with CTS, but differences include palm numbness), absent Tinel's at the wrist and Phalen's test

negative, whilst mid-forearm compression causes pain
- 50% of patients require formal decompression

Anterior interosseus (AIO) syndrome   AIO syndrome has similar symptoms, except for the absence of finger numbness. There are no sensory signs in AION syndrome. There is weakness of the FPL, FDP to index and middle and PQ, with a vague pain in the proximal forearm. The patient complains of difficulty in writing or picking up small objects ('O' pinch).

- Causes include compressions by the deep head of PT, Gantzer's muscle (accessory head of FPL) and aberrant radial arteries
- EMG/NCV may be diagnostic
- The usual management is observation: 3 weeks of rest followed by a review. Decompression (of potential points as discussed above) is offered if there is no improvement. Alternatively, some believe that delay of treatment is unnecessary and ultimately hinders recovery

Carpal tunnel syndrome   CTS is median nerve compression at the wrist (first described by Paget, 1853) that affects approximately 1% population. The incidence increases with age, most commonly affecting middle-aged females with a high rate of bilaterality. Most cases are idiopathic but there may be identifiable risk factors, such as swellings, inflammation due to rheumatoid, fractures/surgery in others. The role of repetitive trauma/work related is more controversial. CTS is more common in smokers, diabetics and hypothyroidism, although routine screening of thyroid function is not useful.

- Note that the palmar cutaneous branches arise proximal to wrist
- Recurrent motor branch has variable origins but usually arises just beyond (extra-ligamentous) or within the tunnel, piercing the ligament (trans-ligamentous) on the radiopalmar side of the nerve. It is often found at the intersection of Kaplan's cardinal line from first web to hamate and proximal palmar crease. Thus, the surgical incision line is usually on the ulnar side.

The main symptoms are numbness and dysaesthesia in the radial three and half digits and in severe cases; there is also weakness of the thenar muscles (some complain of weak pinch and dropping things) and sympathetic dysfunction. When assessing the patient, the entire upper limb should be examined and more proximal compression, e.g. in the neck, should be excluded. Diagnostic tests include:

- Tinel's sign (direct percussion test) is rather insensitive but specific. Strongest in middle two fingers (Tinel was a French neurologist)
- Phalen's test: Flex wrists for 30–60 seconds (George Phalen, American Orthopaedic surgeon), which increases tunnel pressure (modestly, to 4 mm Hg plateauing after 30 seconds). This compresses the nerve between the tunnel edge and anterior border of distal radius. Reports vary on its accuracy, sensitivity and specificity (up to 90% but as low as 50%). It is more specific than Tinel's sign, but less sensitive
- Reverse Phalen's test: Full finger and wrist extension for 2 minutes. The tunnel pressure increases after 10 seconds and increases further to 34 mmHg and 42 mmHg at 1 and 2 minutes respectively
- Direct pressure. McMurty and Durkan's direct carpal compression test is said to be more sensitive and specific than either Phalen's or Tinel's but not universally agreed. Its main advantage is that it can be used in those who cannot flex their wrists
- Others:
  – 2pd
  – Diminished light touch: The most sensitive test is threshold testing, such as the Semmes–Weinstein filament tests
  – Abductor pollicis brevis (APB) power
  – EMG/NCS: The latter is reduced due to demyelination and is better (85% sensitive, 87% specificity)

CTS is a clinical diagnosis. Nerve conduction studies can be useful to confirm the diagnosis when there is doubt (e.g. diabetic neuropathics), dual pathologies (e.g. coexistent higher nerve compression), to determine severity, to localise the level of problem and to monitor postoperative improvement (expected within 2 weeks of surgery). Electrophysiological studies are not needed in every case. In addition, there is a significant false negative/positive rate. When compression is severe, NCS may not record a sensory action potential. Between 10–15% of CTS patients with classic clinical signs will have normal tests.

Treatment of carpal tunnel syndrome
The usual treatment consists of decompression by either open or endoscopic techniques. Non-surgical treatments may be suitable for those with mild, intermittent symptoms in the early stages.

- Conservative: Splint, analgesia, anti-inflammatory medication
- Steroid injection: Up to 2–3 ml of dexamethasone (4 mg/ml) just ulnar to PL and just proximal to distal wrist crease. The effects are temporary and thus useful if the cause of CTS is reversible/temporary, e.g. pregnancy. The response to steroids is diagnostic and is may predict the response to surgery
- The results of diuretics and vitamin B are unconvincing

Indications for surgery include:

- CTS with tactile sensory changes or thenar muscle atrophy
- Signs for more than a year
- Flexor tenosynovitis
- Injection benefit less than 2 weeks (maximum three injections)
- Pain during day

Endoscopic versus open versus mini incisions   Surgery provides superior results and is generally safe. The key to success is complete release regardless of incision type. Opponensplasty may be needed in chronic cases.

Open release is commonly performed under GA or regional block with tourniquet. Numerous incisions have been described, but many advocate the 'ideal axis' from the centre of the wrist at the distal wrist to the radial border of fourth digit (supposedly the watershed between ulnar and median territories). The incision is linear or slightly curved without crossing wrist crease, whilst others prefer the ulnar aspect of the middle finger as a reference point. The ligament is divided from proximal to distal under direct vision, while protecting the motor and palmar branches. A light plaster or bulky bandage to prevent wrist flexion but allowing finger flexion is used for 2 weeks, and then used at night or whilst driving for another month. However, some randomised studies have shown no benefit in postoperative splintage and leaving the wrist unsplinted may be better. Furthermore, formal rehabilitation accelerates recovery but the final function and outcome is the same as home exercise programs.

Indications for open surgery include:

- Revisional surgery
- Other surgery planned, e.g. opponensplasty or synovectomy (rheumatoid). Neurolysis is of little benefit with risks of scarring and further tethering and is usually combined with other procedures to reduce adhesions, e.g. vein wrap, muscle flaps, steroids or early motion

There is a 92% overall patient satisfaction rate. Complications include: Pillar pain (persistent discomfort in hypo/thenar eminences that may be caused by sensory nerve damage or widening of carpal arch and is also possible after endoscopic surgery), persistent symptoms, wound infection, hyperaesthesia, scar tenderness and neurological complications, e.g. pisitriquetral pain syndrome, chronic regional pain syndrome (CRPS), stiffness and nerve injury/neuroma. The average time for a return to work is 3–5 weeks. In general, the longer symptoms preoperatively, the longer it takes to recover.

Endoscopic surgery with its shorter incisions aims to reduce postoperative pain/scars, to allow faster recovery (pinch and grip strength) but has not consistently shown significant difference in terms of outcomes, e.g. sick leave, time to ADL/work.

- Earlier recovery of grip strength at 3/52 but no difference at 3 months (80%)
- More blind dissection. The learning curve is steep and other complications especially nerve injury are higher

There are many modifications, making objective comparison of the literature extremely difficult. There are no randomised trials. In simple terms, the surgery uses a single portal 3 cm proximal to distal palmar crease incision and a 4 mm obturator, cutting the ligament from distal to proximal with a hook. Smaller windows increase the risk of injury to the palmar arch and the motor branch of the median nerve as well as incomplete division. Complications include:

- Conversion to open surgery 14%
- Incomplete release 4%
- Ulnar nerve injury

Recurrent symptoms may be due to incomplete division, scar tissue or flexor tenosynovitis, whilst persistent symptoms are more commonly due to misdiagnosis e.g. thoracic outlet or root compression.

Ulnar nerve

The ulnar nerve arises from the medial cord (C8–T1, sometimes C7) that runs down the arm medial to the brachial artery and pierces the medial intermuscular septum 10 cm from the medial epicondyle (ME) to reach the posterior compartment. From here, it passes under the arcade of Struthers (found in three quarters of the population), a band from septum to the medial head of triceps to the biceps. The nerve runs posterior to the ME, and then into a fibrous cubital tunnel adjacent to the attachment of the head of FCU then between the heads of FCU into the forearm. The volume of the cubital tunnel is greatest in extension. A 55% volume decrease in full flexion raises the pressure from 7 to 11–24 mmHg in cadaveric models. In addition, there is traction excursion of 10 mm proximal to epicondyle with full range of motion.

In the forearm, the nerve runs with the artery as it becomes more superficial and at the FCU tendon, divides into a superficial sensory branch to the dorsal ulnar hand 5 cm proximal to the wrist. It may also give off an inconsistent palmar cutaneous branch, while the main branch continues over the carpal tunnel more radially into Guyon's canal (about 1–2 cm long, radial to pisiform and ulnar to artery), dividing into further branches. These include a superficial branch that is mostly sensory but supplies palmaris brevis, and motor branches to the intrinsic muscles of hand except LOAF (except deep head of flexor pollicis brevis).

Entrapment of the ulnar nerve

Several connections with the median nerve may lead to underestimation of the severity of ulnar nerve injury.

- Proximal or Martin-Gruber anastomosis found in 10–20%, is a connection in the forearm, often from AION branch to FDP, i.e. median to ulnar
- Distal or Riche-Cannieu anastomosis, which is a communication between the palmar cutaneous branches

Common ulnar nerve entrapment syndromes are:

- Cubital tunnel syndrome at the ME is the most common cause. There is medial forearm pain that is often ill-defined, numbness to ulnar wrist and ulnar one and a half fingers. Eventually, there is wasting of the hypothenar eminence and the first web, with a weak key pinch and Wartenberg's sign (an abducted little finger due to a weakened adductor). Symptoms are typically worse at night or with elbow flexion (stretching along epicondyle and decrease cross sectional area of tunnel). Typical compression sites are the FCU fascia/Osborne band, medial intermuscular septum, arcade of Struthers, anconeus epitrochlearis, cubitus valgus, ganglion/lipoma, arthritic bony spurs, direct trauma and fracture
  - Absence of claw hand (above branch to FDP) and presence of numbness on dorsum of hand helps to distinguish it from distal compression
  - Froment's test (thumb MCPJ hyperextension with IPJ flexion due to FPL recruitment) when attempting to hold a piece of paper between thumb and radial border of index metacarpal is the best test
  - Tinel's test has 70% sensitivity, while elbow flexion for 1 minute (Phalen test analogue) has 30% sensitivity
  - Confirm with NCS/EMG (to rule out cervical lesions) and then treat with splintage but not steroid injections (too tight), decompress or transpose if needed
- Wrist compression is less common and may due to repetitive trauma, ganglion/ lipomas and anomalous muscles, e.g. hypothenar insertion or accessory PL. The dorsal sensory branch is spared from entrapment as it arises in the distal third of the forearm
  - Motor involvement is common; the best test is Froment's test. Weak key pinch and ulnar claw hand (MCPJ hyperextension, IPJ flexion due to unopposed EDC action) are late signs
  - Less commonly, pain in the wrist and paraesthesia radiating to the ulnar fingers that is exacerbated by sustained hyperextension of wrist
  - Tinel's is the best provocation test
  - Confirm with EMG and treat the cause. Divide the canal roof and splint in slight extension for 3 weeks

Management of cubital syndrome

Treatment options include:

- Conservative therapy including using a 45° elbow flexion splint, rest and anti-inflammatory medication may resolve mild cases, but surgical decompression is often needed
- Good results are expected from surgery (90% response but one third recur). Options include:
  - In situ decompression (split tunnel) for mild and intermittent symptoms
  - Transposition surgery: Subcutaneous over FCU, sub-muscular under FCU (for more severe forms, reoperation and in the very thin) and intramuscular transposition. Transposition surgery risks devascularisation of nerve, whilst subcutaneous transposition may exacerbate the pain as the nerve subluxes back and forth across the epicondyle. Anterior sub-muscular transposition is probably best choice
  - Medial epicondylectomy may be useful if the problem is related to fracture non-union and deformity, with risk of damaging ulnar collateral ligament and causing elbow instability
- Clawing in low ulnar palsy with loss of thumb adduction and index abduction (first web closure) may be treated:
  - Clawing: Zancolli I or II procedure, but only if correctable by the Bouvier manoeuvre

– Thumb adduction: BR and tendon graft through third and fourth space to adductor insertion
– Index abduction: Strip of APL to the interosseus insertion

Screening for peripheral nerve palsy

Screening for peripheral nerve palsies of the arm is shown in **Table 54.**

Table 54 Screening for peripheral nerve palsies of the arm		
Nerve	Sensory loss	Motor testing
Radial	Dorsum 1st web	Thumbs up [extensor pollicis longus (EPL)]
Median	Tip of index finger	'OK' [flexor pollicis longus (FPL), flexor digitorum profundus (FDP) and opponens pollicis (OP)]
Ulnar	Tip of little finger	Cross and abduct fingers

Further reading

Assmus H, Antoniadis G, Bischoff C, et al. Cubital tunnel syndrome—a review and management guidelines. Centr Eur Neurosurg 2011; 72:90–8.

Neurofibromatosis

Neurofibromatosis (NF) is a subset of the hamartoses, which are a large group of multi-system disorders that exhibit autosomal dominant inheritance or sporadic occurrence. NF is a genetically inherited disorder of neural crest cells (Schwann cells, melanocytes, endoneurial fibroblasts) that is characterised by neurofibromas.

A neurofibroma is a benign nerve-sheath tumour of the peripheral nervous system (PNS) that arises from non-myelinating Schwann cells (NMSC). The normal role of NMSCs is to encapsulate small diameter PNS axons of <1 μm with their cytoplasmic processes, forming Remak bundles. NF NMSCs fail to form Remak bundles but also exhibit biallelic inactivation of the NF1 gene. This causes complete loss of expression of the NF1 gene product, neurofibromin, which is a tumour suppressor.

Types of neurofibromas:

- Dermal (typical): Arises from a single cutaneous nerve bundle. Size limited. They have no malignant potential and typically develop at puberty
- Plexiform: Arises from multiple nerve bundles that are not limited to cutaneous nerves nor size. They may grow into multiple tissue planes and cause pain, severe cosmetic and functional deformity. Wound healing problems typically follow excisional surgery. Since the scope for cosmetic improvement is limited, especially in craniofacial lesions, surgery is highly goal-specific (functional preservation or malignancy). They develop earlier than dermal neurofibromas. There is a 10% risk of transformation into a malignant peripheral nerve sheath tumour (MPNST). MPNSTs display loss of CDKN2A or TP53 genes in NF NMSCs

Types of neurofibromatosis:

- Neurofibromatosis type 1 (NF1): Multiple neurofibromas. Low risk of central nervous system (CNS) tumours and hence better prognosis than NF2
- Neurofibromatosis type 2 (NF2): Characterised by vestibular schwannomas and other CNS tumours. Sensorineural hearing loss is the most common presentation

Neurofibromatosis type 1 (von Recklinghausen's disease, 1882)

The incidence of NF1 is 1 in 3000, of which 50% are sporadic de novo mutations of the NF1 gene on chromosome 17. Prenatal diagnosis is possible but is not widely available. However, only two-thirds of NF1 patients have a demonstrable NF1 gene defect.

Patients may have a variable combination of short stature, scoliosis, macrocephaly and learning difficulties (40%), but most patients lead productive lives. Life expectancy is reduced by approximately 15 years, due to:

- Hypertension: Although the incidence of phaeochromocytoma and renal artery stenosis is increased, most cases are idiopathic
- Spinal cord tumours: Dumbbell tumours causing spinal cord compression
- Malignant tumours: MPNST

The onset of symptoms is gradual but diagnosis is usually achieved by the age of 10. Late onset NF1 has been described but is rare. The diagnostic criteria are two or more of the following features:

- First-degree relative with NF
- Six or more café au lait spots of >5 mm in diameter in a child of 10 years or under, or >15 mm in diameter in an adult. This is often the first finding. The treatment response to laser (typically Q-switched 532 nm) is variable but the spots tend to fade with age
- >2 dermal neurofibromas or 1 plexiform neurofibroma
- Optic nerve gliomas typically present as visual loss before the age of 5 years. However, they tend to be less progressive than non-NF gliomas. Periorbital and orbital tumours are at risk or intracranial extension through a widened superior orbital fissure

- Axillary and inguinal freckles generally appear later in childhood
- Lisch nodules (iris hamartomas). A hamartoma is a focal growth that resembles a neoplasm but is a result of a developmental abnormality of an organ
- Sphenoid dysplasia (usually asymptomatic). Other bony abnormalities such as intramedullary fibrosis and cortical thinning may be present. Long bone abnormalities such as tibial bowing due to pseudoarthroses are rare

Investigations

Imaging is reserved for selected indications such as for suspected CNS or optic nerve tumours. Slit lamp examination is a useful screening tool to detect Lisch nodules in family members of the affected.

Neurofibromatosis type 2

NF2 is less common than NF1 and its genetic abnormality is a deletion on chromosome 22, for which a diagnostic gene test is available. Vestibular schwannomas are the most common, followed by trigeminal schwannomas but any cranial may be affected. The diagnosis of any cranial nerve schwannoma should prompt screening for NF2. NF2 is also known as MISME (multiple inherited schwannomas, meningiomas and ependymomas), reflecting the predominant features and highlighting the relative

rarity of true neurofibromas. Malignant transformation is rare (1%).

Most patients (45%) present in the fourth decade, with symptoms of disrupted vestibulocochlear function. These include sensorineural hearing loss, tinnitus, vertigo and loss of balance. Small vestibular schwannomas are likely to be symptomatic due to nerve compression within the confined space of the auditory canal. Resection is difficult and the facial nerve is also at high risk of injury. Most patients require a multiple operations. Radiotherapy is an alternative if surgery is not a viable option.

The diagnostic criteria are:

- Bilateral vestibulocochlear schwannomas are the hallmark (5–10%), typically delineated best on MRI. Biopsy is unnecessary. Lesions are typically mushroom or ice-cream cone shaped. Necrosis may be seen in large tumours. They may extend from the internal auditory canal into the posterior fossa to compress the fifth and seventh, rarely the ninth and tenth cranial nerves
- NF2 in a first-degree relative and
  - Early onset vestibulocochlear schwannoma or
  - Any two of the following: meningioma (often multiple and affects the thoracic spine), glioma, schwannoma (may be cutaneous), and juvenile posterior subcapsular lenticular opacity/cataracts

Further reading

Uygur F, Chang DW, Crosby MA, et al. Free flap reconstruction of extensive defects following resection of large neurofibromatosis, Ann Plast Surg 2011; 67:376–81.

Related topic of interest

- Facial reanimation

Nipple areolar reconstruction

This is usually undertaken at a period > 3 months after breast reconstruction in order for the breast mound to achieve an acceptable stable shape and position. The symmetry of nipple position is very important and may take priority over placement of the nipple on the top of the breast mound. Symmetry is often well judged by eye, and confirmed by measurement. If bilateral reconstruction is required, the nipple is positioned along the breast meridian (MCL to IMF) on the most projecting part of mound, avoiding scars if possible.

Nipple reconstruction

The main challenge is to achieve longevity of projection. Many different flaps have been described, strongly suggesting that there is no single perfect option. On an average, one should expect 50% reduction with most techniques, thus overcorrection by 25–50% is often advocated.

Common options

Nipple sharing

Nipple sharing (tip or inferior part): The arguments against this option are that it damages the other (usually intact) side, causing scarring and possibly loss of erogenous function. However, it is suitable for patients with a large nipple who desire its reduction and has excellent aesthetic match in colour, texture and symmetry that surpass those achievable with local flaps.

Local flaps

The design of local flaps needs to take into consideration the following:

- Construction of the base and its relative position, it has a tendency to contract/retract due to a combination of scarring and lack of vascularity. Early techniques often had a central base. The Maltese cross pattern was used to form a raised lump and similarly, multiple pinwheel flaps around a central base. The results were not sustained over time and hence a gradual

evolution towards non-central base techniques occurred
- Flap thickness: Split thickness/dermal or full thickness
- Need for skin grafts: Reconstruction of a nipple of significant size is likely to leave a donor defect that requires grafting. Techniques that avoid this tend to give less projection
- Additional materials have been inserted to augment the result with variable and inconsistent success. Stacked cartilage grafts, buried dermis, acellular dermal matrix stacks and calcium hydroxyapatite (lasts about 6 months) have been used in addition to local flaps (**Figure 15**)

There are many different techniques described.

- Skate flap: The lateral wings are raised at a subdermal level, while the central portion includes a core of fat. The designed height is approximately two times final desired nipple height. Typically, small FTSGs are required to close the donor defect as primary closure with tension results in flattening. This technique is the most popular technique for reconstruction of larger nipples (**Figure 15**)
- Star flap: This is similar in design to the Skate flap, but is designed for direct closure of the donor site and thus more limited in its dimensions. It is a good alternative for small to medium sized nipples
- CV flaps: One 'C' for the top of the nipple and two 'V's that interlock to form the sidewalls. It is similar to the skate flap but does not require skin grafts
- S flap: This was one of the first double pedicle techniques that initially used de-epithelialised U-flaps with skin grafts to cover both nipple and areola. A similar technique is the double opposing tab flaps and its variants. A circle with a diameter three times the nipple is required. The flaps are raised at the subdermal level with 10 mm of fat. A key suture is used to appose the midpoint of the base of each

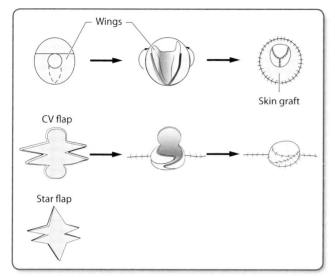

Figure 15 Different methods of nipple reconstruction. Some involve the use of skin grafts (top) whilst others do not (CV flap and star flap).

flap so they come together like hands in prayer. The flaps can be centred on the scar with less vascular compromise but greater tension. There may be a tendency to distort the breast and thus are most suited for reconstruction of smaller nipples on larger breasts

- Bell flap: The bell-shaped random pattern flap has a central portion that is raised with fat, while the triangular segment is subdermal, with a size approximately one sixth of the circumference and is made 15–20% larger than opposite side. Permanent purse-string sutures are used to create the shape. The technique also recreates the areola

Areolar reconstruction

Nipple/areolar sharing: There can be significant donor site morbidity, with the potential to adversely affect erogenous sensation and interrupt the lactiferous ducts and thus breastfeeding)

Skin grafts: Labia minora FTSG, labia majora SSG or inguinal perineal skin (although the donor site scar is usually easily hidden, the propensity for wound infection can make it an inconvenient place to harvest from). An interlocking Gore-Tex suture for the control of

the areolar diameter and shape (popularised by Hammond): A 5 mm dermal rim is left on the outer flaps for suture-holding along with some undermining of the breast flaps for 1–2 cm in the subdermal plane. Using a Gore-Tex CV2 straight needle in dermal layer, eight double bites are taken in wagon wheel configuration, and gradually cinched down until the NAC in the centre is mildly herniated. An interrupted Vicryl 4–0 and a running subcuticular suture are then placed. This aims to pull de-epithelialised dermis slightly under the edge of the areola with mild 'vest-over-pants' protection for the suture line, which is also reinforced with tape for 6 weeks.

Returned skin graft (elevated from the same site as the recipient, i.e. around the reconstructed nipple): Gruber used ultraviolet light to enhance pigmentation, but the results were not sustained.

Tattoo: Timing is variable, but most wait 6–12 weeks after nipple reconstruction to allow tissues to recover and reduce the risk of overstressing the vascularity. However, some suggest tattooing before nipple reconstruction for more uniform colour, as scar does not take pigment well. Some fading is normal and to be expected and touch-up treatments are often needed. Tattooing is generally safe and avoids the need for donor sites that are pigmented. Allergic reactions are rare but have been described. The lack of surface texture (of Montgomery glands) may limit aesthetic results and some have attempted to reproduce this by placing diced cartilage under the skin with variable success. Dermabrasion to induce hyperpigmentation has been described but the long-term results are unclear. Advanced artistic tattoos that draw in the Montgomery glands have good aesthetics but are limited in availability.

Postoperative care

- Support with noncompressive bra
- Antibiotic ointment to suture lines
- Protective dressing, e.g. a stack of gauzes with a hole cut out to accommodate the reconstructed area and then covered with a small plastic cup. Maintain for 2 weeks

Complications are uncommon except for flattening out, which is to be expected. The risk of tissue necrosis may be increased in smokers.

Further reading

Katerinaki E, Sircar T, Sterne GD. The C-V flap for nipple reconstruction after previous skin-sparing mastectomy and immediate breast reconstruction: refinements of donor-site closure. Aesthetic Plast Surg 2011; 35:624–27.

Related topic of interest

- Breast reconstruction

Oral cancer

Head and neck cancers constitute 15% of all cancers and one third of all head and neck tumours that arise within the oral cavity. The oral cavity starts at the lips and ends at the line marked by the junction of the hard and soft palates, and the circumvallate papillae. It has a crucial role in taste, swallowing and speech. The vast majority of oral cancers are SCCs (90%), adenocarcinomas are the second commonest, whilst the other tumour types (e.g. minor salivary gland) are uncommon. The cancers in different sites display different behaviour and prognoses, with the outlook often worse for posterior lesions. Patients (males predominate 3–4 times) usually present with a painless ulcer or cervical lymphadenopathy.

Smoking is the most important risk factor for oral cancer. Those who do not give up smoking have a greater risk of recurrence and of developing a second primary SCC (40% vs. 6% risk in those who give up). Chewing tobacco (verrucous SCC) or betel nuts also increases risk, but susceptibility to this may be partly determined by genetic factors. All forms of tobacco have an additive effect with alcohol, and show a linear association with cancer risk. Leukoplakia and erythroplakia are premalignant lesions that are found in association with up to 20% of oral cancers and can progress to frankly invasive SCCs that tend to be more aggressive. Iron deficiency anaemia and Plummer-Vinson syndrome (atrophic/fibrotic tissues) are also associated with an increased incidence of oral cancer.

Specific areas

- Tongue (20–30% of oral cancers, of which >75% occur anteriorly): The lesion is usually painless and significantly larger to palpation than inspection. Over one third of lesions will have occult nodes (most commonly submandibular, jugulodigastric, upper jugular), even in early tumours. Tumour depth has been shown to be predictive of neck node involvement and elective nodal dissection has been recommended for lesions thicker than 10 mm. Nodal disease is closely related to patient survival: 70% for N0 reduced to 30% for N1
  - Posterior one third cancers are often advanced and have frequently metastasised at presentation
  - There is a high risk of perineural invasion and perivascular spread if more than half the tongue is involved, thus total glossectomy is advisable under such circumstances
- Floor of the mouth (FOM) (30–35%, but > 50% in some Asians due to betel nut chewing): This is strongly associated with heavy alcohol intake. One fifth of T1 tumours have occult neck nodes (submental/submandibular) at presentation. The 5-year survival is 30–60% and is related to stage and nodal status
- The retromolar trigone is the area behind the lower third molar. Tumours here drain to the jugulodigastric and submandibular nodes. Early bone involvement is common, as is spread to neighbouring structures such as the inferior alveolar nerve and muscles of mastication (trismus). Tumours of the tonsils behave similarly but rarely involve bone and they spread laterally to the pterygoid muscles and medially to tongue and FOM
- Buccal mucosa cancer (10%) is strongly associated with tobacco use and tends to occur in an older age group

Subtypes

- Ulcerative subtype is most common. Infiltrative types require careful palpation to determine the extent
- Exophytic: Rare but less aggressive
- Verrucous (of Ackerman, exophytic with papillary morphology) carcinoma is a rare subtype that most often involves the buccal or gingival regions. It is generally treated with excision rather than radiotherapy

The grade of tumour is less important than the size and depth/thickness.

Assessment

History taking and a thorough systematic examination of the whole oral cavity, including bimanual examination, will provide a diagnosis in 90% of cases. Specific investigations include:

- Tissue diagnosis is provided by biopsy. Panendoscopy is essential to exclude synchronous tumours (i.e. within 6 months, otherwise called metachronous) that occur in 15% of patients (vs. 10% metachronous due to field change) in the oesophagus, oropharynx and lung
- FNAC of any neck masses on the first visit. Tongue and FOM tumours have nodes in 30–40% of cases at presentation
- Imaging with MRI and CT is useful to define the extent of the tumour (T stage). Soft tissue characterisation is better with MRI and is more reliable for detecting lymph nodes and extracapsular spread in nodes < 2 cm in size. CT is superior for determining cortical bone involvement and distinguishing malignant nodes. Orthopantomograms may also provide useful information. The most widely accepted method of defining the extent of the disease is TNM staging (Table 55). For different head and neck cancers, the T stage often differs between locations whilst N and M are consistent
  - USG FNA or FDG-PET can be used to increase the accuracy of nodal status, but are not routinely used
  - Distant metastases are rare (most common in lung and bone) and usually occur in the context of persistent or recurrent neck disease. Chest CT is suggested for recurrent cases or Stage III/IV cancers
- Tis: In situ cancer
- T1: < 2 cm
- T2: 2–4 cm
- T3: > 4 cm
- T4: > 4 cm with invasion
  - Adjacent structures including bone
  - Masticator space

This also applies to tumours of the lip and oropharynx.

- N1: Single ipsilateral mobile node < 3 cm
- N2a: Single ipsilateral node 3–6 cm
- N2b: Multiple ipsilateral nodes < 6 cm
- N2c: Bilateral or contralateral node/s < 6 cm
- N3: Fixed, multiple nodes > 6 cm

Treatment

For Stage I or II tumours, either surgery or radiotherapy alone works well. The choice is usually related to patient preference and local expertise. The other modality is still available for treatment of persistent or recurrent disease. Some adopt an approach where anterior lesions are excised whilst posterior lesions are irradiated. For more advanced tumours, surgery and radiotherapy may be combined, but overall response is generally poor.

Surgery should be radical where possible to improve survival. Gross margins of 1–2 cm should be taken. Frozen-section analysis of the resection margins has been used, but is less reliable in previously irradiated tissues. The propensity for perineural spread along the lingual and inferior alveolar nerve dictates that these should be divided as proximally as possible, if sacrificed. Surgery debulks

Table 55 Staging of oral cancers and associated survival rates		
Stage	TNM	5-year survival
Stage I	T1N0M0	90%
Stage II	T2N0M0	50–70%
Stage III	T3 or T(1–3)N1	40%
Stage IV	T4 or N2/N3 or M1	25%
T corresponds to stage except for: • Nodal disease: At least Stage III • Metastasis: Stage IV		

most of the tumour (> 99%) and provides staging information, with radiotherapy is still available as a back-up option if the excision margins are involved. Resection of large posterior tongue tumours may require concomitant laryngectomy or a laryngeal suspension to prevent aspiration.

Radiotherapy in the form of external beam irradiation with or without brachytherapy is as effective as surgery for small lesions, with surgery as a salvage option. Radiotherapy preserves function to a greater extent than surgery (thus may be preferable for posterior third of tongue tumours), and the neck can be treated simultaneously. Contraindications include previous radiotherapy, close proximity to bone and those with poor healing. Treatment causes xerostomia, decreased taste and mucositis, all of which may lead to reduced feeding and weight loss. Local recurrence may be difficult to detect on a background of RT changes.

- Adjuvant radiotherapy should be considered for patients with positive nodes, large primary tumours or where excision is incomplete or those with other clinical and pathological features suggestive of a high recurrence risk

The role of chemotherapy as a primary treatment in oral SCC is unclear and this situation is not helped by the lack of standard protocols. It is useful as an adjunct.

- Neoadjuvant or induction chemotherapy aims to decrease the size of massive tumours, which may then become operable. Resection should still be based on the size of the original tumour
- Consolidation chemotherapy (usually cisplatin) can be utilised after surgery for advanced tumours. Intra-arterial (IA) chemotherapy aims to deliver a large localised dose to the tumour area. It is typically given as four weekly doses with concurrent radiotherapy. Its exact usefulness has not been fully determined
- Those unfit for chemotherapy should be considered for IV cetuximab (Erbitux) combined with radiotherapy. Cetuximab is a monoclonal antibody that acts against the epidermal growth factor receptor (EGFR)

The popularity of adjuvant therapies has led to smaller post-excisional defects. However, the tissue damage from these therapies, such as irradiation, makes the import of healthy vascularised tissue in the form of pedicled or free flaps, more appropriate.

Nodal disease

Treatment of neck disease may be:

- Therapeutic: To treat detectable nodal disease with a MRND. Neck dissection and irradiation are both effective
- Prophylactic/elective: No cervical neck nodes detectable clinically. Elective ND of the contralateral side should be considered if the tumour is advanced (T3 or more), extends into neck, or if midline or multiple ipsilateral nodes are found. Unreliable patients, who will be difficult to monitor, such as obese necks, should also be considered for elective node dissection

Even if node negative on pathological examination, the (nodal) recurrence rate is:

- 8% for surgery alone (vs. 20% if nodes are positive)
- 3% for combined surgery and postoperative radiotherapy (vs. 15% if nodes are positive)

FOM cancer

- 50% of patients with tongue cancer have Stage 2 disease at presentation. Even when clinically N0 (i.e. Stage I and II), 30% have occult nodal disease
- Fukano (1997) found that tumours < 5 mm thick have a 6% chance of positive nodes, but this increases to 60% if > 5 mm
- CT/MRI and other imaging modalities may help to reduce the false negative neck

The choices for a clinically N0 neck are:

- Observation: Not generally advocated as even T1/2 lesions have a significant risk of occult nodal involvement, but may be reasonable in carefully selected patients, e.g. lesions < 4 mm
- Radiotherapy
- Supraomohyoid selective neck dissection, followed by adjuvant radiotherapy if two or more involved nodes are found

Although significant differences in survival have not been found, active treatment is encouraged. The choice of radiation or surgery for the neck depends on the treatment mode of the primary, patient preference and local facilities.

- For tumours T1–3 N0, comparison between elective ND (END) and a 'wait and see' policy with a therapeutic ND performed when needed, showed that 49% of ENDs had positive nodes and 53% of observation-only group subsequently developed clinically apparent nodes
- A T1–2 tongue cancer study in India, comparing hemiglossectomy with hemiglossectomy and END, demonstrated a 52% versus 63% disease-free survival but with no significant difference in overall survival

FOM tumours naturally progress to eventually involve the mandible, as the tumour grows over the alveolus and penetrates the dental sockets (via the periodontal ligament). Note that cortical bone does not regenerate over the sockets after dental extraction, hence cancellous bone is in direct contact with the mucosa at these points.

Loose teeth are clues to bony involvement. X-rays may demonstrate invasion, including new bone formation and loss of marrow. However, the absence of these signs is unreliable, as adenoid cystic carcinoma often invades bone with few radiological signs.

- Rim resection only: In non-irradiated tissue (irradiated periosteum is not a good barrier to tumour spread) for early tumours that abut without invasion, preferably below the level of nerve canal
- Segmental: For T3/4 tumours, irradiated tumours or any tumour showing direct invasion

Tumour resection

Lesions are excised per oral where possible. A lip and mandibular split will provide good access and facilitate *en bloc* resection with the neck nodes (though this is strictly not necessary as in transit metastasis rarely occurs). The osteotomy choices include symphyseal, paramedian (canine and second incisor), straight or step. Tongue stability can be maintained by keeping the osteotomy anterior to mental foramen as genioglossus and geniohyoid are still attached.

Functionally important structures that contribute to airway, speech or swallowing may require sacrifice or may be exposed during surgery. The choice of reconstructive method depends on the patient, the surgeon and the defect (prior irradiation and replacement needs e.g. coverage/lining, bulk or bone). There is currently no true dynamic replacement for the native tongue. Attempts at functional reconstruction have generally been disappointing.

- Direct closure or healing by secondary intention is suitable for small defects in areas such as the buccal mucosa or FOM
- The buccal fat pad can be mobilized taking care to avoid excessive stretch to preserve the plexus, to cover defects of 4–5 cm^2 around the buccal mucosa, maxilla and RMT. Epithelialisation occurs over 3–5 weeks. It is contraindicated with exposed bone or post-irradiation
- Skin grafts are simple and reliable and can be fixed by fenestration and quilting, but tend to contract and may cause tethering. They may be no better than secondary healing in the long-term for small lesions, and is thus of limited application. They may be suitable for large superficial defects such as those of the hard palate but not the soft palate
- Local (mucosal) flaps such as the tongue and buccal mucosa are primarily reserved for salvage. The nasolabial flap can provide small (6×3 cm) but reliable pieces of tissue, but requires two stages and a risk of salivary fistula formation. The temporalis can be raised as either a muscle or fascial flap and may be suitable for small volume deficits. The donor is reasonably well hidden but requires rather extensive dissection with a small risk of facial nerve damage
- Choices of pedicled flaps include the deltopectoral, pectoralis major (PM) and LD. The PM flap is very reliable and can be raised with a rib segment (more a graft than flap), but requires a large amount of dissection with poor donor cosmesis.

This is particularly the case in females, as it produces a bulky tunnel in the neck. Furthermore, the flap itself is often too bulky for the tongue and FOM. LD flaps are more versatile but require more extensive dissection and tunnelling, and is generally a poor choice for intraoral reconstruction. The trapezius flap can be used based on the transverse cervical branch. The upper half is more useful for intraoral reconstruction but lower half can be raised with less risk to the accessory nerve.

- Bone can be included with trapezius, latissimus dorsi/serratus anterior and pectoralis major (with decreasing reliability of the bone blood supply)
- Free flaps can be tailored to the requirements

- For bulk: Muscle flaps such as the RA.
- For coverage: Thin fascial flaps such as the FRFF, lateral arm flap, medial sural flap or ALT flap are better.
- Swallowing function depends more on laryngeal preservation, laryngeal suspension and the amount of functional tongue remaining, than the actual flap used.

Complications

Orocutaneous fistulas are more common with prior irradiation. Residual disease or recurrence must be ruled out. It can be treated with drainage and nutritional support in most, although debridement and vascularised tissue coverage may be required in some cases.

Further reading

Chiu T, Burd A. Our technique of 'tongue' folding. Plast Reconstr Surg 2009; 123:426–27.

Related topics of interest

- Head and neck cancer
- Neck dissection

- Premalignant lesions

Orbital fractures

The orbit is made up of seven bones. It is shaped as a modified pyramid with the optic foramen at its apex, 45 mm from the inferior rim. Low energy trauma will usually fracture the orbit at its weakest point, the medial wall and floor. The lateral wall and the supraorbital rim are strong and thick.

- Floor: Thin, especially medial to the infraorbital canal and nerve
- Medial: Thin and weak bones including lacrimal bone and lamina papyracea, with numerous vulnerable structures here including the lacrimal sac and medial canthal tendon. CT is important for diagnosis although visual symptoms and enophthalmos may be clues
- Isolated lateral wall fractures are rare and usually occur in the context of a zygomatic fracture complex
- Orbital roof fractures are rare and almost never occur in isolation in adults. They usually occur in the context of multiple fractures, particularly those of involving the frontal sinus. Urgent CT and neurosurgery input is required. Large displaced fractures need reduction. In children (up to age of 7), isolated fractures may occur as the frontal sinus is not well developed and cannot disperse the forces as effectively

There is a 10–20% risk of ocular injury in facial fractures. Although most are minor, there is a risk of blindness from retrobulbar haematoma (pain, proptosis, CN III palsy and gradual decrease of visual acuity). Careful eye examination is needed: Screen with pupillary reaction, extraocular muscle movement and visual fields, but the threshold for requesting an ophthalmology opinion should be very low.

Radiology

The Waters view is the most common view requested but is inadequate if used alone. CT is the current standard of care for orbital fractures, with 1.5 mm axial and coronal cuts.

- Current CT technology may be capable of visualising coronal reconstruction adequately from axial cuts alone
- Reformatted oblique sagittal cuts are useful to visualise the orbital apex

CT also allows determination of orbital volume.

- Check for telecanthus, defined as increased intercanthal distance from the normal range of 30–32 mm to > 35 mm
- Check the medial canthal tendon by palpation and distracting lids laterally

The indications for surgical treatment are controversial. Suspected entrapment is an indication for surgery but is not urgent per se, as it may resolve spontaneously. It may be reasonable to perform a trial of conservative treatment for a week, prior to surgery. Other indications include a positive forced duction test, enophthalmos > 2 mm and vertical dystopia and CT evidence of a floor defect greater than 2 cm^2. Delaying treatment of diplopia for > 2 weeks is less likely to be successful (75% vs. 93%)

Blowout fractures

Orbital floor fractures are indicated by symptoms of diplopia and enophthalmia. The mechanisms of injury include (probably mixture of):

- Indirect transmission of force along the bone (conduction/buckling)
- Direct transmission of pressure from the intraorbital contents (hydraulic)

The bone recoils faster than soft tissue and may thus trap it. The floor usually fractures in the midportion, medial to the nerve (bone is thick/thin/thick from anterior to posterior). A medial wall fracture is often posterior to the globe and may cause significant volume disturbance and risk of enophthalmos (> 5 mm is disfiguring).

Blow-in fractures are rare, but may cause proptosis and an increased risk of eye injury, including rupture of globe. Early decompression may be necessary.

Diplopia

Diplopia due to restriction of eye movements can be caused by a variety of mechanisms but is most commonly due to contusion. It may also be due to entrapment or prolapse (a downward displacement > 5 mm is required before diplopia occurs). It most commonly affects the up and down gaze, with the latter the most disabling for reading and walking down steps. A third of cases will be permanent if left untreated.

- Mild diplopia is often transient and may be treated conservatively only if it is confined to the extremes of gaze. Steroids may accelerate recovery. Primary diplopia persisting more than 2 weeks is most likely due to entrapment
- A forced duction test is recommended (see below). If normal, conservative treatment is usually reasonable (in these cases, the alteration of EOM may be due to oedema, muscle contusion or neuropraxia). As the test can be unreliable in the first week, it may be acceptable to wait 1–2 weeks (for oedema to subside) and only proceed to surgery if it fails to improve. On the other hand, some surgeons perform routine early exploration, particularly if diplopia affecting functional fields of vision is present, or there are signs of entrapment on CT
  - Anaesthetise with topical anaesthetic and grasp conjunctiva at a site away from cornea with fine forceps. Test the passive movements of the globe in all directions, especially elevation. Apprehension may reduce value of test under LA
  - Repeat under GA before starting surgery and at the end of surgery

Causes of diplopia in trauma

Mechanical causes: Incarceration of muscle, ligaments, capsule or fat. Most commonly, fine ligaments to the muscles tether the fat. Relative change in mechanical line of inferior rectus is also a cause.

Non-mechanical causes are less common. These include injury to muscles or nerves., such as a nonspecific abducens injury due to blunt head trauma or a direct contusion of the oculomotor nerve.

Enophthalmos

Some important definitions:

- Exorbitism: Normal orbital tissue with decreased bony orbital volume, e.g. congenital, space occupying lesions, fibrous dysplasia, osteomas or post-traumatic bone fragments. There is a risk of eye complications and requires corrective osteotomies for definitive repair. Eye lubrication and tarsorrhaphy are used as temporising measures
- Exophthalmos: Excess of tissue with a normal bony orbit, such as thyroid eye disease. Resecting the excess tissue can be difficult and a three-wall expansion through a reverse-Z osteotomy with inferomedial blowout is often needed
- Enophthalmos: This most often due to post-traumatic intraorbital volume increase, especially after zygomatic fractures. Milder degrees can be treated with bone/cartilage grafts or alloplastic material inlaid to reduce volume without osteotomy. These must be placed behind the equator of the globe; otherwise they will migrate superiorly instead of anteriorly as is required (see below)

The AP position of the globe depends on:

- Volume of bony orbit posterior to vertical axis of globe. Fractures that tend to involve the medial wall and floor tend to increase this. One millimetre of bony displacement causes a corresponding 1 cc of volume change. Shifts of the globe that do not exceed 2–3 mm are usually not deforming. CT analysis is used to assess and monitor this. If there is > 13% increase in volume at 1 month, the risk of enophthalmos is high
- Contents of orbit: These may be displaced, scarred or shrunken by processes such as fat necrosis. Enophthalmos may only become evident after initial swelling has settled
- Attachments of globe to the orbit. Check ligaments and muscle tone, as if intact, are capable of maintaining a normal globe position even if the orbital floor is not. If disrupted, the globe position may be significantly altered

There is no direct correlation between enophthalmos and diplopia. Volume correction may not reduce diplopia and in chronic cases, may exacerbate it. Fractures > 2 cm^2 in area or > 3 mm displacement will cause significant globe displacement and a high risk of developing enophthalmos, and thus are indications for surgery.

Incisions for access

The aims are to expose the orbital floor, reduce herniated soft tissue and repair the bony defect.

- Subtarsal (Converse 1981): This offers the most direct access. The incision is made along the natural fold below the tarsus approximately 5–7 mm from lid margin, with an inferolateral cant. Dissection then proceeds through the orbicularis oculi to orbital septum. The inferior tissue flap is then raised down to the orbital rim where the periosteum is incised before it is elevated off the orbital floor. There is less bruising with this technique and it leaves a reasonable but external scar, with the risk of mild ectropion
  - Compared to subciliary incisions, the transcutaneous subtarsal approach causes less scleral show and ectropion but greater oedema and a more visible scar
- Subciliary: The skin incision is made just below the lash line, through muscle and to the orbital septum. It is often modified to include a lateral extension below lateral canthal ligament, allowing access to lateral orbit and ZF suture, thereby avoiding a separate upper lid incision. It has the highest risk of ectropion, with potential problems related to denervation of pretarsal orbicularis and more ecchymosis
  - Stepped (Converse 1981) skin incised 2–3 mm below lash line and the skin is raised off the muscle to just below tarsus, which is then divided down to the septum and followed to the orbital rim. The periosteum is incised anteriorly on the orbital rim to avoid vertical lid shortening. Stair stepping may reduce scar inversion but still has

a 10% transient ectropion and 30% permanent scleral show rate
  - Skin only: High incidence of skin necrosis, bruising and ectropion
  - Skin-muscle: Non-stepped
- Transconjunctival: The internal incision is made below the level of the tarsus, through the septum, to reach the plane anterior to this. Orbital rim dissection proceeds as previously discussed. Lateral canthotomy may improve exposure but if performed, requires a canthoplasty. There is no external scar and less ectropion (3% permanent scleral show vs. 28% in subciliary)

Repair of floor

The aim is to perform an anatomical repair. Care is required during exploration to avoid dissection into the maxillary sinus. The fracture may first require enlargement to free entrapped tissue and to visualise the entire defect. Options for repair materials include:

- Autologous: Requires a donor site and an associated risk of resorption, e.g. split calvarium, cartilage, split rib and fascia lata. The resorption rate is lowest in the former
- Alloplastic: Avoids donor sites but the risk of infection is theoretically higher. Choices include: Supramid sheet implants (made from thin woven polyamide), Teflon, silastic, titanium mesh (expensive) and MEDPOR (porous polyethylene). The latter two have been used with a low infection rate. The use of absorbable implants is popular in paediatric fractures

Complications

- Infection especially with alloplastic materials
- Persistent diplopia: This may be due to or be exacerbated by muscle damage during surgery
- Persistent enophthalmos: Usually due to increased orbital volume or less commonly due to loss of ligamentous support (which allows further soft tissue contraction), fat atrophy, fibrosis or muscle contraction (check with forward traction test). The risk is higher if the initial surgery was delayed

- Ectropion: Typically due to scar contraction, especially with subciliary incisions (though the scar itself tends to heal well). A Frost suture in lower eyelid is left for 24–48 hours taped to forehead or sutured posterior to hairline. Initial management consists of lower lid massage, eye lubrication and taping, with which most cases resolve. For persistent cases, a transconjunctival scar release can be considered at 6 months, unless the cornea is at risk, in which case earlier intervention is needed. Other options include skin grafting in severe cases. Steroid injection into the lower lid is not recommended
- Superior orbital fissure syndrome (SOFS) and orbital apex syndrome (OAS)
  - SOFS results from fracture line extension from the orbit into the fissure. It usually follows high velocity trauma, injuring CN III, IV, V1 (motor) and VI, producing ophthalmoplegia, upper lid ptosis, proptosis, a fixed dilated pupil and sensory loss over V1 (sensory), including the corneal reflex. Unless there is radiographic evidence of nerve compression or local bony injury, treatment is conservative (steroids can be considered)
  - OAS is similar but with optic nerve involvement, mostly due to direct trauma to the optic nerve or retrobulbar haemorrhage causing ischaemic neuropathy. Surgical decompression for fracture-related OAS is increasingly popular
- Postoperative blindness: This is fortunately rare and may be caused by many mechanisms, including nerve impingement or direct damage. Pressure on the globe or nerve accounts for 5% of cases, and are commonly from haematoma, manipulation, fracture extension to the optic canal or usage of an implant that is excessively large. An urgent CT is required prior to re-exploration
- Sensory loss: 95% recover spontaneously

Further reading

Brucoli M, Arcuri F, Cavenaghi R, et al. Analysis of complications after surgical repair of orbital fractures. J Craniofac Surg 2011; 22:1387–90.

Related topic of interest

- Eyelid reconstruction

Paediatric burns

Paediatric burns are commonly accidental (90% are avoidable) and >60% are scalds. The group most at risk are males in their second year of life as they have the physical capability to explore their environment but lack awareness of its dangers. There are significant characteristics that distinguish the paediatric burn and its management from the equivalent burn in an adult.

Acute care (ABC)

- Airway: As the airway of a child is narrower and more irritable, it is more prone to obstruction. Any degree of swelling will have a relatively greater obstructive effect
- Breathing: Children are more reliant on diaphragmatic breathing. Inhalational injuries may have prolonged adverse effects on the respiratory function
- Circulation: Intravenous access may be difficult due to the small vessel size and high amount of subcutaneous fat. Options include the femoral vein, a cutdown of the long saphenous vein or an intraosseous line. Blood pressure is generally well maintained even with severe hypovolaemia. Overt shock is usually a late feature

Depth of burn

The skin thickness significantly influences the histological depth of burn sustained. Deeper burns are sustained by an infant compared to an adult with the same injury due to thinner skin in the former. Water at 60°C will cause a full-thickness burn in

- <1 second in an infant
- Up to 5 seconds in older children
- 20 seconds in an adult

Burn depth, particularly after scalding, is more difficult to judge in children, and is often of mixed depth and can progressively deepen over 48 hours. LDI may provide more accurate and an objective measure of burn depth but requires specialised scanning equipment. An alternative is the selective use of test shaves under anaesthesia, which may

help to identify those who are most likely to benefit from (earlier) surgery. It is often best to pursue a trial of healing for 10–14 days before embarking on surgery.

Surface area

Use a paediatric Lund and Browder chart. Due to the different body proportions in children, Wallace's rule of nines in its basic form cannot be applied. It can be modified to account for the patient's age, but the formula becomes unwieldy.

- From birth up to 1 year of age, the surface area of the head and neck is 18% and for the leg it is 13.5%
- For each year after, the head loses 1% and each leg gains 0.5%
- The adult proportions are attained by age 10

Children have a greater surface area to volume ratio than adults, and this has several effects:

- Increased metabolic rate: Adequate calorific nutrition differs from adults, especially in large burns. The Galveston formula a one method for calculating such nutritional requirements. The Curreri formula can be used in both children and adults
- Increased heat loss (less fat and shivering): The child should be kept warm and the ambient temperature raised, if necessary (this is particularly important during burns surgery)
- Increased evaporative water loss

Adequate analgesia is important (oral morphine 0.1 mg/kg/q6h), particularly before dressing changes. Morphine can be given intravenously 0.2 mg/kg/q6h, if needed.

Resuscitation

The Parkland formula is a suitable guide for the resuscitation of paediatric burn patients, but must be supplemented with maintenance fluids (**Table 56**).

Fluid administration should be adjusted to maintain urine output at 1 ml/kg/h or more. The renal tubules have a reduced capacity to

Table 56 Fluids in paediatric burns	
Resuscitation	**Maintenance**
2–4 × BSA (%) × body weight (kg)	100 ml per kg for the first 10 kg 50 ml per kg for the next 10 kg
Lower threshold: 10% burn	20 ml per kg for the rest
Ringer's lactate	5% Dextrose water or 5% Dextrose with 0.45% saline and 10 mmol KCl

concentrate urine and hence urine output tends to be maintained even when volume depleted. Weighed nappies can be used to monitor the output of babies and infants (generally defined as up to 1 year old, but the upper limit is discretionary in this context). During resuscitation, children are particularly prone to problems with hypoglycaemia and hyponatraemia.

Long-term effects

It is important to consider the sequelae of a major life threatening and disfiguring injury on the body and psyche of a growing patient. The effect of growth on the effects of scars and contractures should be anticipated and treated early.

- Psychological upset is difficult to deal with and requires a great deal of support
- Major burns cause growth delay that never fully recovers
- Breast burns have the potential to recover well, even if the NAC appears badly burnt. Acute burn management should be conservative to maximise survival of the breast bud. Allow the burn to demarcate before carrying out tangential debridement. However, subsequent contractures should be managed aggressively, with timely release and reconstruction with graft or flap repair, to allow the greatest potential for normal development

Toxic shock syndrome

Staphylococcus aureus colonises burns wounds within 1–2 days. On rare occasions, some strains produce toxic shock syndrome toxin (TSST-1, 75%) or staphylococcal enterotoxins (25%), which are absorbed.

TSST-1 is a super-antigen (see 'Necrotising fasciitis') as it overstimulates T-lymphocytes and an exaggerated and deleterious response. The burn areas themselves are often small and patients typically present within 2 days.

- Prodrome: 24–48 hours of diarrhoea, vomiting, malaise and pyrexia > 38.9°C
- Rash
- Change in clinical condition
- Shock (50% mortality)
- Raised leukocyte count, raised INR, low calcium and low albumin

Management involves:

- Aggressive resuscitation and invasive monitoring (CVP is recommended)
- Clean the infected wound
- Administration of antibiotics: Clindamycin is first line for invasive group A streptococcal infections. Some recommend a combination with a β-lactamase resistant anti-staphylococcal antibiotic
- FFP/blood
- Specific antitoxin (commercial preparations of pooled immunoglobulin, reserved for refractory cases)

The role of prevention with prophylactic antibiotics is controversial and is not common practice. It is more important to have a high index of suspicion and to educate parents to be vigilant for it.

Non-accidental injury (NAI)

There are characteristic features of burns that should raise suspicions of a non-accidental aetiology. No single marker is entirely predictive.

- History inconsistent with injury. Children cannot usually climb into baths unaided before 10–18 months

- Changing story: Siblings often blamed
- Delay in presentation
- Presentation at locations illogically distant from the home. Check with A&E departments near home for previous attendances
- Previous or other injuries including fractures and cigarette burns
- Glove and stocking distribution, symmetrical scalds with clear upper margins and absence of splash marks (although this may occur with lower temperature injuries below 54°C)

- Scalds: Immersion injuries usually involve hot tap water, affecting the extremities especially the lower limbs, buttocks or perineum. Total surface area involved is not predictive
- Skin fold sparing, doughnut ring pattern with central sparing of buttocks

Scalds due to neglect outnumber those from intentional injury by >10 fold, with features similar to accidental scalds. The child is often passive, introverted and fearful. There is a risk of subsequent injuries (up to 70%) and late mortality up to (30–40%).

Further reading

Khorasani EN, Mansouri F. Effect of early enteral nutrition on morbidity and mortality in children with burns. Burns 2010; 36:1067–71.

Related topics of interest

- Acute burns
- Necrotising fasciitis

Parotid gland tumours

The most important relation of the parotid gland is the facial nerve. The superficial and deep lobes of the parotid are demarcated arbitrarily by the facial nerve, resulting in 80% of the gland lying superficial to it. The lobes of the parotid are not true anatomical demarcations and are histologically indistinguishable.

- 80% of salivary gland tumours are in the parotid
- 80% of parotid lumps are benign
- 80% of benign parotid tumours are pleomorphic adenomas (less)

While lumps of the parotid are likely to be benign, lumps of the increasingly smaller salivary glands are more likely to be malignant (50% submandibular, 80% sublingual are malignant). Parotid lumps in children are also more likely to be malignant. Most parotid tumours are well-circumscribed masses. More diffuse lumps may be due to inflammation, lymphoma or deep lobe tumours. The features suggestive of parotid malignancy include:

- Invasion of the facial nerve giving rise to facial palsy or pain. Pain is not as significant a sign as expected, due partly to its subjectivity and its lack of specificity. Benign conditions such as inflammation, infection or haemorrhage into a cyst, such as that after FNA, can cause discomfort
- Invasion of the parotid duct causing obstruction, infection or bleeding
- Invasion of the muscles or temporomandibular joint, causing trismus

Up to 75% of patients with these features have positive nodes at the time of presentation and on average they survive less than 3 years. Other features include fixation to the deep structures or to skin, and rapid increase in size. The presence of a parotid mass with enlarged nodes is nearly 100% predictive of malignancy. The presence or absence of cysts is of little value for delineating the nature of the lump. Overall, the clinical picture is only 30% predictive of the nature of a parotid lump. The precise diagnosis is often made after surgery, reinforcing the view that a superficial parotidectomy is an excisional biopsy.

The classification of parotid gland tumours is rather complex and only the commonest benign and malignant lesions are discussed below. There is a wide range of histopathology and benign tumours may be locally aggressive. For TNM staging, T staging is similar to other head and neck cancers (2 cm and 4 cm as limits) with further assignment of a or b to denote local extension to skin, soft tissue, muscle and bone.

Benign parotid tumours

Pleomorphic salivary adenomas

Pleomorphic (pleomorphic) salivary adenomas (PSAs) are sometimes called mixed tumours due to the presence of different epithelial and mesenchymal components within it. These are the commonest benign parotid tumours, usually presenting as a slow-growing painless firm, but slightly compressible mass in the parotid, most often in the tail of the gland, which is often noticed coincidentally while shaving or washing. Typical patients are 40–50 years old with a slight female predominance.

The standard treatment is a superficial parotidectomy. The delicate pseudocapsule around the tumour is formed by compressed normal glandular tissue and may harbour some pseudopodial tumour projections. Simple enucleation leads to recurrence rates of > 25%. Excisional surgery with a cuff of normal gland will reduce the recurrence rate to 1–5%.

- The risk of malignant transformation to a carcinoma ex pleomorphic adenoma (CXPA) is 2–10% and usually presents as a sudden increase in size, pain, palsy and fixity. After 10–15 years, the transformation risk may be high enough to warrant excision of PSA
- Risk of facial nerve damage
- Risk of recurrence: This is more common if there was tumour rupture or close tumour proximity to the facial nerve. The best chance for cure is at primary surgery, as recurrences may be multifocal

and reoperation has an increased risk to the facial nerve. The chance of cure with recurrent tumours is < 25%

Adenolymphomas (Warthin's tumour)

Adenolymphomas are classically soft cystic lumps in the tail of the parotid (rarely other glands) in elderly (60–70 years) males (5–10 times more common than in females). The risk is increased by up to 40-fold in smokers. The commonly quoted 10% rule is: 10% bilateral, ten times risk in smokers, ten times in males, 10% malignant risk, although this inaccurate. Tumours are usually well defined with a lymphoid stroma. Despite its name, it is not a lymphoma. There tends to be a higher incidence in the Eastern Asian population, and in some studies exceeds that of PSAs (25–40%); cyst infection is also common. Recurrence is uncommon (2%) after treatment with a superficial parotidectomy. Some of the reported recurrences may be due to multifocal disease.

Malignant parotid tumours

Malignant parotid tumours occur mostly in the body of the parotid. They can either be primary or secondary (SCC 40% and melanoma 45%, particularly from the scalp or ear). The diagnosis of malignancy can only usually be made on biopsy, which necessitates a parotidectomy. The outcome of malignant salivary tumours depends more on tumour stage than specific histopathology.

Mucoepidermoid carcinomas

Mucoepidermoid carcinomas comprise one third of malignant parotid tumours and 8% of all parotid tumours. The degree of histological differentiation influences its behaviour and prognosis.

- Most are well-differentiated carcinomas that behave like pleomorphic adenomas, and thus rarely metastasise. It has a 90% 5-year survival rate after excision with margins
- Poorly differentiated tumours behave more like adenoid cystic carcinomas and are prone to local invasion and regional spread. Treatment is aggressive excision with adjuvant radiotherapy. The 5-year survival rate is 10%

Adenoid cystic carcinomas

Adenoid cystic carcinomas only make up one-fifth of malignant parotid tumours but are the commonest malignancy of the minor salivary glands. There are a number of histological subtypes: Cribriform tumours have the best prognosis and solid tumours the worst, with tubular tumours lying in between. The clinical behaviour of the lesion is unpredictable. It is locally invasive but may remain stable for many years. Haematogenous spread to the lungs is more common than nodal spread.

These tumours do not have a capsule. Aggressive excisional surgery and radiotherapy is the typical treatment. If the superficial parotidectomy specimen shows high-grade malignancy, a large tumour or nodal involvement, a complete total parotidectomy should be performed. However, there is a tendency for perineural invasion with skip lesions along the facial nerve and the observed propensity to recur, often after many years, raises some doubt whether a true cure is possible.

Lymphomas

Parotid lymphomas occur in 5–10% of Warthin's tumours and often occur in patients with Sjögren's syndrome or Hepatitis C infection. Chemotherapy is the treatment of choice.

Investigations for parotid masses

The pathology of the parotid gland is complex and ideally, a dedicated parotid pathologist should examine the sections. Investigations may help to allow differentiation of:
- Non-parotid from parotid, e.g. lymph nodes in Chinese patients with nasopharyngeal carcinoma
- Neoplasm from inflammation of parotid
- Malignant from benign

Imaging

Imaging is generally unnecessary unless there is suspicion of malignancy, parapharyngeal space involvement or deep lobe/dumb-bell tumour. Imaging is especially useful in assessing recurrent disease that may be multifocal. MRI and CT provide nearly the same information with nearly 100% sensitivity, although the T2-weighted MRI is better than CT

- For assessing tumour margins
- For distinguishing between benign and malignant disease with 93% sensitivity
- For delineating a poorly-defined boundary with evidence of local invasion
- Not affected by the amalgam artefact
- More useful for larger tumours > 3 cm, especially where deep lobe involvement is suspected

CT provides better detail of surrounding tissue including the duct. Overall, CT provides useful information in 14% of cases, primarily the extent (deep lobe), parapharyngeal involvement and lymph nodes.

Fine needle aspiration cytology (FNAC)

The role of FNAC is controversial. One view is that biopsy (and imaging) is unnecessary, as all parotid gland tumours require excision (except lymphomas). It provides little information that will alter management. However, it is simple, cheap, has high patient acceptance and can simplify discussions. It may be useful in providing confirmatory results in:

- Poor surgical candidates or those who wish to avoid surgery. It can distinguish between benign and malignant tumours with 90% specificity. Howler found that it changed management in 35%, mostly from an altered diagnosis of an inflammatory condition
- Parotid lumps in patients with other malignancies (possible metastases) or with lymphoma (non-parotid causes)
- Parapharyngeal masses

FNAC is very operator-dependent and the best results are achieved by experienced cytopathologists. Repeated non-specific results have a higher risk of eventually being malignant. It is of little use in epithelial lesions, for which the architecture is needed for diagnosis. Sensitivity is relatively low (75%), but specificity and overall accuracy is over 90% (97%). The false negative rate is around 10%. Therefore, only positive results should be accepted.

Frozen sections are at best 93% accurate, with a false positive rate of 10%, and highly dependant on the experience of the pathologist. They should not be totally relied upon. Clinical impression is paramount and is most useful for checking margins and neck nodes. FNA and FSs may complementary, providing information on cellular details and cellular architecture, respectively.

Superficial parotidectomy

Superficial parotidectomy with facial nerve preservation can be viewed as a biopsy procedure (involving a nerve dissection) for parotid lumps that will also serve as adequate management in over 80%. The tumour can be 'peeled off' the facial nerve unless it demonstrates definite invasion. Postoperative radiotherapy can clear the nerve of tumour contamination while preserving adequate nerve function. Due to the 'bare area' over the facial nerve, the operation approximates a near-total conservative superficial parotidectomy and long-term follow-up is mandatory.

For benign or low-grade malignancies, superficial parotidectomy (or total parotidectomy with nerve preservation if the mass is in the deep lobe) is adequate treatment. However, high-grade malignancies should be treated with radical parotidectomy with nerve sacrifice (if invaded) and excision of masseter, medial pterygoid, styloid process and muscles, posterior digastric, skin, and a neck dissection. Tumours should be excised with a cuff of normal tissue whenever possible so that surgery is definitive treatment.

- Surgery is performed under a GA and muscle relaxant is avoided. The use of nerve stimulators is common but not universal. It useful to check the integrity of the nerve branches at the end of the operation. The commonly used incisions are the lazy-S or Blair incisions
- The skin flap is elevated from the parotid anteriorly
- The parotid tail is separated from the muscles (sternomastoid and posterior belly of digastric). The great auricular nerve should be spared if possible (success

rate of 69% and only costs an additional 10 minutes). Temporary deficits of the greater auricular nerve territory still occur but are less severe and recover quickly. If sacrificed, the sensory loss may lead to problems with putting on earrings, shaving and general increased vulnerability to injury. Recovery may take up to 2 years but occurs incompletely and in < 50%

- Injury to the large veins will lead to congestion of the gland and increased bleeding
- The facial nerve is normally approached in an anterograde manner using the tragal pointer as a landmark (see below). The facial nerve described as being 1 cm inferior and deep to it. In practice, this is often more in both respects. Some studies have found the nerve 23.6 mm deep, and it is dependent on ear configuration and retraction. A large deep lobe can distort the nerve position. Do not operate down a deep hole. Mobilise more of the posterior border if needed. The parotid is gradually dissected away from the nerve. Retrograde dissection may be required in very large, and proximal lesions that are difficult to retract for trunk visualisation or for reoperations. The distal branches are identified and traced back. Useful landmarks include:
  - Buccal branch: Above the parotid duct
  - Marginal mandibular branch: Over the facial vessels
  - Retromandibular vein: Inferior aspect of the gland
- Neck dissection: FNA nodes >10 mm, primary tumour > 4 cm

Other proposed landmarks for the facial nerve:

- Tympanomastoid fissure: The suture between the posterior bony EAM and mastoid portion of temporal bone. This has the advantage of being a true bony landmark. The nerve is 6–8 mm below its lowest point
- Mastoid origin of sternomastoid: The two finger technique, where nerve is 1.5 cm deep to index fingertip placed on lateral surface of mastoid perpendicular to other index on sternomastoid along its fibres,

and flush with lower border of mastoid
- Retromandibular vein (nerve runs over it)
- Styloid process, stylomastoid foramen, stylomastoid artery
- Posterior belly of digastric
- Antitragus

The role of radiotherapy in PSA (a benign disease) is controversial and there is a general lack of agreement on its indications and usefulness. The response rate is low and there is a concern that it may cause malignant change. Radiotherapy may be useful for multifocally recurrent pleomorphic adenomas, but is more often used for malignant disease in an adjuvant fashion for adenoid cystic carcinoma, high-grade tumours or low-grade tumours with suspicious margins.

Complications

These need to be carefully explained to patients:

- Frey's syndrome is sweating over the parotid area when eating. It is due to severed secretomotor parasympathetic fibres (glossopharyngeal nerve, lesser petrosal nerve) from the auriculotemporal nerve that connecting with the cutaneous nerves to sweat glands. It may occur in 10–50% of cases, although subclinical disease is more common (the incidence is > 90% when tested objectively with Minor's starch iodine test tapes). There may be a long delay since it does depend on nerve regeneration through scarred tissue. To reduce its incidence, a thick skin flap or muscle (SMAS or sternomastoid) flaps have been used. Treatment for symptomatic disease can be as simple as antiperspirants or topical scopolamine, while surgical options include interpositional flaps or grafts (may increase the rates of fistulae) or neurectomy (transmeatal tympanic neurectomy of tympanic branch with parasympathetic fibres of glossopharyngeal nerve, with variable success and largely temporary). Botulinum toxin injection is effective and is gaining popularity, with effects that may last > 6 months

- − Dr Lucia Frey a French neurologist described gustatory sweating in a Polish soldier after a bullet wound of the parotid (1923) calling it 'auriculotemporal syndrome'. The condition can, though uncommonly, follow other facial traumas or without a known cause
- Facial nerve palsy is usually only temporary (20% or more, usually recovering over 2 months but may last up to a year on occasion) but is permanent in a small number (0.5–1%). The risk is increased with reoperation
- Parotid mucocoele or sialocoele: Treat with aspiration and pressure, botulinum toxin
- Parotid fistula: These tend to heal up with conservative treatment. Radiotherapy, if indicated for the disease, will also hasten resolution. Fistulae may have a greater chance of spontaneous closure if the parotid duct is patent. Some distinguish between fistula from the gland (minor duct transection) or the duct. Sialograms may help assess the site of injury

Further reading

Yoo YM, Lee JS, Park MC, et al. Dermofat graft after superficial parotidectomy via a modified face-lift incision to prevent Frey syndrome and depressed deformity. J Craniofac Surg 2011; 22:1021–23.

Related topics of interest

- Botulinum toxin
- Facial reanimation
- Hidradenitis suppurativa and hyperhidrosis

These are benign lesions that show cellular changes, such as dysplasia or atypia that are not yet frankly malignant.

- If left untreated, there is a recognised risk of progression to frankly invasive malignancy, although not all cases will become malignant
- If adequately treated, overt cancer can be prevented
- Cancers that arise from premalignant lesions may be more aggressive than *de novo* cancers (actinic keratoses being an exception)

Actinic keratoses (AKs) or senile keratosis are the commonest premalignant lesions.

- These are rough, scaly, slightly raised and well-demarcated red lesions that show cellular dysplasia and atypia. These are fairly common in the elderly in sun-exposed areas. They almost universally caused by chronic sun exposure although there is weak link to high fat intake. Some lesions may regress with sun avoidance, but this is controversial
- A relatively large proportion will progress eventually to SCC in situ, with 10% becoming frankly invasive. These figures vary widely and the risk may be related both to the number of lesions as well as duration. SCCs arising from actinic keratoses tend to be less aggressive with a lower metastatic potential. However, transplant patients have a greater risk of transformation and are treated more aggressively
- AKs can be treated non-surgically with topical 5% 5-fluorouracil (5-FU, applied twice daily for 4 weeks). While an effective treatment, its numerous and common side effects, such as pain, erythema and erosions, reduce compliance and hence its effectiveness. The overall cure rate is up to 93% vs. 50% for those who complete treatment and prematurely stop treatment respectively. The recurrence rate is approximately 50%
- Other options include cryotherapy (99% cure rate but with scarring and hypopigmentation), phenol peeling, imiquimod, photodynamic therapy (PDT,

90% response rate with good cosmesis, but at the cost of increased recurrence rates) or surgery (may be offered for lesions that remain after topical therapy). The results with topical diclofenac (Solarase) are inconsistent. Some who have used ablative lasers, claim simultaneous prophylactic treatment of the remaining skin

Leukoplakia and erythroplakia

Leukoplakia or white patch

- These are slightly elevated and sharply defined white patches of hyperkeratosis, parakeratosis, keratosis and acanthosis found commonly on the oral mucosa or vulva. Most are idiopathic, but may be related to recurrent irritation from sharp teeth and tobacco smoke in some (risk factors for head and neck SCC). Leukoplakia may regress if the identifiable cause is removed, but 10–20% will progress to SCC, indicated by ulceration, nodules or verrucous change. Tumours that arise from leukoplakia tend to be more aggressive
- Biopsy is mandatory and excision is recommended. Toluidine blue vital staining can be used as an adjunct to guide biopsy of the most dysplastic areas (10% false positive staining). Relapses are common

Erythroplakia

- These are flat, slightly raised red velvety lesions. The colour is due to the loss of orthokeratin. Lesions may be granular or mixed with leukoplakia. There is greater malignant potential than leukoplakia, with the risk of transformation approximately 50%. In addition, there is a 30% risk of an occult focus of carcinoma-in-situ in these lesions
- Early excision is recommended

Bowen's disease

- This is a disease of the elderly and presents as scaly, itchy, red-pink and

well-demarcated plaques (usually isolated). Although they may affect any body location, they are commonly found on the trunk, legs and arms, and are often non-sun-exposed parts. It may also be mistaken for psoriasis. The cause is unknown although there is an association with UV exposure. Very rarely, multiple lesions may be related to chronic arsenic poisoning (Fowler's solution was once commonly used as a tonic and general panacea for malaria, chorea and syphilis)
- The suggested link with an internal malignancy is not strong enough to justify routine investigation. Most cases are idiopathic
- Bowenoid papulosis is a different disorder and related to HPV16 (genital warts)
- John Templeton Bowen was an American dermatologist who described it in 1912
• This is squamous cell carcinoma-in-situ and therefore technically not premalignant. Three to eleven per cent of cases progress to frankly invasive SCC (greater in genital lesions) and such lesions tend to be more aggressive, with a tendency to metastasise early. There is also a tendency for poral invasion. Erythroplasia of Queyrat (SCC in situ of the penis) is more likely to become invasive and lead to metastasis

• Surgery with or without Mohs is preferred, as it provides histopathological material for examination. It can also be treated with daily 5% 5-FU (can be combined with DNCB for better penetration but this treatment is often limited by the irritant effect), cryotherapy (90% success but slow healing may be a problem), PDT (limited availability and no consensus on technique), curettage or laser. Radiotherapy is not useful. The successful use of imiquimod has been reported but is usually regarded as an option only if other modalities including surgery are contraindicated. Good sun protection is recommended to reduce the risk of recurrence, estimated to be about 10%
- Imiquimod is FDA approved for superficial BCCs, actinic keratoses and anogenital warts. Other indications are off-label

Giant congenital naevus (see 'Melanoma') and sebaceous naevus (see 'Basal Cell Carcinoma') are known to have risks of malignant transformation. There has been a reported case of melanoma developing in an area of Becker's naevus (Fehr 1991). The majority of evidence suggests that the naevus itself does not have an increased risk of developing malignancy, and any treatment should be regarded as cosmetic.

Further reading

Sciallis GF, Sciallis AP. Becker nevus with an underlying desmoid tumour: a case report and review including Mayo Clinic's experience. Arch Dermatol 2010; 146:1408–12.

Related topics of interest

- Basal cell carcinoma
- Melanoma
- Oral cancer
- Squamous cell carcinoma

Pressure sores

This condition is often called a decubitus ulcer from the Latin '*decumbere*' meaning 'to lie down'. This is a misnomer as the commonest sores are ischial that occur in the seated position (wheelchair bound). For similar reasons, the term 'bed sore' is not applicable in all cases. Pressure sores occur most commonly in the elderly (70% are in the over 70s) and neurologically impaired. It accounts for 6% of deaths on geriatric wards and 7–8% of the deaths in paraplegics.

In decreasing order of frequency, ischial sores are most common (30%), followed by sacral and greater trochanteric (20% each) and heel (10%), with the remainder consisting of sores on the malleoli and occiput. Note that the distribution between paraplegic patients and acute patients differ. Sacral and heel sores are more common in the latter.

Causes

The most important causative factor is prolonged excessive pressure. When the extrinsic pressure exceeds the capillary pressure of 32 mmHg, vessels are occluded and blood flow to the tissue stops. It is not an instant effect and the time needed to cause ischaemic necrosis is inversely related to pressures involved, and also varies between different tissues. This ischaemia causes pain or discomfort in the sensate and unimpaired, prompting a rectifying positional shift. Impairment of this protective action occurs in the insensate and obtunded.

Kosiak's principle states that tissues can tolerate an increased pressure if interspersed with periods of relief. This period of relief should be a minimum of 5 minutes every 2 hours if supine, or 10 seconds every 10 minutes if seated. This is the basis for turning patients every 2 hours in pressure sore prevention. If the pressure is persistent, then necrosis and ulceration will result. Muscle and fat is more susceptible to ischaemia than skin, hence the skin injury seen is often just the tip of the iceberg.

In clinical situations, sores are unlikely to be due to pressure alone and other contributing factors include friction and shear, low-level bacterial infection (increasing the susceptibility of skin to pressure, and in turn pressure may also reduce resistance to infection), as well as maceration or traumatic desquamation. In addition to pressure and the other extrinsic factors above, certain intrinsic features of the patient will also increase the risk of developing pressure sores:

- Malnutrition: This also contributes to general debilitation and loss of protective padding. However, nutritional support has not been shown to prevent the development of sores
- Incontinence
- Immobility
- Altered sensation and consciousness: cannot recognise or respond to pain
- Advanced age

The importance of these risk factors is reflected in their inclusion in the numerous risk scales that exist, such as the Norton (for geriatrics), Braden (original cutoff of 16, but depends on the setting) and Waterlow scales (> 20 very high risk). It is important to realise that these scales are dependent on the competence of the assessor and only assess the general condition of the patient and their risk of developing pressure sores. It is the administration of a good standard of care that has the greatest contribution. However, it is inappropriate to blame all pressure sore on poor care, as not all are preventable in the susceptible patient. Paraplegics often have additional problems, such as recurrent urinary tract infections, contractures and soft tissue calcification.

Grading of pressure sores

It is common to grade the sore by the extent of visible destruction. The common schemes are based on Shea 1975. The National Pressure Ulcer Advisory Panel (NPUAP) was updated in 2009 and the definition more restrictive. A pressure sore is a localised injury to skin and/or underlying tissue usually over a bony prominence as a result of pressure. Denudement due to maceration or shearing is *not* included.

- Stage 1: Non-blanching erythema only (may not be obvious in pigmented skin, rather a difference in colour may be seen). Other staging systems have suggested 'erythema that does not recover after 30 minutes of pressure relief', but this is not included in the latest classification. This roughly correlates to 1 hour of pressure

- Stage 2: Partial-thickness skin loss, with a shallow ulcer or serum-filled blister. There is no slough (nor blood blisters) that would indicate deeper injury (2–6 hours)
- Stage 3: Full-thickness skin loss into the subcutaneous layer that does not expose bone, muscle or tendon. The depth of the ulcer will depend in part of the thickness of the subcutaneous layer that varies between anatomical sites (>6 hours)
- Stage 4: Extensive deep destruction may involve bone, joints, muscle or tendon (visible or palpable). These are often extensively undermined or tunnelled

Note that if there is an intact eschar or slough layer that prevents adequate assessment of the base, the ulcer is unstageable until debridement. Dry intact eschars should be left alone in most cases as a biological dressing. There is an extra category of deep tissue injury (DTI), where bruised but intact skin is associated with deeper tissue necrosis. This diagnosis is often made retrospectively after debridement. The potential for recovery of DTI by conservative means is unclear.

The mechanism of shear and pressure sores are very different. In the former, the injury is due to friction/drag on the superficial layers (sometimes deeper injuries) usually sustained during patient transfer. In the latter, the problem arises in the deeper layers of the muscle adjacent to bone, where the pressure is the highest. However, the presence of perpetuating factors for the latter may cause the former to appear as the initiating factor.

Management

Prevention is important and infinitely preferable. However, preventative measures, even if implemented correctly, cannot absolutely guarantee pressure sore prevention. The aim is to distribute weight evenly over a larger area. Static padding such as standard mattresses is suboptimal. Specialised beds and mattresses (low air loss, air fluidised, and alternating air cell) dynamically alter the bed to the static patient. No RCTs exist that validate their use. The use of a low air-loss bed will reduce the risk of pressure sores *developing* but the effect on *healing* improvement compared to a normal bed is less obvious.

Treatment

Treatment of pressure sores can be difficult and prolonged. It is important to investigate fully and to identify and correct any correctable predisposing factors, which will also be important in reducing recurrence:

- Optimise nutrition especially protein (some suggest normalising the albumin)
- Correct anaemia
- Treat spasm (common in spinal cord injury) as sores will inevitably recur if the spasm is not relieved. Diazepam, baclofen and dantrolene may be useful. Surgical release may be required to relieve spasm and contractures in selected cases
- Treat infection (commonly *Staphylococcus aureus, Proteus, Pseudomonas, and Bacteroides*) with oral antibiotics. Colonisation is common (swabs only represent surface contamination only) and proof of actual infection requires deep biopsy. A pressure sore can cause sepsis, but sepsis is most commonly due to a urinary tract infection
- Osteomyelitis must to be actively excluded using a combination of investigations, although bone biopsy is the most sensitive
- The role of HBOT is largely unproven. Ultrasound is not useful
- The role of growth factors has not been fully elucidated, although some studies claim improved healing with bFGF and PDGF

Stage 1 and 2: Dressings with pressure management

The aim of dressings is to keep the wound moist for healing, and simultaneously remove excess exudate. There is a wide range of dressings available but without properly controlled trials it is difficult to establish relative efficacy. Antiseptics are unnecessary as they may kill healing cells. Pressure sores often improve despite the antiseptic rather than because of it. Common regimes include alginates and foams, sequentially followed by hydrogels/hydrocolloids. Negative pressure wound therapy (NPWT) is often useful to clean up a wound and as a temporising measure.

Stage 3 and 4: Surgery

Surgery may not always be appropriate and is not usually indicated in deteriorating or terminal patients or where the inciting and perpetuating factors are not reversed. Surgery is most useful for young patients who are motivated, clinically stable and where post-operative prevention of recurrence is possible. Incontinent patients may require faecal or urinary diversion to improve wound care.

The NPWT can be useful but requires careful patient selection. Recurrence rates even in the best series with adequate follow-up are 20% after 4 years. Reusable reconstructive options or those with incorporated redundancy are useful. Tissue expansion for closure of sores, particularly those without a large dead space, has been advocated. However, the wisdom of having a foreign body in a contaminated wound seems questionable.

Principles (after Conway 1930)

- The wound must be clean prior to surgery. The use of whirlpool baths and pulsatile lavage is currently undergoing evaluation in controlled trials. This will make the wound appear bigger. Send material for culture
- Formal debridement is needed to remove dead tissue, bursae and calcified tissue and to smooth down bony surfaces. Pseudotumour excision with methylene blue and gauze packing (alternative use methylene blue and dilute peroxide) to excise the ulcer and wall en-bloc, often including a segment of bone, may be more effective than simple debridement and curettage of the cavity
- Patient should be positioned so that the defect is at it largest, so that after closure, the tension will not be any higher. Suture line tension is the commonest reason for dehiscence
- Large flaps should be used, but always preserve future options. Use flaps that can be readvanced (rotation and V-Y) in cases

of recurrence. Dead spaces should be filled in a tension-free manner. Osteomyelitis is associated with a higher risk of dehiscence
- Primary closure is tempting but almost universally fails as there is a deficiency of tissue that almost always leaves a subcutaneous dead space
- There is evidence that fasciocutaneous flaps are better, with less recurrence than myocutaneous flaps (muscle is more sensitive to ischaemia and will atrophy with time). However, they have limited bulk and are less able to fill in large dead spaces. Donor areas should be covered with a thick split-skin graft if they cannot be closed primarily
- Suture lines should be placed away from direct pressure. Sutures should be left for 3 weeks or more
- Large drains are kept in place for a minimum of 2 weeks
- Optimise nutrition and avoid pressure on flap for 4 weeks. Evaluate the flap after each sitting session, watching for erythema that lasts more than 30 minutes

The postoperative period is prolonged but is an important part of the procedure. Traditionally, the patient was immobilised for up to 8 weeks (based on animal studies that show maximal wound strength after 6 weeks), but prospective trials in 1997 have shown no difference between 2 or 3 weeks of immobility before gradual mobilisation. Stage IV sores can take a year to heal. There is an increased risk of recurrence as the scarred tissue only has 40% of the original strength.

Sacral sores

Ironically, while these patients often lack protective sensation, sacral sores can very painful. There is usually only a small dead space and thus fasciocutaneous flaps are suitable. In general, non-surgical methods and SSG coverage is successful in selected patients:
- Sacral: 29% and 30%, respectively
- Trochanteric 41% and 33%
- Ischial 18% and 17%

Gluteal and lumbar flaps are commonly used.
- Gluteus maximus musculocutaneous flaps can be used as a large rotation flap (can be raised again, see above) or as bilateral

V-Y advancement based on the SGA (but cannot be reused). The insertion to the greater trochanter can be sacrificed to increase flap excursion in non-ambulatory patients. The trend is to use gluteal tissue flaps based on perforators (pedicled SGAP flaps or its variants). Musculocutaneous flaps were popular in 1970s, but there are fewer current indications for their use, except for large cavities or intractable osteomyelitis

- Transverse lumbosacral artery flap: This fasciocutaneous flap utilises fascia of the paraspinous muscles and based on perforators from lumbar and posterior intercostals arteries. The SSG of the donor site is often required
- ALT flap pedicled subcutaneously or trans-thigh. It may require sacrifice of the descending branch and vastus lateralis (an option for future trochanteric reconstruction)

Ischial sores

Ischial sores are often seen in paraplegics and have larger dead spaces. They are more likely to require muscle bulk for obliteration and are some of the most difficult sores to treat. Excessive excision of the ischial tuberosity is not beneficial and will lead to increased pressure on the contralateral side. Recurrence is likely (75% Conway, the most likely of the pressure sores) therefore flaps that can be readvanced are favoured. Common options are the inferior gluteus maximus island and gluteal thigh flaps, which are most reliable. Operating in the jack knife flexed position is favoured.

- The first choice is often the gluteal thigh fasciocutaneous flap, which is an axial fasciocutaneous flap (descending branch of inferior gluteal artery) along midline of back of thigh, with the pivot/axis halfway between the ischial tuberosity and greater trochanter. A large flap (15 × 34 cm) can be raised subfascially, from distal to proximal
- Muscular V-Y flaps that can be harvested with overlying skin are also common, such as the semitendinosus, based on the first profunda femoris perforator, or the biceps femoris flap. While a single muscle flap is sufficient in the ambulatory, a larger posterior thigh flap (V-Y hamstring) can be used in paraplegics. These flaps can be readvanced if the sore recurs
- Tensor fascia lata (TFL), which is supplied by the terminal branch of the LCFA from the profunda femoris, can be used to provide sensate coverage of the ischium in some paraplegics (T12 to L3 innervation). However, the distal part of the flap can be thin and vascularly tenuous. A gracilis flap works similarly from the medial aspect
- Pedicled ALT

Greater trochanter

The bursa and bony prominences should be trimmed down. SSGs are used to close the donor site in most flaps.

- TFL is the most useful, either as a V-Y or transposition flaps. Its lack of distal bulk makes it more suited for trochanteric ulcers rather than ischial
- The vastus lateralis flap is based on first descending branch of the lateral circumflex artery and may be combined with TFL
- Gluteal thigh flap, distally based gluteus maximus

Further reading

Yang CH, Kuo YR, Jeng SF. An ideal method for pressure sore reconstruction: a freestyle perforator-based flap. Ann Plast Surg 2011; 66:179–84.

Related topics of interest

- Breast reconstruction
- Groin dissection
- Vacuum wound closure

Prominent ears

Prominent ears have no functional impact but may cause psychological distress especially in the younger age group due embarrassment and teasing. The degree of acceptability varies with local culture and consequently the rates of corrective surgery vary greatly.

Management

The preoperative assessment is vital.
- It is important to establish the reason for surgery. This is straightforward in adults and children where the wishes of the parents and child concur. It is inadvisable to operate on children who object or are indifferent to surgery, despite parental pressure otherwise. In such situations, defer reassessment until the patients are mature enough to comprehend and desire treatment for themselves. The minimum age for surgery is usually 6 years in the UK that corresponds to school age. Surgery at an earlier age risks growth impairment with no additional psychological benefit, although the situation should be individualised for each patient
- Surgery targets the precise anatomical deformity causing the prominence. The most common are:
  - Flattened antihelix
  - Excessively deep conchae
  - Flat conchoscaphal angle
  - Problems that give an illusion of prominence include a prominent mastoid, isolated protrusions of the upper or lower poles, constricted ears (small prominent ears) and Stahl's ear (third crus)

Non-surgical treatment

Neonates have malleable cartilage that begins to progressively stiffen beyond the 72-hour post-partum time point. This has been attributed to high maternal oestrogen levels and high hyaluronic acid levels that dissipate rapidly after birth. Non-surgical splinting and moulding is effective for correction if applied before the second week and maintained continuously for a minimum of 6 weeks

(Matsuo). It is most effective for deformities without deficiencies of skin or cartilage. While its effectiveness may be variable, it is low risk and only a minor inconvenience.

Surgery

The key otoplasty techniques are
- Cartilage shaping (antihelical fold)
- Cartilage suturing (antihelical fold, concho-mastoid)
- Conchal reduction

The technique used (or its combination) is determined by the pathology presented and surgeon preference. Surgery may be performed under LA in the compliant patient.

Cartilage shaping

Cartilage shaping is divided into cartilage scoring and cartilage breaking techniques.
- Cartilage scoring causes it to permanently and predictably bend when weakened on one side. The Gibson principle dictates that it will bend away from the scored surface, supposedly due to release of the interlocked stresses. This is exploited in a variety of open (anterior degloving and scoring) and closed (closed rasping through a distant port) techniques, of which the former is most common
- Cartilage breaking techniques (Luckett) incise the cartilage full-thickness at the desired area of bending. The resultant fold is often sharp. Adaptations to combat this include tubing of a bipedicled segment to create a round fold, but have been largely superseded by scoring and suturing techniques
- Note that techniques that use posterior abrasion aim to thin down the posterior cartilage similar in principle to a subtotal wedge excision, so that the cartilage may be folded back. This is closer to a cartilage breaking technique than a scoring technique and does not utilise the Gibson principle
- Cartilage shaping techniques are difficult to revise and precision at primary surgery is paramount

Sutur

The sole   nique is
associat   rence rate,
especiall   ore rigid
cartilage   es carry a risk of
suture sp   uced with use of
a posteri   lap. Proponents
argue tha   cartilaginous
damage   degloving and
scoring i   avoidable.
Howevei   ıg techniques
does not   ;equent use of
scoring t   rence can also be
addresse   turing relatively
easily.

- Antihe   are full-thickness
  cartila   only (Mustarde)
  horizo   utures tied only just
  tight e   ate the antihelical fold
  (not to   surfaces). Temporary
  trans-   ng (Bonnie's blue or
  methylene ᴗᴗ, ʋy be used to guide
  placement. Knots are tied on the posterior
  surface
- Suture use is variable but should follow
  basic principles: If the sutures are used
  to primarily create the correction (e.g.
  suturing technique alone), a permanent
  suture such as Ethibond is used. If the
  sutures are used to splint the correction
  (e.g. help maintain a scoring or minor
  adjustments to it), an absorbable suture
  may be used
- Conchomastoid: This suture reduces
  the projection of a deep concha. The
  postauricular tissue between the concha
  and mastoid periosteum is dissected away
  and mattress sutures are placed between
  them
- The earlobe behaves like a pan that is
  adjustable by its antitragal panhandle.
  Residual earlobe prominence can thus
  be addressed with Furnas-type sutures
  between the posterior antitragal cartilage
  and the mastoid periosteum, tensioned
  appropriately

Excision

- Posterior skin is resected primarily for
  access and to a lesser extent addresses
  the post-correctional redundancy. The

superior and inferior poles are the most
difficult areas to access. The commonly
used dumb-bell shaped incision gives
the best access. Variations such as
the postauricular groove incisions
compromise access for a better scar
location and a lower anecdotal risk of
hypertrophic and keloid scarring

- Excision of excess conchal cartilage can
  be performed by either an anterior (at
  the junction of floor and posterior wall)
  or posterior approach. Mild conchal
  bowl excess can often be managed with
  conchomastoid sutures alone

Postoperative care

- Soft splint dressings such as proflavine-
  impregnated wool are moulded to
  conform to the newly created anterior
  contours. Tight conchal dressings (and
  EAM) can contribute to postoperative
  nausea and should be avoided (Ridings
  1994). A head bandage is often used
  for comfort but does not affect the final
  outcome (Ramkumar, 2006)
  - Headbands or other support are worn
    for variable lengths of time (weeks to
    months) but is particularly important
    in children. Avoid contact sports for
    6 weeks or more
- Check for bleeding or displaced dressings

Complications

The complication rate is 4–8% and includes
the following:

- Haematoma (1%): Failure to recognise
  and drain a haematoma may lead to late
  calcification and cartilage deformity, termed
  a cauliflower ear. Adrenaline infiltration can
  be safely used intraoperatively without any
  increase in complications
- Infection is rare. Prophylactic antibiotics
  may be given to reduce the risk of chondritis
  and its severe sequelae, but is not universal.
  Early pain is more likely to be caused by
  haematoma (1 day), whereas chondritis
  usually presents several days later
- Scarring problems are less common
  in Caucasians (2%) compared to
  Afro-Caribbeans (11%)

- Undercorrection and overcorrection (4%), asymmetry and recurrence. A 10–25% revision rate is quoted in the literature
- Anterior skin necrosis particularly in techniques involving anterior degloving (1–2%)

- Iatrogenic deformities: Sharp antihelix, hidden helix (overcorrection), Spock ear (pointy upper pole), telephone ear (undercorrection of upper and lower poles) and reverse telephone ear (undercorrection of middle third)

Further reading

Byrd HS, Langevin CJ, Ghidoni LA. Ear molding in newborn infants with auricular deformities. Plast Reconstr Surg 2010; 126:1191–200.

Ptosis of the eyelid (blepharoptosis)

Ptosis (general definition) is abnormal gravitational displacement of a body structure relative to a fixed reference point, when in the anatomical position.

Blepharoptosis is drooping of the upper eyelid (*blepharon* is Greek for eyelid) such that the lid margin is in an abnormally low position. Ptosis can be congenital or acquired due to muscle/ ligament weakness by injury, disease or nerve damage but most cases are due to aging (senile ptosis). It is not uncommon after cataract surgery.

Ptosis may cause visual impairment and can be a cause of cosmetic concern alone. Patients may complain of a tired appearance, blurred vision and increased tearing. In severe cases, patients may need to tilt their head back, manually lift their eyelids or consciously raise their brows to be able to see. The continuous activation of the forehead and scalp muscles may cause tension headache. The following may resemble ptosis:

- Dermatochalasis: Involutional skin laxity and redundancy
- Pseudoblepharoptosis/pseudoptosis: Excess skin and tissue depressing upper lid, due to a problem with the lid weight rather than a fault with the levator mechanism
- Fat protrusion: Orbital septum attenuation allowing anterior fat prolapse
- Pseudoptosis may also be secondary to enophthalmos

Congenital ptosis

This is present at birth or within the first year of life. It is unilateral in 75% and tends to be associated with lagophthalmos. Major ptosis may be due to localised myogenic dysgenesis (improper development of the LPS, which is stiff; muscles are either fibrosed with fatty infiltration or do not work) or abnormal innervation.

- Bilateral congenital ptosis may be due to myasthenia gravis or myasthenic maternal antibodies

- Ptosis may also be seen in Sturge-Weber syndrome

A frontalis sling fashioned from fascia lata is a common definitive treatment, but there are many variants. Mild/moderate congenital ptosis may improve with time; hence a trial of conservative treatment may be instituted for up to 5 years, unless there is amblyopia or impending corneal scarring. Alternatively, monofilament nylon can be used satisfactorily as temporary suspension material.

Mechanisms of ptosis

The LPS muscle originates from the muscle cone and is 45 mm long, with an aponeurosis of 15 mm length. With congenital ptosis, muscle function is generally poor whereas with acquired ptosis, muscle function is usually good (except myasthenic/neurogenic ptosis). Mild ptosis with good levator function is usually due to aponeurotic disinsertion or dehiscence.

- Myogenic ptosis: Most commonly myasthenia (signs only in 20% of patients), myotonic dystrophy, myopathy and oculopharyngeal muscular dystrophy and chronic progressive external ophthalmoplegia. It is generally progressive and has a high risk of recurrence, despite repeated surgery
- Neurogenic ptosis is rare and is usually due to malfunction/damage to oculomotor nerves (e.g. diabetes), sympathetic nerves (Horner's syndrome) or CNS. Botulinum toxin causes a neurogenic ptosis
- Aponeurotic ptosis is synonymous to senile ptosis, and is the most common cause of acquired ptosis. Gravity effects and ageing causes stretching and attenuation or disinsertion and dehiscence of the aponeurosis, resulting in the superior displacement of the upper lid crease. It may also be related to chronic inflammation, surgery, hard contact lens use or severe eye infections

- Mechanical ptosis: Eyelid is too heavy (masses or scarred) to lift. Skin tends to stretch due to its thinness. Vision may be blocked
- Traumatic ptosis: Various degrees of trauma causing levator disinsertion, scarring and interruption of nerve supply

Evaluation

Previous traumas, surgery, contacts lens wear are important. Be vigilant for stroke, diabetes and myasthenia, in particular.
- Acquired or congenital (check family history)
- If acquired, is it aponeurotic, myogenic or neurogenic?
- Ptosis measurement (see below): MRD1—mild (2 mm or less), moderate (3–4 mm) and severe (> 4 mm) is probably the most useful clinical test along with levator excursion

Examination

Preoperative assessment should include:
- Acuity test (best corrected)
- Eyelid tone, look for a lid crease
  - Upper lid margin to crease measurement: 8–9 mm in men, 10–11 mm in women. A higher crease or deeper sulcus may suggest aponeurotic disinsertion. Even if the lid moves poorly, the presence of a crease suggests that there is some levator function, whilst an absent lid crease is usually accompanied by poor levator function (note ethnic differences)
- Others:
  - Schirmer's test in selected patients
  - Bell phenomenon with forced eye closure, brow ptosis
  - EOM and pupil reactivity
  - Lid retraction (if sclera is seen above the superior limbus, thyroid testing should be considered)

Investigations are not routinely required, unless specifically indicated by clinical suspicion.

Ptosis measurement

In normal adults, the upper lid margin lies 0.5–2 mm below the superior limbus.
- MRD 1: Distance from papillary light reflex to upper lid margin (severity see above); normal > 2.5 mm
- MRD 2: From light reflex to lower lid margin
- Levator excursion is the best clinical test of levator function and is mandatory if considering surgery. It is the distance from the extreme downward to extreme upward gaze with the brow immobilised (with the examiner's fingers). A distance of > 10 mm represents good function, 5–9 mm fair and < 4 mm poor function. The excursion is usually correlated with degree of ptosis
- Phenylephrine (PE) test to assess the action of Müller's muscle is performed by instilling 10% phenylephrine (for near maximal stimulation of the smooth muscle) or 2.5% phenylephrine (to reduce complications) in those with minimal ptosis, into the eye. Measured after 5 minutes, a rise in the MRD 1 of > 1.5–2 mm is positive and surgery, particularly Müller's conjunctival resection, is indicated

The choice of treatment depends on patient appearance, eyelid function and cause (myasthenia treated medically).
- Ptosis surgery can often be performed under LA and sedation, with or without a frontal nerve block
- The precise surgical options are influenced by the levator function and the severity of ptosis (**Table 57**), but the desired outcome is the same. The target lid position is 1 mm below the limbus, or if unilateral 1–2 mm above contralateral lid. In general, the best results are achieved in patients with mild ptosis and good muscle function
- Common complications include bruising, asymmetry, incomplete correction or lagophthalmos, and may require revision
- Contraindications: Loss of blink reflex, loss of corneal sensation, dry eye, absent Bell phenomenon and squint

Table 57 Choices for ptosis correction surgery	
Minimal ptosis (< 2 mm)	Müller's muscle conjunctival resection—good for PE test positive. Fasanella-Servat—often best results in PE negative. Levator aponeurotic surgery—can set eyelid height during surgery.
Moderate ptosis (2–4 mm) Usually PE negative	Levator aponeurotic surgery
Severe ptosis (> 4 mm) Usually poor levator function	Frontalis suspension/ sling

Mild ptosis

Mild ptosis is repaired with upper lid shortening techniques. The exact ratios of tissue resection to effective shortening (and thus treating ptosis) depend on the exact technique.

Müller's muscle conjunctival resection is suitable for patients with minimal ptosis (thus usually normal levator function). Those that also have a positive PE test (and thus an active Müller's muscle) give the most precise and predictable results, though studies have shown reasonable results are possible even in those with negative PE. Advancement of the muscle strengthens the posterior lamella and appears to cause plication of the aponeurosis with subsequent scarring that maintains the elevated eyelid position.

The eyelid is reflected over a retractor with the aid of a suture placed through the tarsus at the eyelid margin. The amount of resection is measured. The various formulae described generally follow a 4:1 ratio. This means a 4 mm of resection of conjunctiva/muscle is required for 1 mm of expected ptosis correction. Three sets of traction sutures are used to grab the conjunctiva and Müller's muscle (but not LPS), which are placed into a special resection clamp. The tissues above the clamp are cut flush, while tissues below the clamp are stitched with a 6–0 running suture. Complications are uncommon, but include corneal abrasions. Late failures are rare.

Fasanella-Servat: The lid is everted over a Desmarres (French ophthalmologist 1810–1882) retractor and two sutures are placed through the conjunctival tarsal border. The tarsus is marked centrally and the proposed resection measured (conjunctiva/

muscle to ptosis, 4:1). The tissues to be resected are elevated with traction sutures and positioned in the Putterman clamp. An imbricating 6–0 Prolene is passed back and forth through the tissues just below the clamp and exteriorised through the skin. The clamped tissues are excised with a knife angled at 45°, by running the blade against the clamp. The suture is removed after 1–2 weeks.

The Fasanella-Servat is in effect, a partial tarsectomy with some Müllerian resection and thus can be used after a negative PE test. The amount of tarsus removal is based on the PE result in a 1:1 ratio, with relatively predictable results. It can also be used in patients with a positive PE test, but such patients will usually have better results with a Müllerectomy. Excision of > 2 mm of tarsus may lead to loss of the accessory lacrimal glands, exacerbating pre-existing dry eye conditions more than other techniques. Overall, the Fasanella-Servat ptosis repair has a 70% success rate. The commonest complications are undercorrection and overcorrection.

Moderate ptosis

For moderate ptosis with reasonable muscle function, the lid can be shortened via open approaches with resection, plication or advancement.

- Lesser degrees of ptosis can be treated by simple plication of the aponeurosis: 3 mm plication per 1 mm elevation (plication is not suited for ptosis due to dehiscence, as it will continue to deteriorate)
- Advancement techniques: Resection should be avoided in those with poor muscle function and the full length should be preserved. The muscle is detached at

its aponeurotic insertion and reattached lower down to the tarsal plate

Levator aponeurotic repair is the operation of choice for mild ptosis where a concomitant blepharoplasty is required, or simply for moderate ptosis. By shortening the levator, the mechanical advantage of the muscle is strengthened. A 2 mm difference may result after the operation, although in selected patients with minimal ptosis, symmetry within 0.5 mm can be achieved. It is best performed under LA with minimal sedation. More severe ptosis may be treated with maximal levator advancement or a Whitnall sling with an optional tarsectomy.

Frontalis suspension

Congenital ptosis is usually treated with various slings (see below). There are variable problems with donor sites, prosthetic materials, lagophthalmos and a tendency for the lid to lift away from globe.

These are forms of lid suspension with attachment to the eyebrow muscles, so that brow elevation produces synchronous lid elevation. A degree of overcorrection is expected at the end of the procedure and eye protection is required for up to 6 months.

- Fox: Single sling
- Crawford: Double sling of fascia lata, four holes in the tarsus, two laterally and one above

Alternatives to slings include the inferiorly based trapezoidal orbital septum flap raised through a blepharoplasty incision (5–6 mm from lash line, at superior border of tarsal plate). A second superiorly based frontalis flap is raised via an incision above the brow with a medial limit 5 mm lateral to supraorbital notch to reduce nerve damage. The septal flap is tunnelled up, overlapped with the frontalis flap and secured with three permanent sutures. This is the modification of the frontalis-only flap, which may be too short to attach to the tarsal plate by itself.

Materials for slings

- Fascia lata is commonly used and provides more predictable and longer lasting results. The fascia (6 mm × 10 cm) is harvested via a 3–4 cm incision along the lateral mid-thigh, halfway between fibular head and the ASIS, with the foot pronated slightly to place the fascia on stretch. The fascial donor defect does not require repair. The use of lyophilised fascia lata is associated with a high recurrence rate
- Palmaris longus (PL) (absent in 15–30%) may be used in circumstances where fascia lata harvest may be difficult, such as in those under the age of 3. The PL presence is verified with the lotus pinch test and harvested via a 0.5 cm incision in wrist fold and a second 1 cm long incision 7–10 cm away. The tendon can be taken partially, or split and doubled up. The plantaris is an alternative
- Silicone rods (1 mm solid) can be used for patients with disorders that are either progressive (myogenic) or if fascia lata is unavailable. It offers comparable results with the additional advantage of adjustability and easy removal. Limited height adjustment of height is possible after the LA effects have worn off, but this is only practical within 24 hours

Complications

- Undercorrection is most common (10–15%) and may require revision
- Overcorrection may cause a dry eye. Mild degrees will often settle with massage and gentle traction. If it persists, surgical exploration may be required
- Lagophthalmos may be secondary to adhesions (may be increased with haematoma)
- Loss of eyelashes due to traumatic dissection

Further reading

Sokol JA, Thornton IL, Lee HB, et al. Modified frontalis
    suspension technique with review of large series.
    Ophthal Plast Reconstr Surg 2011; 27:211–15.

Related topics of interest

- Blepharoplasty
- Eyelid reconstruction

Rheumatoid arthritis and osteoarthritis

Rheumatoid arthritis

Rheumatoid arthritis (RA) is a chronic idiopathic bilateral symmetrical inflammatory polyarthropathy affecting small joints in particular. It tends to be progressive, is monocyclic in a minority (10%), but polycyclic in the majority. It may either follow relapse-remission pattern (45%) or follow a relentless progressive course (45%). The disease process causes synovitis with inflammation and pain that leads to secondary bone and joint destruction, deformity and functional loss. There are also extra-articular manifestations. RA tends to affect females aged 20–40 years most frequently. Other arthritides include:

- Psoriatic: Seronegative with skin changes that may be unnoticed. Pain is less severe
- SLE: Seropositive, with rash and multi-organ involvement. The synovitis is less florid and soft tissue repair is usually problematic
- Gout: Affects men (9:1), particularly the MTP of the hallux. Surgery is restricted to the removal of large tophi or arthrodesis

Stages in RA

- Proliferative: Synovitis, pain, stiffness and nerve compression
- Destructive: Tendon rupture (enzymatic destruction, tendons become attenuated to the point where a simple act, such as lifting a cup may snap them), subluxation and erosions
- Reparative: Fibrosis, adhesions, ankylosis and fixed deformities

Alternatively, the disease process can be staged:

I. Synovitis
II. Narrowing of the joint space and bony erosion
III. Moderate joint destruction and limited ulnar volar subluxation of the MCPJ
IV. Severe destruction and deformity

Treatment is primarily medical, but surgery can be performed with the following aims:

- Preventive: Prophylactic synovectomy has been shown to reduce the chance of tendon rupture and is indicated if the synovitis or inflammatory masses have not responded to 6 months of medical treatment.
- Reconstructive
- Salvage

In general terms,
- Stage I: Splinting and steroids.
- Stage II: Synovectomy.
- Stage III: Splinting and soft tissue reconstruction if adequate articular surfaces.
- Stage IV: Arthroplasty to relieve pain and improve hand function.

It is important not to operate for deformity alone, in the absence of pain or functional loss.

Hand deformities

The typical hand deformities of RA include swan neck, boutonnière and subluxation of the MCPJ (due to attenuated lateral ligaments, weakness of stretched dorsal expansion and dislocation of extrinsic extensors). There is also ulnar deviation of MCPJ with ulnar inclination of the metacarpal heads, radial deviation of the wrist, ulnar shift of the extensors, ulnar flexor forces and thumb pressure. The characteristic X-ray features are a narrow articular space, periarticular osteoporosis, marginal erosion, and swollen soft tissue shadows. Joints may be subluxed, dislocated or in contracture. PIPJ complications are particularly disabling. The diseased soft tissue compromises repair and arthroplasty. Arthrodesis may often be the best option (formal arthrodesis is usually not required as pinning for 4–6 weeks works just as well).

- Ulnar drift due to radial sagittal bands and radial collateral ligaments
- Thumb: Z-deformity that is analogous to a boutonnière/swan neck of the thumb

- Wrist: Caput ulnae. Dorsal subluxation with the piano key sign

Boutonnière (DIPJ hyperextension)

This deformity characterised by DIPJ hyperextension and PIPJ flexion, may be due to:

- Divided central slip of the extensor. This is the commonest cause and precipitating factor that arises from either complete disruption or attenuation from the underlying synovitic process. The path of least resistance to synovial expansion is dorsal, with the weaker parts on either side of central slip allowing the lateral bands to slip sideways
- Tear of triangular ligament

Initially, there is full active flexion and passive extension of IPJs. As the lateral bands displace volarly, they shorten and become fixed. When this occurs, the deformity can no longer be passively corrected as the oblique retinacular ligament (ORL) tightens and the triangular ligament stretches. Contractures and arthritic changes then result. It is important to determine if the joints are fixed or supple. Surgery for the boutonnière deformity can be very difficult and is usually reserved for patients who do not respond to splintage. The aim of surgery is to divert the increased tone at the DIPJ to the PIPJ, either by:

- Division of extensor mechanism transversely over the MP, between the middle and proximal thirds, preserving the ORL. This allows the lateral bands to slide proximally
- Littler: Divide the lateral bands, and then shift them dorsally to be sutured to central tendon. The finger is then immobilised with a K-wire. The ORL is kept intact to control DIPJ

Swan neck (PIPJ hyperextension)

The swan neck deformity results from the imbalance of forces at the PIPJ that favours its hyperextension, with a flexion deformity of DIPJ. The problem may originate at either the DIPJ or PIPJ. Most cases are related to volar plate laxity, intrinsic tightness (effects mimic intrinsic muscle activity) or mallet finger (or combinations of). In RA, the first two are the most important.

It may either be a dynamic deformity seen during attempted full finger extension or a fixed deformity with underlying contracture. The swan neck deformity does not usually respond to splintage or exercise. While splintage does not improve tendon imbalance, it may improve contractures. In general, surgery can be used for cases of early deformity due to dynamic imbalance with normal joints. Intrinsic tightness release, capsulodesis and tenodesis with tendon synovectomy is performed. Late deformity with contracture and arthritis should be treated with arthroplasty or arthrodesis.

- Type I: PIPJ is flexible in all positions. Treat with splintage
- Type II: Deformity is position-dependent (correcting MCP drift). Treat with intrinsic release
- Type III: PIP flexion limited in all positions. Treat with dorsal band release
- Type IV: Bony changes. These occur late. Treat with arthroplasty or arthrodesis

Extensor tendon rupture

Extensor rupture is not uncommon and tendons tend to rupture in sequence, from ulnar to radial:

- EDC and EDM: Rupture over the ulnar styloid and distal radioulnar joint, which is affected first by RA (Vaughan Jackson lesion). The ring finger EDC or EIP tendons can be used to reconstruct these, with interposition of extensor retinaculum (ER) under the tendons. Alternatively, synovectomy or the Darrach procedure
- EPL on Listers tubercle: Direct repair or graft, FDS transfer

Osteoarthritis

Osteoarthritis (OA) is a common degenerative arthrides where the underlying problem is primary articular destruction. This is in contrast to the inflammatory arthrides (rheumatoid) where inflammation is the underlying problem with joint destruction being secondary.

The radiological appearance does not correlate directly with symptoms and many will have asymptomatic radiological changes. Articular cartilage degeneration with bone hypertrophy may be present at the articular margins. Inflammation is minimal and although anti-inflammatory medication may ameliorate early symptoms, there is no possibility of spontaneous recovery once the articular cartilage has been destroyed. Treatment is based on symptoms, mainly pain, which affect patients differently. In the hands, OA primarily affects the CMCJ of the thumb and the DIPJs of the digits.

Traumatic arthritis is often considered separately from primary OA (regarded as 'wear and tear' and most commonly affects the weight bearing joints and certain joints of the hands), although the appearance, and histological findings are identical. However, the distinction is not usually clear-cut and the association with occupational factors controversial. Patients with OA tend to be older than RA patients.

- Thumb: Pain and swelling at base of thumb that is aggravated by use and may have loss of strength. Crepitus of the affected joints and subluxation is common, but reduction of the subluxation is painful. The thumb will eventually collapse in a zigzag manner. Treatment is based on disability and symptoms:
  – Conservative treatment
  – Trapeziectomy and implant arthroplasty: When the joint surfaces are destroyed, permanent relief can only be obtained by separating the damaged surfaces. Both trapezial resection with ligament reconstruction and implant arthroplasty achieve this, but the former is the most common
- DIPJ: Heberden's nodes are hard nodules of connective tissue over the DIPJ osteophytes. Gross joint destruction may be surprisingly pain free. The mainstay of treatment is rest. Joint replacements have limited success and arthrodesis is a common option. There may be a dorsal mucous cyst that may become infected
- PIPJ: Bouchard's nodes. Joint fusion relieves pain but at the cost of loss of mobility at the joint. This is less important for the index finger, which functions mainly as a post for the thumb for pinching. PIPJ mobility is not essential but stability is. By contrast, the little and ring finger require PIPJ mobility for power grip. PIPJ silicone spacers (Swanson) generally work well as there is little axial stress on the joint. Stability is of a lower priority for the ulnar digits

Further reading

Burke FD, Miranda SM, Owen VM, et al. Rheumatoid hand surgery: differing perceptions amongst surgeons, rheumatologists and therapists in the UK. J Hand Surg Eur Vol 2011; 36:632–41.

Related topic of interest

- Extensor tendon injury

Rhinoplasty

The bony and cartilaginous framework, and the enveloping skin determine the shape of nose. Rhinoplasty has both aesthetic and functional goals. Patients may present with objective structural abnormalities causing nasal dysfunction or deformity, or cosmetic concerns that may either be objective (obvious deformity or asymmetry) or subjective. The nose should be consistent with the patient's ethnic identity and be in harmony with rest of the face. The attempts to objectify harmonisation include the use of:

- Proportions such as the Thirds rule: From the frontal view, the nose roughly occupies one third of the vertical height of face (hairline to brow, brow to end of nose, nose to chin) and one fifth of the horizontal width
- Angles (see below) and proposed ideal nasal lengths
  - If the face is of equal proportions, the RT (radix to tip) distance should equate to the SMe (stomion to menton) distance
  - Ideal tip projection = 0.67 × RT
  - Radix projection = 1 cm

History

Patient expectations are key and should be elicited in detail. Only contemplate surgery if patient expectations are realistic and surgically deliverable. Common complaints include issues with the dorsum (hump or saddle) or tip (bulbous or cherry). Specific details in the history that should be ascertained include:

- Previous trauma and surgery
- Evidence of nasal disease, such as epistaxis, rhinitis, nasal obstruction or anosmia
- Use of nasal drugs, both prescribed and recreational

Be cautious of the male rhinoplasty patient, particularly those with pure aesthetic concerns. Up to 15% have narcissism and may have unrealistic expectations. SIMON (single immature male over-expectant and narcissistic) is an acronym commonly used to summarise the features of a stereotypical patient to avoid surgery on.

Examination

A systematic assessment of the skeleton and soft tissue envelope is performed and preoperative photographs are important. There are ethnic differences in nasal shape. In general, there is less skeletal support in non-Caucasians that produces a broad and flatter nose, wider-based alae, flared horizontal nostrils and less tip projection.

- Overall shape of the nose, comparing it to the skeletal proportions of the face, including the dentition and forehead. A lateral smiling view tends to accentuate the problems for easier detection
  - Dorsum: Height/width and humps/saddles
  - Angles: Septal, tip-columella, nasolabial (90–95° for males, 100–105° for females); nasofacial angle (from nasion to tip relative to vertical is 36°); a straight dorsum for males and a 34° slight concavity of the dorsum for females
  - Tip: Nasal tip projection (from nasal spine to tip), nasal length (from root just below eyelash line to tip) and tip definition
- Skin quality: Thicker nasal skin can conceal underlying structures including subtleties of the cartilaginous framework. Thin nasal skin is less forgiving of underlying irregularities
- Inside
  - Septum: Deviation and availability of cartilage for grafting, size of the inferior turbinates
  - Assessment of nasal obstruction and internal valve
  - Internal valve: This is the area between the septum and the caudal border of the upper lateral cartilage that narrows on inspiration and widens on expiration. The angle formed is 10–15° in Caucasians. Potential collapse can

be assessed with lateral traction (Cottle manoeuvre, although false positives are possible in those with alar collapse due to excessive resection of alar cartilages or due to scarring) and is usually treated with a spreader graft placed in between the septum and upper lateral cartilage. It is shaped like a matchstick and wedged in to widen the middle third of the nose
- In Afro-Caribbeans, the narrowest point is usually at the inferior turbinate

Surgery

The nose grows significantly until at least age of 16 and it is unusual to operate before this. Rhinoplasty can be performed under LA and sedation, although GA is more common. In either case, it is usually a day surgery procedure. Intraoperative bleeding can be reduced by hypotensive anaesthesia and vasoconstriction with adrenaline injection (using only small amounts along incision lines and dissection planes to avoid distortion) and topical xylometazoline or cocaine paste (5 ml of 5%).
- Local anaesthesia for nerve block: Infratrochlear and external nasal branch of anterior ethmoidal (V1) and infraorbital (V2) by injecting along boundaries of nose, from radix to nasolabial fold
- Infiltrate soft tissue for haemostasis
  - Supraperiosteal/perichondrium: Nasal dorsum and upper lateral cartilages
  - Submucosal intranasal incision line and nasal septum

Types of incision
- Intercartilaginous (retrograde): Standard route to the nasal dorsum, in between cartilages where the alar meets upper lateral cartilage (**Figure 16**). Part of the upper alar cartilage may be subsequently removed
- Intracartilaginous or transcartilaginous aka cartilage splitting: Provides better exposure for tip work. The incision line cuts through the alar cartilage parallel to and 4–5 mm above its caudal edge. It is thus higher laterally. The portion of alar cartilage above the incision is usually discarded

- Infracartilaginous (marginal): Incision along the lower border of the alar cartilage, used primarily for domal suturing and scoring. It is often combined with a columellar incision for the open approach. This has been mistakenly labelled a 'rim' incision, which actually applies to a rarely used incision that stays close to the alar rim
  - Delivery incision combines infracartilaginous with an intercartilaginous incision. The lateral crura can be freed from the skin and delivered through the upper incision
- Transfixion: Allows elevation of soft tissue of columella from the cartilaginous septum. It cuts into the membranous septum, which is the part between cartilaginous septum and medial crura
- Transcolumellar: This is used in the open approaches (see below). Gruber – step, Toriumi – central peak transverse or V or W. Some propose an inverted-V with lateral transverse components to reduce the vertical component

Surgical techniques
- Closed (endonasal): This was the most frequently used approach and is regarded as the traditional approach. The skin flap is raised subcutaneously up to the nasal bones, where it is dissected subperiosteally. It provides adequate access for most patients, typically with a transcartilaginous incision or a delivery incision. The disadvantages include limited exposure (often requiring retraction that may distort assessment of tip/symmetry) and limited flexibility
- Open: Transverse columellar and marginal incisions with degloving, gives excellent exposure. This is especially useful for extensive nasal tip work. It allows accurate visualisation of the cartilages, especially where they are distorted, such as in the cleft nose, and allows the precise placement of grafts. It is commonly used for difficult rhinoplasties, such as secondary rhinoplasty and for rhinoplasty in non-Caucasians. Although the operative time is longer, the open technique may be better for the inexperienced with a shorter learning curve. However, it involves extra

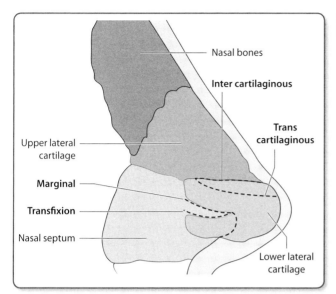

Figure 16 Types of nasal access incisions.

Labels: Nasal bones; Inter cartilaginous; Trans cartilaginous; Upper lateral cartilage; Marginal; Transfixion; Nasal septum; Lower lateral cartilage

dissection and is probably unnecessary if no nasal tip work is required. The resultant tip oedema can persist for months and there is also a columellar scar.

Dorsum

Reduction

The male nasal dorsum has a straight profile, whilst in females it is slightly lower with a supratip break.

- Elevate skin off the bone subperiosteally. Smooth down humps with a rasp, if less than 4 mm high (it is also easier to use for beginners) or an osteotome. If this leaves an open-roof deformity, the edges are brought together again with lateral osteotomies (see below)
- A broad bridge can be narrowed, or if there is an open book deformity, the sides are in-fractured after weakening the base with osteotomies (transnasal or transcutaneous) or a Joseph saw

Augmentation

Whilst Caucasians tend to need reductions, Orientals tend to request augmentation. There are different methods of augmenting the dorsum. Prior infection is a contraindication to augmentation as the infection rate nears 40%. Although

some inject modern tissue fillers, the more common choices are solid materials:

- Bone: Iliac bone, calvarium and rib. The tenth and eleventh ribs have naturally straight segments. However, the rib may be more prone to resorption due to its endochondral origin as compared to calvarial bone, which is membranous
- Cartilage: Ear (curved cartilage can be difficult to shape, may warp or crack, but is made up of elastic cartilage and is more resistant to infection and resorption), nasal septum (limited amounts available, risk of collapse), costal cartilage (tendency to warp and donor site morbidity)
  - Cartilage has a strong memory, although this can be disrupted and altered with scoring, sutures or stacking. Cartilage, with its low metabolic activity tends to have far less volume loss and resorption
- Synthetics: Silicone/silastic, MEDPOR (porous high-density polyethylene, PHDPE, is more rigid, providing more support and also encourages vascular ingrowth, but reports on long-term results are lacking). With alloplastic materials, the procedure is quicker with no donor site morbidity, but it can be complicated by (late) extrusion and infection. It may

be less suited for use in less favourable recipient beds, such as secondary rhinoplasties

In the US/UK, autologous grafts are generally preferred due to fewer complications and better long-term outcomes. In the East, the use of synthetics is much more widespread as they are well tolerated. The thicker Asian skin and the relative lack of autologous tissue may explain this.

Nasal tip

The tip-defining points and the lateral projections of the left and right domes define the nasal tip. In females, a supratip break of 1–2 mm (dorsum is set back from the tip-defining point) is desirable, but not in males. A higher dorsal line is often called a supratip deformity or parrot's beak.

Tripod concept of nasal tip: Two lateral legs and one medial (conjoint). Shortening the lateral legs will cause rotation and reduce tip projection. Strengthening the medial leg with columellar struts will increase tip projection and rotation. Excess volume can be corrected by resection of the cranial edge of the lateral crus (need to preserve at least 5 mm). There has been a trend against such resection to preserve as much support as possible. Tip suturing is used to improve tip definition (see below). The two main techniques of suturing and cartilage grafts are often combined (suture before grafts).

- Suture techniques
  - Between domes
    - Interdomal at middle crura level to narrow tip
    - Domal definition suture: Transdomal mattress sutures make the domes more convex and the adjacent ala more concave. The extent is determined by how tight the suture is tied
  - Between medial crura to stabilise and narrow columella
  - Between medial crura and membranous septum to adjust tip projection
- Cartilage grafts (5% will have graft visibility)
  - Onlay graft on the top of tip: A double layer of cartilage can often be fashioned from the excised alar cartilage

- Columellar struts: Fixed floating (septal, costal or double layer auricular) or fixed (K-wire through costal cartilage graft that sits in a drill hole in the nasal spine)
- Variety of T-shaped grafts combining a vertical columellar strut between the medial crura with a flattened transverse section on the alar tip. Examples include the umbrella, anchor and shield or Sheen grafts

Postoperative care

- Expect bruising and swelling. Bed rest, a head-up position and ice packs may help. Nasal blockage may persist for 2 weeks, whilst tissue swelling may be prolonged for up to 6 months
- Nasal packing is a common practice, which is kept for 24–48 hours. It is not strictly necessary, but if used, does not need to be inserted very deeply into the nose. Nasal packs can also function as internal splints
- External splints, if used, can be removed after 1–2 weeks. Avoid contact sports or wearing glasses for 4–6 weeks
- Antibiotics coverage is required if an implant has been used. The routine use of antibiotics (prophylactic and up to 5 days) in cases without implants is debatable, but common

Complications (4–20%)

The early risks of the procedure are those of GA, bleeding (4% and usually minor) and infection (particularly, if alloplastic materials have been used, may occur late). Late complications include:

- Under/overcorrection, asymmetry, irregularity and postoperative deformities requiring secondary surgery occur in 5–10%. The most common cause of patient dissatisfaction is lack of tip definition, although it does improve with time
- Numbness of the nasal tip due to injuries to external branch of anterior ethmoidal nerve, which usually recovers over several months
- Nasal obstruction: 10% have a vasomotor-type rhinitis and dryness
- Septal perforation: 1%

Specifically, for patients with implants:

- Infection can occur many months or years after surgery. It may be possible to clear the infection with broad-spectrum antibiotics and irrigation, but many eventually need removal of the implant. Further surgery should ideally be delayed for 6–9 months
- If an implant is extruding, the sterility has been compromised and it should be removed

Further reading

Ismail AS. Nasal base narrowing: the alar flap advancement technique. Otolaryngol Head Neck Surg 2011; 144:48–52.

Related topic of interest

- Nasal reconstruction

Rhytidectomy

The cumulative effects of ageing, sun damage and gravity contribute to the formation of deep wrinkles and facial creases that are most prominent at the cheek, and loose folds of skin and fat, most prominent around the neck and jaw line (jowls). The facelift (rhytidectomy) and necklift aims to reverse some of these effects. In the classic operation, skin is lifted up, redraped and the excess is removed. It is most suited for those with loose skin that still remains its elasticity. Surgery will not prevent on-going changes and thus like all rejuvenation surgery, is temporary and it may be necessary to repeat the procedure.

Ageing face syndrome

Although the causes of ageing can be intrinsic (atrophy and loss of structural components) or extrinsic (related to environment, particularly sunlight, smoking and gravity), the two are interrelated. A simple and practical conceptual view of ageing is:

- Weathered skin, i.e. ageing skin, in terms of its superficial features
- Loss of structure, i.e. sagging face. The laxity of the soft tissue envelope can be caused by volume resorption, tissue laxity and thinning of the skeleton

The ageing face of an individual will have different relative contributions of these components and thus rejuvenation needs to be tailored to account for these. The issues that need or can be corrected fall into the following categories:

- Soft tissue descent: Resuspension. The skin should be addressed separately from the underlying soft tissue (similar to breast surgery). The majority of modern facelift techniques focus on the precise method of resuspension (sutures, excision, plication, elevation) and tissue plane for its execution (skin, SMAS, subperiosteal, composite). Skin-only techniques have poor longevity as the viscoelastic skin stretches with tension, causing early recurrence
- Volume loss: Volumetric rejuvenation. This is volume replacement/augmentation

in the correct anatomical location. Facial fat is organised into compartments (Rohrich).
- Dermal elastosis: Treat with resurfacing

Note that the mid-facial ageing (medial to the nasolabial folds) is poorly addressed with facelifts.

Relevant anatomy

The facial soft tissue has five clinically important layers:

- Skin
- Subcutaneous fat
- Superficial musculoaponeurotic system (SMAS, Mitz and Peyronie 1976) and its analogous layer: platysma, facial expression muscles, frontalis and temporoparietal fascia. It is a mobile fibrous support layer lying between facial skin and bone that is the key element for suspension in most facelifts. Understanding of the planar relationship of SMAS to the surrounding structures (facial nerve) and structures in contiguity with it are key to effective surgery and avoiding iatrogenic damage
- Loose fascia
- Facial nerve branches: The parotid protects the facial nerve branches during dissection of the pre-parotid area. The temporal (frontal) branch of the facial crosses over the zygomatic arch to lie under the temporoparietal fascia superior to it

These layers are compressed in some areas, e.g. zygomatic arch, but they are still present in the same fashion. Thus, subcutaneous dissection is safe as is above the SMAS layer (nerves supply muscles from the deep aspect except for buccinator, levator anguli oris and mentalis).

Retaining ligaments

These are found at specific locations (e.g. zygomatic and mandibular), directly attaching the skin to bone. They form an inverted L-shape that tends to restrict the benefit of traction of SMAS outside or lateral to the 'L', and may require release during a facelift (controversial, disputed by Little).

Facelift surgery

Before a facelift surgery, the eyes and brows should be dealt with first (forehead and brow lift, followed by blepharoplasty).

The face should be assessed in thirds. It is important to counsel patients comprehensively that some areas of wrinkling will be improved, but not eliminated (nasolabial folds, malar bags, forehead and glabellar creases and marionette lines). Fine wrinkles respond better to resurfacing rather than rhytidectomy. The surgery can be performed under LA with sedation, although GA is often used. The most common facelifts involve both skin and SMAS dissection in-continuity and combinations of:

- Skin resection
- SMAS plication/transposition
- Fat resection (conservative), e.g. buccal fat pad or transposition, malar fat
- Platysmal tightening
- Liposuction: Part of the necklift component. Chin liposuction or supraplatysmal liposuction to facilitate redraping of neck skin after platysmal plication/transection

Incisions

- Incisions are preauricular with superior extension into the temporal scalp (at or within the hairline) and posterior extension into the postauricular sulcus and onto the occipital scalp
  - There has been a recent trend for short scar lifts that may be suited for selected patients
- Tragus
  - Pretragal: Males, smokers, older patients, those with a definite crease and/or a protruding tragus
  - Retrotragal: Females, young, no crease or non-protruding tragus

Planes

The plane of the undermining and lift has been debated. Skin-only lifts have a direct tension effect on the skin only, with no effect on deeper tissues. Deeper lifts affect the entire soft tissue mass, but the effect is dissipated. Most modern facelifts involve the SMAS layer and currently, the main surgical choices are:

- Skin and SMAS: This is the standard operation for many. The traditional/original SMAS lift could not treat the medial cheek, and thus became unpopular. The revised extended SMAS lift includes dissection over medial cheek over the zygoma and nasolabial areas
  - The skin is lifted with a thin layer of fat up to the NLF. The SMAS is then lifted as a separate flap up to the NLF. Resection of a 2 cm ellipse or plication with a superolateral vector of pull is performed (Little disputes this and advocates a superior vector). Overlapping skin is excised closed tension-free
- Deep plane: Cheek dissection under SMAS with skin-SMAS in a single flap (also called composite). Better for smokers, as there is less risk of necrosis. This is the preferred option, when there is a redundant NLF, but it carries a slightly higher risk of nerve injury
- Subperiosteal lift for midface laxity. There is an increased risk of nerve injuries and prolonged facial oedema. Endoscopic subperiosteal lifts have been described. There is a steep learning curve
- Minimal incision rhytidectomy (short-scar technique): Lateral SMASectomy for less retroauricular scarring due to the truncated postauricular incision. It is ideal for patients with changes primarily in the mid and lower face with moderate jowls

Postoperative care

- Patients are advised to sit up and sleep head up early in the postoperative period to reduce swelling. Ice packs/compresses are occasionally used but some argue it potentially compromises the tenuous skin-flap circulation
- Strenuous activity should be avoided for 2 weeks, during which the face will become less tight and feel better

Complications

In most patients, the risk of complications is small, but caution is required in smokers (some surgeons enforce smoking as a contraindication to surgery) and those on anticoagulation.

- Haematomas, especially behind the ear, are the commonest complications (4%). Most occur in the first 12 hours after surgery (often in the recovery room), presenting as pain and should be evacuated
  - Vomiting may increase the risk of bleeding/haematoma. Hypertension is the most common predisposing factor, although causes are multifactorial
  - Haematomas are more common in males
- Numbness around the incision is almost universal and will fade (4–6 months) in most, but not all cases. Nerve injuries are mostly sensory. Facial nerve branches, such as the buccal are often cross-innervated and injuries are usually well compensated, asymptomatic and often unrecognised. Less commonly, injuries to temporal or marginal mandibular branches are more obvious and may be permanent
- Hypertrophic scar, tragal or ear distortion of tragus and 'drapery swag' due to inappropriate lift vectors
- Hairline distortion: Stepping of the occipital hairline, transient alopecia. Repeat lifts are more likely to distort
- Flap necrosis and skin slough are more common in smokers, and may be exacerbated by tension, thin flaps or haematomas. Superficial slough eventually heals relatively well, even for larger areas, but full-thickness slough will scar albeit to a size smaller than anticipated. Sloughing is generally treated conservatively, followed by secondary scar revision
- Infections: The incidence has been reduced by the routine use of perioperative antibiotics

Further reading

Lihong R, Daping Y, Zhibo X, et al. Longevity of SMAS facial rejuvenation and support. Plast Reconstr Surg 2011; 127:989–90.

Related topics of interest

- Liposuction
- Skin rejuvenation
- Tissue fillers

Scalp reconstruction

Reconstruction of the scalp may be required after tumour extirpation, burn injury or traumatic avulsion. The procedure of choice depends on the hair/hairline, contour and donor site morbidity. Simple coverage (of the bone) is the minimum target, but reconstruction should aim for a cosmetically appealing result, ideally by replacing like with like. Hair transplantation is an effective fine-tuning procedure to adjust the hairline or camouflage incision scars.

Scalp anatomy

A commonly used mnemonic for the layers is SCALP—skin, connective tissue, aponeurosis, loose areolar tissue and periosteum:

- Skin. The hair follicles often extend deep into the fat layer, complicating FTSG from the scalp. If the graft is too thin, the hairs will be damaged, and if the graft is too thick, there will be reduced take. As a result, scalp FTSGs are rarely used in its conventional form
- Vessels, nerves and lymphatics are in the subcutaneous connective tissue layer. The connective tissue also splints the vessels open when transected, preventing vasoconstriction and retraction, causing significant haemorrhage if not controlled. The arterial supply comes from vessels at the periphery with good anastomoses between vessels, but less so across the midline. The entire scalp can be raised on single major pedicle (in theory) and although, successful replantation of scalp avulsions has been reported after single set of anastomoses, having more anastomoses is probably advisable
  - Superficial temporal artery is the main supply, with frontal and parietal (larger) branches located 2 cm above the zygomatic arch
- Aponeurosis (galea) is continuous with frontalis, occipitalis and the temporoparietal fascia (and at same level as SMAS layer)
- Emissary veins lie in loose areolar layer

Scalp surgery

- Haemostasis is important and should be achieved with judicious use of cautery to reduce damage to the follicles. Strategies that may help include using dilute adrenaline infiltration, haemostatic clips (Raney clips) and haemostatic sutures (1 cm from edge)
- Incisions should be made parallel to the hair direction and the skin closed with minimal tension to minimise damage to the follicles
- Kazanjian showed that galeal scoring incisions 1 cm apart (with a knife and not cautery) allows advancement of 1.67 mm each without damaging the vessels. Skin staples are the least ischaemic way of closing the skin

Scalp reconstruction

If bone is exposed, a flap is required needed for coverage. Local flaps (Orticochea) may be used for small areas, but larger distant flaps are preferable if loss exceeds 30%.

Bony defects

Reconstruction of bony defects is not always necessary, but it is often desirable (particularly, the frontal region for cosmesis). Bone (heals well, is resistant to infection in the long term and may grow in children) is available from a variety of sources:

- Split calvarium: Parietal, just behind the coronal suture
- Rib (additional morbidity): Which can be split and contoured
- Iliac bone can be harvested unicortically, but donor pain can be severe

Alloplastic material such as titanium/steel mesh or MMA (with or without mesh) can be useful to avoid a donor defect, but may suffer from late infections/extrusions. Vascularised flap coverage of the alloplast is desirable.

Options for soft tissue reconstruction

Secondary healing may be a satisfactory option under certain circumstances, particularly if the pericranium is intact, such as donor sites in forehead flaps:

Direct closure is easier in the temporoparietal region where there is greater mobility. Strict elliptical ratios are not vital, as dog-ears tend to be less of an issue in the scalp. Differential undermining can be used to reduce distortion of landmarks, such as the hairline.

Skin grafting: Direct grafting on pericranium or exposed bone is feasible for fresh non-desiccated wounds. The grafts must be thin, but may be rather unstable. Skin grafts can be used as a temporising measure until definitive cover with flaps or tissue expansion. If periosteum has been lost, the surface can be burred until a punctate bleeding (5–7 mm apart) surface is encountered. Alternatively, the outer table can be removed and the graft placed onto medullary bone. NPWT can be used to hasten granulation as well as to secure the SSG.

- Flaps of pericranium or subgaleal areolar tissue can cover small areas of bare bone. These should be made large (contract quickly), but should not cross the midline (neighbouring territories are not well vascularised through anastomotic vessels)
- The use of Integra with HBOT for irradiated tissues has also been reported. This combination works well as Integra, unlike skin grafts, can be vascularised at a slower rate. Integra has also been used independent of HBOT for the same indication with success

Local scalp flaps (raised above the periosteum) are generally required for closure of areas 2–25 cm² (or up to 5 × 5 cm). Local flaps are limited by amount of remaining skin available and thus the size of defect.

- Rotational advancement flaps are the most common. The flap needs to be eight times the size (margin) of the defect to move well. Particular attention is paid to the hairline and dog-ears (which should

be kept, as they tend to resolve; resection reduces vascularity, adversely affecting the width-length ratio)
- Other choices include V-Y and rhomboid flaps, particularly multiple flaps that are useful in parietal/vertex defects
- Orticochea described multiple (4 and then 3) flap techniques based on known arterial territories. The central defect is closed with bilateral flaps based on the superior temporal arteries, which have been relaxed with galeal incisions. A larger posterior flap bearing the remaining scalp, based on an occipital vessel, is moved forward by advancement and rotation. Extensive undermining and scoring is needed. For larger defects, tissue expansion or free flaps will produce better results. Orticochea flaps will be cosmetically inferior to tissue expansion in most cases and should be a second choice, unless single-staged reconstruction is important
- Transplant techniques have largely replaced need for hair bearing flaps, such as the Juri flap, temporoparietooccipital (needs delay) or single-stage island flaps based on superficial temporal artery

Tissue expansion is ideal for the scalp as the fixed base (skull) and thick tissues offer the potential for the best cosmetic result. It should be considered when local tissue is inadequate for local flaps. Approximately 50% of the scalp can be reconstructed in this manner at the expense of staged procedures, long total treatment time and complications in up to 25%. Expanders are placed in the subgaleal plane.

Pedicled flaps: Tubed pedicle flaps are of historical interest only. The commonest modern option is the latissimus dorsi that can potentially reach the temporal and forehead regions. The trapezius can be used for lateral and posterior defects (see 'Chest Reconstruction').

Free flaps: A wide variety has been described in the literature. Although most are non-hair bearing and offer relatively poor colour matching, they are the only practical choice in near total defects.

- Omentum (Buncke 1972) with SSG provides a large pliable flap that is suited to cover large surfaces
- Muscle flaps are classically recommended for infected wounds. Latissimus dorsi is a workhorse as it is both a large flap and has a long pedicle making it extremely versatile
  - ALT flaps offer a good fasciocutaneous alternative
- The recipient vessels around the scalp can be an issue. The superficial temporal vessels are the first choice (if palpable preoperatively), but concerns include small diameter, inconsistent vein and questionable ability to support large flaps. The alternative is an anastomosis in the neck, in which case, vein grafts are likely to be needed

Further reading

Corradino B, Di Lorenzo S. An algorithm for oncologic scalp reconstruction. Plast Reconstr Surg 2011; 127:2506.

Related topics of interest

- Chest reconstruction
- Tissue expansion
- Hair restoration

Skin grafts

A skin graft is a piece of completely detached skin that has to pick up a new blood supply from its recipient site. It must be sufficiently thin to permit vascular reestablishment before necrosis and graft failure results. Grafts become incorporated and this feature distinguishes it from dressings.

- Autograft: The donor and recipient is the same individual
- Allograft: Graft from an individual of the same species but of a different genotype
- Xenograft: Graft from an individual of a different species

Stages of graft take:

- Adhesion: This is due to fibrin
- Serum imbibition (24-48 hours): Nutrients are delivered to the graft passively from the recipient bed. The graft increases in weight and volume during this stage and remains pale
- Inosculation: Some vascularity is re-established as blood vessels in the recipient bed connecting to pre-existing vessels in the graft dermis. This has been demonstrated in experiments with Indian ink. The graft begins to look pink at this stage
- Revascularisation: After 4–7 days, new vessels form with host endothelium ingrowth into the graft either along existing channels or new ingrowths (neovascularisation)
- Maturation: Increased mitoses from the third day onwards, with partial regeneration of appendages, reinnervation and repigmentation

Since the recipient bed must be sufficiently vascular to support a graft, relatively avascular structures such as bare bone, bare tendon and bare cartilage, will not support grafts reliably. However, the privileged areas of the orbit and temporal calvarium will support a SSG on their bare bony surfaces. In the presence of an adequately vascular bed, the commonest reasons for skin graft failure are:

- Haematoma/seroma: The fluid that dissects the graft off the vascular bed will severely limit the passive transfer of nutrients. This can be reduced by careful haemostasis, making fenestrations in the graft or a tie-over dressing
- Shearing will disrupt developing vascular connections. Immobilising the graft reduces this problem. Securing the periphery with sutures, glue or staples, and fixing the graft to bed, such as with quilting sutures or a tie-over dressing achieve this. A splint may be used to reduce joint-related movement, if applicable. NPWT dressings are useful for securing grafts in difficult areas, such as the perineum and axillae
- Infection: A clean bed is required. Small colonisations of most bacteria are generally not clinically important, but heavy growth of bacteria (> 10^5 organisms per gram of tissue) or small to moderate growth of β-haemolytic *Streptococcus* (lysins) will lead to graft failure. Wound swabs can be used to detect the latter and to guide treatment prior to grafting

Complete graft failure is rare and usually due to the graft being placed upside down on the recipient bed. The waterproof stratum corneum does not allow nutrient passage to the graft cells. Methods to determine the correct graft orientation:

- The graft has a dull and shiny side. The former is the top and the latter the bottom. The graft should be placed shiny side down
- The edges of the graft naturally curl towards the bottom

Thickness of grafts

Skin grafts consist of epidermis and a variable amount of dermis. Depending on the amount of dermis taken, skin grafts can be classified as:

- Partial thickness or split skin grafts, usually called SSGs (Thiersch graft) where only a part of the dermis is taken along with the epidermis. The donor site will usually heal spontaneously, since the epidermal regenerative capacity resides in the appendages (sebaceous glands, sweat glands and hair follicles) in the remaining dermis. The donor area can be reharvested a number of times, depending on thickness of the grafts taken and thickness of the donor dermis (which does not regenerate to a significant degree)

- Full-thickness skin grafts (Wolfe graft – classically postauricular) contain the entire thickness of the dermis along with its appendages. The donor area will not re-epithelialise and consequently requires formal closure

The advantages and disadvantages of both skin graft types guide its use. The FTSGs have the following properties:

- The final appearance of the graft approximates normality better, but the donor site will leave a scar
- The graft is more durable and general skin functionality is more likely to be preserved:
  - SSGs are typically very dry due to loss of glands and may require emollients
  - Reinnervation also leads to sensory return that begins after around 4 weeks, with pain recovering before light touch, temperature or vibration, but final results may take months to years. Reinnervation of SSG occurs more quickly, but is less complete as compared to FTSGs
- There is less contraction
  - Primary contraction is the immediate recoil or shrinkage of a graft, once taken and is due to elastin in the dermis
  - Secondary contraction is late contraction after the skin graft has taken and healed. It is related to myofibroblast activity that may be inhibited by dermal components. Note that it is the wound bed that contracts not the graft itself
  - Therefore, SSGs will have less primary contraction (10% vs. 40%), but more secondary contraction than FTSGs. Overall, SSGs contract more than FTSGs

Colour match for the pinker skin of the face is best achieved with skin from the head (and scalp), and skin from the neck/supraclavicular area is still acceptable. However, skin from below the level of the clavicle will have a significant colour discrepancy. The amount of available FTSG is limited.

Meshing

Skin grafts can be meshed to
- Expand the area of coverage
- Improve contouring
- Allow drainage of exudate

Multiple regularly spaced holes are made that allows the skin to open out like a net. The maximum ratio of expansion can be varied by machine or by meshing board. The amount of traction or spreading of the graft on the bed adjusts the actual expansion. With a wider mesh (> 3–4 times expansion), the interstices will heal more slowly by re-epithelialisation from the sides, and potential desiccation of the central part. A widely meshed skin can be covered with a biological dressing such as cadaveric skin (the sandwich graft technique), or with cultured keratinocytes.

Donor site

In SSGs, these are clean partial thickness wounds that should heal in 7–10 days. The multitude of dressings may offer advantages in terms of patient comfort and reduced dressing changes, but have very little impact on healing times.

- The commonest method is to dress the donor with alginate and inspect after 10–14 days with or without topical anaesthetic. The dried block of material can be uncomfortable
  - Tegaderm or another clear semiocclusive dressing is prone to form collections of haemoserous fluid, particularly in few couple of days, and thus may require frequent changes early on. However, it is more comfortable
  - Hypafix has been used as a retention dressing (for donor and graft sites)
- In the elderly, the donor site can be overgrafted with a thin/meshed skin graft to accelerate healing

Further reading

Pilanci O, Saçak B, Kuvat SV, et al. Use of outsized composite chondrocutaneous grafts in conjunction with dermal turnover flaps for reconstruction of full-thickness alar defects. J Craniofac Surg 2011; 22:864–67.

Related topic of interest

- Vacuum wound closure

Skin rejuvenation – chemical peels

Actinic changes (photoageing)

- Thick, coarse and wrinkled
- Increased elastosis, increased type III collagen

Note that photoageing in Asians differs to Caucasians. Asians more frequently have acquired (and congenital) dyspigmentation and tend to suffer from lentigines and seborrhoeic keratosis instead of wrinkling. Treatment with light sources should be approached more cautiously in Asian skin types.

Skin pigmentation

Melanocytes export melanin packaged in melanosomes that are transferred to neighbouring cells via cytoplasmic processes. Recipients thus often have more melanin than the original melanocytes. Skin colour is related to melanin content rather than the number of melanocytes.

- Freckled skin has normal melanocyte numbers, but more melanin granules
- Solar lentigo has increased numbers of normal cells (and supposedly explaining their persistence even in the absence of sun exposure)

Different types of pigmented lesions may coexist in a single patient (Table 58). It is important to distinguish melanin pigmentation from non-melanin pigmentation. The latter is termed chromatosis.

Lentigines

These are common and similar in nature to age spots. First line treatments are ablative resurfacing in nature and include:

- Laser ablation or Q-switched (Nd:YAG, KTP 532 nm) is probably closest to the standard treatment. The most common complication is postinflammatory hyperpigmentation (PIH). IPL (micro crusts) may be associated with fewer problems
- Cryotherapy (melanocytes are sensitive to cold injury; a single cycle with liquid nitrogen is usually sufficient)
- Chemical peels/dermabrasion or microdermabrasion

Second line treatment: Combination topical treatment with retinoids and hydroquinone (HQ). This stimulates turnover, while the HQ controls pigmentation. Sunscreens are important.

Naevus of Ota

Naevus of Ota is a relatively common problem in Japanese patients (1 in 200, 80% female) in particular. It is a bluish-grey pigmentation in the mid and upper face, typically periorbital, and represents a benign dendritic melanocytosis of the upper dermis. There is usually a good response (80% reduction) to 4–5, bi-monthly treatments with a Q-switched laser (usually Nd:YAG), which fragments the pigmented cells. The free melanin debris is phagocytosed and transported to lymph nodes. Scarring is rare, but 25% may have temporary hyperpigmentation.

Café au Lait spots

Café au lait spots can be treated with Q-switched laser with good results. Recurrences are common and darkening may occur in a subset. Patients should be counselled carefully.

Table 58 Different types of pigmented lesions	
Epidermal	Ephelides, lentigines, café au lait spot, Becker's naevus.
Dermal	Naevus of Ota/Ito, melanocytic naevus , blue naevus.
Mixed	Post-inflammatory hyperpigmentation (PIH), melasma, naevus spilus.

Melasma

Melasma (from Greek *melas* meaning black), also known as chloasma (from Greek *chloazein* for green) is exacerbated in pregnancy when it is termed 'the mask of pregnancy'. There are more pigmented cells that are more active. Up to 90% of patients are females and is often associated with hormones and sun exposure. It may worsen with thyroid disease and stress (increases melanocyte stimulating hormone, MSH). It often fades after the hormone stimulus has gone but is still poorly understood.

- From a consensus treatment paper (sunblock and ultraviolet avoidance is important)
  - First line treatment is triple therapy (see below). Pre-mixed preparations, such as Tri-Luma may be used (0.01% flucocinolone, 4% HQ, 0.05% retinoic acid)
  - Second line treatment: Chemical peels with or without topical bleaching
  - Third line treatment: Cautious light treatment (lasers or IPL) may be attempted, but with a risk of PIH or conversion of epidermal melasma to dermal melasma (deeper and more difficult to treat)
  - Long-term results from fractional lasers have disappointing

Triple therapy

The classical Kligman formula is a mixture of HQ 5%, tretinoin 0.1% and dexamethasone 0.1%, applied once daily for 8 weeks. Mild local irritation is the commonest side effect. Combination therapy was found to be more effective than single agents. Many modifications and variations of this combination are in current use.

- Hydroquinone (2–4%) Blocks the tyrosinase enzyme (dopamine to melanin) of the melanogenesis pathway. Complications include skin irritation and phototoxicity. Resistance develops with prolonged continuous use and requires treatment breaks to maintain its effectiveness

- Tretinoin (0.05–0.1%) (trans isomer) Increases keratinocyte turnover, thus limiting the transfer of melanosomes to keratinocytes. It may reduce the side effects of steroids, especially epidermal thinning. Retinoids are teratogenic and must not be used in pregnancy or lactation. It should be applied at night due to increased photosensitivity. Tretinoin is a topical treatment
  - Note that the oral form is isotretinoin 13-cis-retinoic acid or Roaccutane, which inhibits keratinisation, thins the stratum corneum and decreases skin appendageal activity. It reduces wound healing and patients should wait at least 1 year before considering skin resurfacing. There is otherwise a high risk of hypertrophic scarring
- Steroids reduce irritation
- Azelaic acid (20%): A dicarboxylic acid found in wheat, rye and barley that inhibits tyrosinase and decreases melanocyte activity in hyperactive cells only

Chemical peels

Chemical peels are methods of producing a chemical burn of controlled depth to the skin surface. The benefit is related to the depth of treatment, which also determines the risk of side effects and complications. Non-facial skin should be treated with extreme caution, as they lack the large numbers of skin appendages that allow rapid healing.

- Superficial peels (epidermal, stratum granulosum to upper papillary dermis) have very little effect on wrinkles and tend to only produce a refreshed look. They are simple to apply and have few complications, if done properly. There is no significant downtime but there may be temporary irritation and thinning of skin requires sun protection
  - Very light: Alpha hydroxy acids (AHA) e.g. glycolic acid, topical retinoic acid, 10–20% trichloroacetic acid (TCA), Jessner's solution, azelaic acid
  - Light: 20–35% TCA
- Medium depth (to upper or papillary dermis), such as 35% TCA peels tend to tighten the skin, but are painful and

recovery takes approximately 1 week. TCA is one of the oldest agents used, but remains very versatile, whilst the lack of systemic toxicity makes it particularly safe. Patients are advised to treat the treated area like sunburn and to avoid sun exposure. There is usually a bright pink erythema that resolves after 7–9 days

- The Obagi Blue Peel is a proprietary TCA peel formulated with a blue dye indicator of depth that allows reproducibility and consistency. The mild blue colouration may persist for up to 10 days

• Deep peels (reticular dermis), such as phenol peels have been largely replaced by lasers (which avoid problems with toxicity) for the treatment of actinic and seborrhoeic keratosis, lentigo/lentigines, melasma and fine wrinkles

- A phenol peel uses either phenol or carbolic acid (C_6H_4OH) with or without croton oil as an irritant to increase inflammation, and soap (glycerine) as a surfactant to decrease surface tension and function as an emulsifier. Phenol peels are painful and conscious sedation is often needed. Hypopigmentation is the commonest side effect and may be permanent. Erythema can persist for 3–6 months
- High levels are toxic to liver, kidneys and cardiac tissues. Cardiotoxicity (arrhythmias) is related to speed of application

Pre-treatment is a common practice and includes prior sun avoidance (and sunblock) for 2 weeks and various combinations of retinoic acid, AHA and HQ (continued for 4 weeks afterwards). There is a tendency to use less retinoic acid due to potential irritation and phototoxicity.

Side effects of medium/deep peels

• Peels will thin out the epidermis. The skin will look pinker due to increased transparency
• Hypopigmentation (usually related to loss of repigmentation from skin appendages and is difficult to treat) is more common after phenol peels, whilst hyperpigmentation (which is more an inflammatory reaction, and often can be treated with bleaching) is more likely to occur after TCA. UV avoidance for 6–18 months is mandatory after peels, as the skin is thinned
• Scarring: Particular caution is needed when using phenol and TCA > 50%. The neck has fewer skin appendages and is at greater risk of poor healing
• Infections are rare, but potentially serious and can generally be prevented by meticulous care

- Folliculitis (streptococcal/ staphylococcal), pseudomonal infections
- Herpes (acute increase in pain) prophylaxis is required in patients with a history of cold sores (from pre-treatment day for 5 days). Frank infections should be treated aggressively with oral aciclovir

Further reading

Ilknur T, Bicak MU, Demirtaşoğlu M, et al. Glycolic acid peels versus amino fruit acid peels in the treatment of melasma. Dermatol Surg 2010; 36:490–95.

Related topic of interest

• Rhytidectomy

Skin rejuvenation – lasers

Resurfacing lasers can be used to treat sun-damaged skin including rhytides (particularly in perioral and periorbital regions) by removal of the aged epidermis and dermis. Rejuvenation is produced by subsequent regeneration, connective tissue contraction and remodelling. Laser is often regarded as the gold-standard resurfacing method, but there is no evidence of its absolute superiority of result to chemical peels or dermabrasion. However, lasers may allow greater control and flexibility. Ablative lasers can also be used for lentigines and selected scars.

- CO_2 laser has a deeper (100 μm) ablation depth compared to Erbium:YAG (10–60 μm)
- Dermabrasion depth: 300 μm
- Phenol depth: 1000 μm (i.e. 1 mm)

Carbon dioxide laser (10,600 nm) provides a precise and predictable depth of ablation. It targets water in skin and a defocused beam ablates the superficial layer with non-selective heating. This thermal effect leads to beneficial collagen contraction, new collagen deposition (3–6 months in papillary dermis) and remodelling, including reorganisation of elastic fibres that become more parallel and tightly bundled. However, this non-specific heating is also responsible for complications. Reepithelialisation occurs through the appendageal structures. The main side is erythema that persists for 2–4 months. Erbium:YAG (2940 nm): Water absorbs 12–18 times more Erbium:YAG laser than CO_2 laser. There is thus less non-specific damage and healing is quicker (erythema lasts for 2–4 weeks). However, the beneficial effects are similarly less profound as it lacks the photothermal effects. Erbium:YAG effects are primarily photomechanical. It does not provide haemostasis.

- Pre-treatment: Laser treatment does not generally require pre-treatment (see 'Skin Rejuvenation – Chemical Peels'), which is typically a consideration in chemical peels
- Treatment: Extensive laser resurfacing is painful. Topical anaesthetics are usually insufficient, thus nerve block or local infiltration with intravenous sedation may be needed for larger areas
- Post treatment: Cool skin and cover with ointment and dressing (hydrogels are very popular). Faces should not be scrubbed and should be left to slough naturally. Antibiotics (for 1 week) are often used, but are not essential. Wounds are healed after 2–4 weeks and become normal after 4 months

Complications of ablative lasers

Patients are strongly advised to avoid the sun and smoking.

- Erythema peaks at 2 weeks and can last for several months (shorter with Erbium:YAG). It is possibly due to increased blood flow and reduced melanin absorption and can be partly ameliorated with topical steroids
- Acne and milia: Small pustules are reported in 10%, and are usually self-limiting. They may be improved by reducing use of moisturisers and occlusive dressings
- Hyperpigmentation: The risk is related to the patient skin type, being more common in darker patients. Sun avoidance may help, as well as bleaching cream regimes. Hypopigmentation is also more common in darker skin types. Delayed hypopigmentation is more likely to be permanent
- Bacterial infections (*Staphylococcus* and *Pseudomonas* are commonest) may be related to occlusion. There are no controlled studies on the effectiveness of prophylactic antibiotics. Viral reactivation (5%) can have serious sequelae and Herpes simplex virus (HSV) prophylaxis is recommended
- Scarring is rare with current equipment and treatment regimes, but may result in ectropion or synechiae. Take particular care in those prone to problematic scarring such as keloids

Other uses of ablative lasers

Ablative lasers are less useful for:
- Rhinophyma

- Tattoo removal
- Seborrhoeic keratosis: No better than other treatments

Non-ablative skin rejuvenation

- Lifts are invasive, as is volume replacement
- Semi-invasive techniques include fractionated CO_2, fractionated Erbium:YAG, radio frequency (RF) and plasma (ionised nitrogen plasma)
- Noninvasive: Infrared, RF, focused ultrasound

Non-ablative techniques are defined as those causing no harm (minimal) to the epidermis, although the actual mechanism(s) of nonablative skin tightening is not entirely clear. The aim of such techniques is to improve the skin with little/no change to the superficial skin by acting primarily on the deeper layers. This avoids the lengthy downtime of ablative techniques and its potential complications, at the expense of efficacy (more treatment cycles required). Non-ablative treatments tend to be less effective for wrinkles, although they may still be reasonably effective for pigments. A combination approach is possible and may be superior for patients of darker skin (who tend to have a higher risk of pigmentary complications). E.g. IPL, followed by VBeam, then QS1064/Erbium:YAG.

Non-ablative lasers include Smoothbeam (1450 nm diode, popular for acne treatment) and Cooltouch (Coolbreeze, 1320 nm). These incorporate cooling that may reduce surface damage, but some believe that the overuse of cooling may cause PIH (Smoothbeam). These lasers may be effective for acne scars/wrinkles and generally require 5–7 sessions. They may work through heat-induced fibrosis, collagen remodelling (which tends to have a slower prolonged effect) and stimulation of fibroblast activity.

Intense pulsed light (IPL) is non-laser light, with a range 530–1300 nm. It has a lower energy and is less specific, but the range can be a limited using a filter. It is generally less destructive and perceived to be safer with less downtime (at the expense of efficacy). There may be slight erythema for 1–2 hours and crusting after treatment of pigmented/vascular lesions. However it is contraindicated in patients with very dark skins, those with recent tans and active skin infections.

- Photo-rejuvenation – Ineffective for coarse wrinkles/scars
- Pigmented lesions require 2–3 sessions of treatment and may crust. IPL is good for superficial pigment such as café au lait, freckles, lentigines, but is less useful for dermal lesions, such as naevi, Naevus of Ota and tattoos. The response of melasma is poor as the superficial pigment may lighten, but dermal pigment may darken. Pigmented scars do not respond well and topical bleaching is preferred
- Vascular lesions require 3–6 sessions. The response is good in lesions with small superficial vessels, such as telangiectasia and rosacea. Moderate results are seen with PWS, where it can be used for PDL-resistant lesions. IPL is poor for thicker lesions and leg veins (big vessels). Crusting is seen sometimes
- Hair removal

Skin tightening

There is a large market for non-ablative skin tightening, and there are a variety of machines with different modalities. Most of them involve collagen denaturation and tightening, followed by new collagen deposition and remodelling.

While some studies claim a biopsy-proven beneficial effect, histological remodelling does not directly correlate with clinical improvement. Consequently, there are currently no FDA-approved devices for skin tightening due to the difficulty in proving results with specific outcome measures. Patients should be advised that wrinkles will reduce but will not disappear, multiple treatments are required and results are seen only gradually. Combination treatments are popular but are difficult to compare.

- Radiofrequency is a non-ablative method (e.g. Thermage) that uses radiofrequency energy. Alternating current 0.3–10 MHz (high) causes non-specific bulk heat production through resistance, transmitted to the mid-deep dermis (2–4 mm; by comparison, lasers penetrate 1 mm) with immediate tightening of existing collagen/collagen damage and new collagen production through increased fibroblast activity and remodelling. It is primarily used for periorbital wrinkles and the effects increase for up to 6 months, but in some cases, up to 2 years

- Focused ultrasound: This has been used in obstetrics and gynaecology for fibroids and in urology for prostate carcinoma
- Infrared (1100–1800 nm) with precooling, heats water to a depth of 1–3 mm with the aim of inducing thermal injury to collagen, leading to shrinkage and tightening. It also activates fibroblasts and induces neocollagenesis

- Fractional laser: The principle of fractional skin resurfacing is the creation of microscopic thermal injures interspersed by normal undamaged skin. The ablative laser is used to create the injury grid with a spacing of 200-300 μm in between. This narrow healing distance permits rapid reepithelialisation within 24 hours. The CO_2 laser is frequently used, but alternatively a 2940 nm Erbium:YAG laser may also be used. The effectiveness is significantly less than with ablative laser resurfacing (2% shrinkage vs. 15%). It may be useful in pigment disorders as it may allow better absorption of bleaching agents due to its barrier disruption effect (melasma, photodamage)

Further reading

Reilly MJ, Cohen M, Hokugo A, et al. Molecular effects of fractional carbon dioxide laser resurfacing on photodamaged human skin. Arch Fac Plast Surg 2010; 12:321–25.

Related topics of interest

- Facelifts
- Lasers
- Skin rejuvenation – chemical peels
- Tissue fillers
- Ultraviolet light

Soft tissue sarcomas

Soft tissue tumours are mesenchymal neoplasms of muscle, fat, fibrous, vascular or nervous tissue that are classified according to the mature tissue that they resemble. Sarcomas are commonly found in the limbs, retroperitoneum and trunk. They generally appear insidiously as painless masses and thus often present at an advanced stage. Most soft tissue tumours are benign, but may still invade locally and have a tendency to recur. Malignant lesions tend to be more locally aggressive and metastasise through the haematogenous route (instead of the lymphatic). Sarcomas are slightly more common in males and constitute 1% of all adult malignancies and 15% of childhood malignancies. Certain types are more common in certain age groups.

- Extremity lesions are generally painless and may be mistaken for a strained muscle or haematoma. The cardinal sign of suspicion is a mass > 5 cm lasting for > 4 weeks. The overall 5-year survival is 75%
- Abdominal (retroperitoneal, 10%) tumours tend to present with vague symptoms with a palpable mass in 80%. The prognosis is typically poor due to late presentation and close proximity to vital structures that make resection or radiotherapy (RT) challenging. The median survival is 72 months, reduced to 10 months in the presence of metastases

Biopsy will cause architectural distortions that hamper radiological interpretation. As such, suspected sarcomas should be imaged first. With the exception of osteosarcomas that may have characteristic radiological appearances, definitive diagnosis can usually be made only by biopsy. Excisional biopsy is recommended if the mass is < 3 cm, using Tru-Cut biopsy for larger tumours. It is important to place the biopsy tract in such as way that it can be incorporated into the resection of definitive surgical specimen. Biopsies should preferably be performed by the definitive operating surgeon and not by the referrer. FNA tends to be uninformative and should be avoided. This combination of factors necessitates investigation at the tertiary centre where the definitive treatment will be instituted as part of a multi-disciplinary team.

Histological grade is often the best predictor of behaviour, with the exception of rhabdomyosarcomas and osteogenic sarcomas. Tumours tend to infiltrate tissue planes, but may have pseudocapsules, leaving major fascial planes generally intact. High-grade tumours have 50% chance of metastasis, compared to 15% in low-grade tumours. Larger lesions > 5 cm also have a greater risk of spread. Nodal metastases are rare and haematogenous spread to the lung is the commonest. CT/MRI with gadolinium enhancement is recommended in the work-up. There are many staging systems including AJCC and GTNM (Grade Tumour Node Metastasis).

AJCC staging

- T1   < 5 cm
- T2   > 5 cm, subdivided into a or b depending on its relation to the muscle fascia (a = superficial, b = deep)
- N0   No verifiable nodes
- N1   Nodes involved

Memorial Sloan-Kettering practical staging

Describes favourable (tumour < 5 cm, superficial, low-grade) vs. unfavourable features (tumour > 5 cm, deep, high-grade):
- Stage 0: 3 favourable features
- Stage I: 2 favourable, 1 unfavourable
- Stage II: 1 and 2
- Stage III: 0 and 3
- Stage IV: 3 unfavourable with distant metastasis

The Enneking staging is most commonly used. It is similar to TNM except that since sarcoma rarely metastasises to lymph nodes, the nodal status is less important and ignored. The T stage describes tumour site and extent rather than just size. The exceptions being rarer types such as epitheloid sarcoma, some rhabdomyosarcoma subtypes and clear cell sarcoma. T1 describes an intra-compartmental lesion and T2 an extra-compartmental lesion, i.e. a lesion breaching periosteum, joint cartilage, joint capsule or fascia. G1 and G2 denote low-grade and high-grade tumours respectively. Most tumours are stage IIB or III at the time of presentation.

- Stage I - Low-grade tumour
  - IA: G1 T1 M0
  - IB: G1 T2 M0
- Stage II - High-grade tumour
  - IIA: G2 T1 M0
  - IIB: G2 T2 M0
- Stage III - Metastasis present
  - III: G1/2, T1/2, M1

General risk factors

- Radiation injury > 10 years after exposure
- Specific environmental factors, e.g. Lymphangiosarcoma in lymphoedema (10–20 years), mesothelioma in asbestosis and liver angiosarcoma with vinyl chloride exposure
- Some lesions are part of a syndrome, e.g. Gardener syndrome, type 1 neurofibromatosis (5% lifetime risk, and patients make up 10% of all neurofibrosarcomas), Gorlin syndrome, tuberous sclerosis, familial polyposis coli and Li Fraumeni syndrome

Other useful definitions

- Reactive zone: This is the discoloured area around a tumour, which is made up of haemorrhagic tissue, scar, degenerating muscle and oedema
- Barrier refers to any tissue with resistance to tumour invasion and can be classified as either thick or thin. E.g. membranous muscle fascia, adult periosteum, vessel sheath or epineurium
  - Thick is equivalent to 3 cm of tissue margin and thin 2 cm. Joint cartilage or a margin of normal tissue before the fascial layer is also equivalent to 5 cm. These are arbitrary and should only serve as a rough guide

Multidisciplinary: O&T, PRS and oncology

General treatment is a wide *en bloc* resection with 2–3 cm margins, followed by adjuvant radiation (external beam or brachytherapy). Radiation is indicated for most sarcomas, with the exception of small, low-grade lesions. Chemotherapy regimens are not first-line and not standardised in adults, but may be given adjuvantly for high-grade and chemosensitive tumours and can be effective as neoadjuvant therapy in many childhood tumours. Chemotherapy may also be used for palliation. Local recurrence is related to adequacy of margins, and recurrence is the rule if margins are involved. Adjuvant radiotherapy is insufficient to prevent recurrence in such situations.

Limb sarcoma excision

Terminology:
- Compartmental—en bloc of entire compartment
- Wide > 2.5 cm, or intact anatomical barrier
- Marginal < 2.5 cm, but clear margins
- Intralesional – disease at margins

There is no consensus on what adequate surgical margins are in soft tissue sarcomas. The two schools of thought are the less-is-more and the more-is-better. The former argues that local recurrence is not directly correlated to survival, is predominantly reduced by radiotherapy and that the extra surgical margins do not prevent margin-specific recurrence. The unifying goal remains obtaining negative margins. How this is achieved, whether by quantification of margin in centimetres or by layers is controversial.

Limb lesions may be treated without amputation for low-grade lesions, if the major vessels/nerves do not need to be sacrificed (i.e. not directly involved), and if useful function can be maintained.
- Curative margins: Normal cuff of 5 cm or more outside of reactive tissue
- Wide: 1–4 normal tissue

- Adequate: > 1 cm
- Inadequate: > 1 cm
- Marginal: goes through reactive zone
- Intralesional: Curettage or debulking

Adjunctive treatments

Neoadjuvant therapy (RT or chemotherapy) aims to shrink the tumour, and thus allowing smaller resections. On average, margins are reduced by 1 cm.

- Sensitivity to radiotherapy is variable. Ewing's sarcoma and liposarcomas are very radiosensitive
- Risk of nodal metastasis is highest in rhabdomyosarcoma and synovial sarcoma. Sentinel node biopsy may be considered

Different types of sarcomas

- Rhabdomyosarcomas (skeletal muscle) are usually malignant unlike other soft tissue tumours, and are the most common sarcoma in those younger than 25 years. They occur mainly in the head and neck, limbs or genitourinary tract. They are very locally aggressive and commonly spread both to lungs and lymphatics. Treatment is multimodal, with excision and nodal dissection for clinical disease, radiation and multi-agent chemotherapy providing an average cure rate of 50%
- Desmoid tumours are aggressive benign fibromatoses (monoclonal proliferation) that can grow to large sizes with diffuse margins that infiltrate aggressively and recur in one third of cases. It tends to occur in young adults, especially females and have been associated with pregnancy, soft tissue trauma and familial polyposis coli, typically presenting as deep painless masses
  - The emphasis has shifted somewhat from aggressive sarcoma-like wide excisions to function-preserving resections
  - Surgery is the treatment of choice where possible. If the margins are negative, RT may be given early or late. Most studies show that although salvage rates are high, the risk of late RT complications is relatively high in young patients

  - Primary RT will cause slow gradual regression as it is a benign tumour, and prolonged follow-up is needed. Adjuvant RT is usually reserved for positive margins or recurrent tumours
  - The role of chemotherapy is less clear and optimal therapies/regimes are unknown. Some good results have been reported with chemotherapy, NSAIDs and interferons
- Fibrosarcoma: The older literature is difficult to interpret due to recent changes in classification and improvements in diagnosis. These tumours are often found deep in the thigh or trunk, and intralesional haemorrhage may cause fluctuance. It is the most common type in adults and tends to be locally aggressive with lung and bone metastases, with a 5-year survival rate of 50%
- Liposarcoma is the commonest sarcoma of middle age. They are usually large at the time of presentation. Prognosis is related to grade, with a high recurrence rate (> 50%), but a reasonable long-term survival rates. They are radioresistant
- Dermatofibrosarcoma protuberans (DFSP) are relatively rare (1 per 1,000,000 per year) low-grade well-differentiated malignant skin tumours of uncertain histological origin. Many variants have been described with mostly indolent growth patterns. The resistance to chemotherapy and radiotherapy makes surgery the treatment of choice. Macroscopic borders may be indistinct and this leads to high recurrence rates. Up to 5 cm margins extending into the muscle fascia are recommended by some. Moh's micrographic surgery may be the best treatment for the face or distal extremities, with recurrence rate of 0–6%
  - There are reports of potential progression into tumours with fibrosarcomatous differentiation [fibrosarcoma (FS) or malignant fibrous histiocytoma (MFH), i.e. transformed DFSP] with greater risk of recurrence and metastasis, but the actual risk is uncertain
  - Dermatofibromas are common benign non-encapsulated nodular lesions in the dermis composed of proliferating fibrocytes. Some are attributed to minor trauma, such as mosquito bites

- Paraganglioma, e.g. glomus or chemodectoma (carotid body), often presents in late middle age as a painless asymptomatic mass (unless impinging on nerves). These may be multifocal or bilateral and may display an autosomal dominant inheritance. Most are benign and are cured with surgery. Pre-operative vascular imaging is recommended
- Malignant fibrous histiocytoma is the most common sarcoma in the elderly, commonly presenting as painless subcutaneous mass in the limbs or buttocks and may involve skin. Some are retroperitoneal. Most are high grade and invasive with haematogenous spread. Recurrence is common. They are both chemo and radioresistant
- Angiosarcomas affect the scalp and face of elderly patients. Microscopic extension beyond the visible limits is common, and thus lesions are particularly prone to recurrence and metastasis

Further reading

Johnson-Jahangir H, Ratner D. Advances in management of dermatofibrosarcoma protuberans. Dermatol Clin 2011; 29:191–200.

Related topics of interest

- Basal cell carcinoma
- Neurofibromatosis

Squamous cell carcinomas

The incidence of SCCs is 4 times lower than BCCs in Caucasians. SCCs typically occur on the sun-exposed skin (75% head and neck) of late middle-aged or elderly males (2:1 ratio). There is an inverse relationship between incidence and latitude. The appearance can be variable, depending on the degree of differentiation. Most lesions tend to fall into either a slow growing exophytic type or a faster growing ulcerating type. Keratin pearls are characteristic histological finding in reasonably well-differentiated SCCs.

Risk factors

- Ultraviolet light B (UVB) leads to the formation of thymidine dimers causing point mutations. p53 mutations have also been reported. The interaction between complexion/skin type and cumulative sun exposure, especially that causing sunburns, is important. Those of a dark complexion have a higher SCC to BCC ratio by comparison. SCCs are most closely associated with total and occupational UV exposure. PUVA (psoralen and UVA) treatment for psoriasis is also a risk factor
- Irradiation was used in the past to treat a variety of benign conditions including acne and ringworm, before its risks were known. It continues to be part of the treatment of many malignancies. The patients are typically younger
- Chronic wounds: Marjolin's ulcer (see below). A high degree of suspicion is required. The prognosis is poor, as the diagnosis is often delayed and the tumours are more aggressive
- Premalignant conditions: Actinic keratosis, leukoplakia and erythroplakia. Bowen's disease and Erythroplasia of Queyrat are both SCCs in-situ
- Immunosuppression: A third of transplant patients develop SCCs (over three times more than BCCs), which are often multiple
- Xeroderma pigmentosum (XP), albinism and epidermolysis bullosa, particularly the dystrophic form
- Keratoacanthoma is an important differential diagnosis. These are fast growing nodular lesions that have a central ulcer with a large keratin plug. They classically involute within months, sometimes with significant scarring. It is regarded by some as a well-differentiated subset of SCC, and is sometimes referred to as SCC, keratoacanthoma type. They are histologically indistinguishable from well-differentiated SCC, thus biopsy is unhelpful. It is generally not appropriate to wait and see, if a potential keratoacanthoma will involute and early surgical excision is preferable
- Carcinogens, such as soot and hydrocarbons. Potts scrotal tumours are largely only of historical relevance

Management

SCCs carry significant risks of nodal and distant metastasis (mortality), particularly if recurrent. The first chance is the best chance of cure and therefore complete resection with adequate margins is the goal.

- History and examination: Neural invasion may demonstrate characteristic patterns of sensory loss. Check for lymphadenopathy. The risk of occult nodes is 2–3% overall. Approximately 5% of SCCs will metastasise. Prognosis is closely related to the TNM stage. SCCs that arise due to risk factors other than UV light, including immunosuppression, XP and Marjolin's ulcers tend to be more aggressive. In recurrent tumours, the rate of metastasis is almost 30%, with a mortality rate of 30%. Recurrent tumours may be multifocal
- High risk tumours have an increased risk of recurrence and metastasis, and display the following:
  - Site: Lip or ear; recurrent; arising from non-exposed sites such as perineum, sacrum and sole of foot
  - Diameter: > 2 cm
  - Tumour depth and invasion: > 4 mm depth or invading beyond dermis
  - Histological features and subtype: Moderately or poorly differentiated (well-differentiated and poorly- 287. differentiated recurrence rate is 7% and

28% respectively); perineural invasion; acantholytic, spindle or desmoplastic subtypes
- Host immune status: Immunosuppressive therapy or chronic immunosuppressive disease (CLL)

Treatment

For selected early lesions, options include:
- Cryotherapy for the elderly, or for in situ disease/actinic keratosis
- Curettage and electrodessication
- Radiation is generally not recommended as a primary treatment modality (90% cure in T1 lesions), but may be suited for selected sites, such as the lip, nasal vestibule and ear. It has a role as an adjunctive treatment, particularly those with evidence of perineural invasion or positive margins

In majority of patients, surgery is the mainstay of treatment. The use of nonsurgical modalities has to be considered very carefully, particularly the increased risk of metastasis. Commonly, margins of 5 mm are taken on the face and 1 cm elsewhere, but there is a little hard evidence to support this. Zitelli suggests 4 mm for low-risk lesions and 6 mm for high-risk lesions giving close to 95% cure. Complete margin control, i.e. Moh's micrographic surgery, is useful for high-risk tumours and recurrences.

Marjolin's ulcer

These lesions are uncommon, occurring in 1–2% of patients with chronic osteomyelitis and burn scars. They constitute only 1–2% of all SCCs. The precise aetiology is unknown, but is possibly related to persistent stimulation of the epithelial margin due to cycles of repair and injury in an unstable epithelium with chronic irritation or immunological changes.

Jean Nicholas Marjolin (1828) described malignant ulcers in chronic burn scars specifically. Currently, the term is more general and includes malignancy in chronic scars, wounds including pressure sores, fistulae especially osteomyelitis and is occasionally described in pilonidal sinuses and hidradenitis suppurativa. Lesions are often overlooked and ignored.

Transformation is typically slow and may take 30–35 years (a recent Turkish series demonstrated an average of 19 years). Some suggest that injury at a younger age takes longer to change. The commonest type of tumour is SCC, but transformation to melanoma; basal adenocarcinoma and fibrosarcoma have been reported. The SCC that arises has a poorer prognosis as compared to other UV-related SCCs (UV related), with a metastatic rate of 30% versus 2%. It requires more aggressive treatment and margins of 2 cm have been suggested (no hard evidence). The need for elective lymph node dissection is controversial and not routine. Five-year survival is 60–70%, with a 30% mortality rate.

Follow-up

Due to the risk of recurrence and metastasis, patients should be followed-up 3-monthly for 3 years and then 6-monthly indefinitely. Perineural and vascular/lymphatic invasion are indicative of more advanced disease and worsen the prognosis.

Further reading

Grampurohit VU, Dinesh US, Rao R. Multiple cutaneous malignancies in a patient of xeroderma pigmentosum. J Cancer Res Therapeut 2011;7:205–7

Related topics of interest

- Basal cell carcinoma
- Melanoma
- Premalignant lesions
- Ultraviolet light

Stevens–Johnson syndrome

Stevens–Johnson syndrome (SJS) share similar clinical signs and symptoms with EM but have been recently recognised as separate diseases. This distinction is not made in older literature. The notable differences are summarised in **(Table 59).**

Drs Stevens and Johnson were paediatricians, who described the syndrome in children after drug treatment (1922).

Toxic epidermal necrolysis (Lyell) is regarded as a severe variant of SJS, in which the extent of blistering is more than 30% of the body surface area. This is in contrast to regular SJS where there is less than 10% involvement; although the two terms are often used interchangeably (10–30% bracket is often referred to as SJS/TEN). TEN is consequently associated with a greater mortality (up to 40%) and with a greater risk of sepsis, renal failure, GI bleeding and pneumonia. It is most often described in adults.

The underlying pathology of SJS/TEN immunity-related and has been described as an immune-complex disorder with type IV (delayed) hypersensitivity. It is associated with other autoimmune disorders such as lupus and there is evidence to suggest a HLA linkage. It may also occur in graft-versus-host disease. The condition is often preceded by a nonspecific upper respiratory tract infection with a prodrome of fever, dullness and malaise. Overall mortality is 3–15%. See **Table 60** for the clinical features of SJS/TEN.

Causes

- Drugs: Almost any drug can precipitate SJS. However, sulpha-based drugs such as sulphonamides, phenytoin, allopurinol and NSAIDs are responsible for 91% of cases. Symptoms may be delayed for up to 8 weeks following administration of the offending drug
- Infections: Approximately one third of patients with SJS have an associated infection. There is anecdotal evidence to suggest that infection-related SJS tends to have a milder clinical course. Infections are commonly viral (herpes simplex, and coxsackie), bacterial (group A β-haemolytic *Streptococcus*) or mycoplasmic. HIV infection significantly increases the risk of developing SJS/TEN
- Malignancy

Drugs and malignancy are more common causes in adults, whereas an infectious aetiology is more common in children. A quarter of cases are idiopathic.

Diagnosis

The diagnosis is largely clinical but a definitive diagnosis can be made with skin biopsy that demonstrates epidermal necrosis, separation at the epidermal-dermal junction, subepidermal bullae and perivascular lymphocytic infiltration.

Table 59 Differences between erythema multiforme (EM) and Stevens–Johnson syndrome/toxic epidermal necrolysis (SJS/TEN)	
Erythema multiforme	**SJS/TEN**
Typically raised target lesions on extensor surfaces and dorsum of hands. They are often symmetrical in distribution.	Larger lesions with more blistering, typically flat. Subcutaneous oedema is rare, unlike burns, and thus fluid requirements are less.
Younger males are more frequently affected than females (3:2).	Female predominance.
Frequent relapse.	Relapse less common.
Less fever.	Fever is more frequently seen.
Less mucosal involvement in general.	Almost universal involvement of mucosal and corneal surfaces.
Associated with infections (*Mycoplasma*).	**Drugs are the most common cause.** The risk increases with age and may be related to polypharmacy. It is often idiosyncratic and unpredictable.

Table 60 Clinical features of Stevens–Johnson syndrome/toxic epidermal necrolysis (SJS/TEN)	
Affected area	**Features**
Skin	Skin lesions appear abruptly and start as a non-pruritic macular rash that develops central blisters or necrosis. Individual lesions heal within 1–2 weeks, but new lesions can appear in crops for 2–3 weeks. Confluent blistering and desquamation results in large open wounds that are vulnerable to infection. Nikolski's sign is present when the epidermis wrinkles or separates with slight lateral pressure. Histology shows necrosis limited to the epidermis. Healing is rapid and behaves like a superficial partial thickness burn. The inability to sweat due to local scarring of sweat glands is encountered occasionally.
Eye (50%)	Anterior uveitis, ectropion and corneal ulceration may lead to blindness in 5–10% of cases.
Gastrointestinal (GI)	Oesophageal strictures
Genitourinary	Dysuria, vaginal stenosis
Respiratory	Bronchopneumonia, respiratory failure
Nasal	Crusting

Treatment

Treatment is supportive and symptomatic.
- Stop the suspected drug and avoid other unnecessary drugs
- Sepsis is the major concern. Active prevention and early treatment is paramount. Manage wounds with simple dressings with minimal trauma. Biological dressings such as Biobrane, Transcyte and Apligraf may be useful for this purpose. Mouthwash is useful for mucosal decontamination. The use of SSD carries a theoretical risk of worsening the problem as it bears a sulphonamide moiety but there is no evidence for this. Prophylactic antibiotics have not been shown to be of proven benefit
- Fluid replacement is administered as determined clinically. The burns resuscitation formula should not be applied
- Early feeding for enteric protection and stress ulcer prophylaxis may be indicated
- DVT prophylaxis

Systemic steroids use is controversial. There is some evidence of benefit if administered early (24–48 hours), but there is an increased risk of complications from immunosuppression, infection and GI bleeding. Furthermore, this may mask signs of sepsis and retard healing. There are no randomised clinical trials for its effectiveness. Current studies in favour of steroids may be confounded by the fact that steroids tend to be used in the more severe cases. The French use supportive care only, whereas the Germans tend to administer steroids.
- The benefits of immunoglobulin use have not been consistently reproducible and there is little data to support its use. It is expensive and carries with it a risk of renal failure and aseptic meningitis. Other complications include anaphylaxis and haemohyperviscosity
- Plasmapheresis has been used to increase the removal rate of the offending drug but there is little evidence of benefit
- Cyclophosphamide and cyclosporin A requires further evaluation
- TNF-α overexpression has been noted and this forms the basis for thalidomide treatment. However, its use is associated with an increased mortality

Further reading

Lin A, Patel N, Yoo D, et al. Management of ocular conditions in the burn unit: thermal and chemical burns and Stevens-Johnson syndrome/toxic epidermal necrolysis. J Burn Care Res 2011; 32:547–60.

Suturing

Optimising results

- Optimise the patient: Treat malnutrition and relevant vitamin deficiencies (vitamins A and C), hypoxia (stop smoking), stop or review drugs that may adversely affect wound healing such as steroids or anticoagulants (including herbal remedies) and treat comorbidities such as diabetes mellitus.
- Minimise the infection risk: Asepsis and prophylactic antibiotics if indicated.
- Gentle tissue handling
- Tension-free closure

Despite this, the individual scar response is variable and unpredictable.

Principles of good suturing

Place incisions within or parallel to relaxed skin tension lines (RSTL) as this will produce a better scar with a lower risk of hypertrophic scarring.

- RSTL (Borges, 1962) are usually, but not always perpendicular to the directional of underlying muscle pull. Scars along RSTLs give better results than those following Langer's lines but RSTLs were originally only described for the face
- Langer's cleavability lines (Karl Langer, 1861) were derived from observations of ink dots cleaving into predictable lines in cadavers (*spaltbarkeit)*. They may **not** correspond to the best line for incisions in areas such as the scalp, forehead, periorbital, glabella and central cheek
- Wrinkle lines were observed in the elderly with folds of loose skin oriented perpendicular to the underlying muscle direction and were described for whole body. They share some similarities to Langer's and RTSLs

Incision

- Mark out the incision before infiltrating with LA (which causes distortion)
- Make incisions perpendicular to the skin plane to avoid shelving

- An ellipse of adequate length (fusiform ellipse) is required to avoid dog-ear formation. The length to width ratio should be 1:3 and oriented parallel to an RSTL. The corner angles should be less than 30°. Although an M-plasty (fishtail) may be used to shorten its length to avoid crossing into an adjacent aesthetic unit, the unsightly appearance of the M should be taken in account before embarking on this

Suturing

- Gentle soft tissue handling is paramount. The skin edges should not be grasped firmly with forceps. Skin hooks are the least traumatic. Avoid undermining unless necessary. Careful differential undermining (undermined side moves more) may be used to reduce pull or distortion on neighbouring structures, especially anatomical landmarks
- Evert the skin edges to allow maximal dermal apposition. Equal depth of tissues should be taken on either side to ensure a level wound. Differential depth suturing can be used level out an intrinsically uneven wound edge
- Avoid tension in wound closure. Dermal sutures provide most of the strength in wound closure and limit the amount of scar stretching after the removal of the skin sutures. Skin sutures should be tied just sufficiently to appose, allowing room for postoperative swelling. Sutures tied too tightly will strangulate. Approximate not strangulate
  - Use the minimum number of sutures possible to achieve adequate wound closure. As a general rule, the distance between simple interrupted sutures should equal their length
- Healing by secondary intention may be suitable for concavities in the face such as the medial canthus, temple, nasofacial, nasomalar grooves and auricle. However, healing times are longer and carry an increased risk of hyperpigmentation and scar contraction. Grooves heal well, but will flatten (shallower)

Classification of suture material

- Material: Synthetic versus natural
- Degradability: Absorbable versus non-absorbable. Absorbable sutures do not require removal, but causes greater inflammation and tissue reaction. Most sutures are degraded by hydrolysis. Catgut is degraded by proteolysis but its availability is limited
- Filament: Monofilament versus braided. Braided sutures handle and hold knots better, but exhibit tissue drag that may cause damage. They have a theoretically higher risk of infection due to bacterial colonisation of the braid crevices. Monofilament sutures exhibit memory and the knots are more prone to unravelling. Extra throws are required
- Antimicrobial impregnated: Vicryl Plus and Monocryl Plus (see below)

Suture material

Selected commonly used suture materials include:

- Vicryl (polyglactin 910) is a synthetic absorbable braided suture that maintains its strength for 2–4 weeks. It is used frequently as a dermal suture. It is usually coated with a lubricant to reduce tissue drag. Newer variants such as Vicryl Plus have a triclosan coating, which provides anti-staphylococcal activity
- Vicryl Rapide (irradiated polyglactin 910) is a fast absorbing suture that retains only 50% of its strength at 5 days. It begins to fall out spontaneously after 7–10 days when used as a skin suture
- Monocryl (poliglecaprone) and PDS are both synthetic absorbable monofilament sutures but differ in absorption rates. Monocryl retains its strength for up to 3 weeks whereas PDS dissolves in 3 months
- Prolene is a synthetic non-absorbable polypropylene monofilament suture frequently used as skin and subcuticular sutures. It elicits little tissue reaction and glides extremely well through tissues, making it the best choice for pullout sutures. However, it is vulnerable to instrument crush and undergoes significant plastic deformation when overstretched. If unrecognised, the suture may snap prematurely
- Ethibond and Ticron are braided and coated polyester sutures

Removing sutures

Some advocate application of regular ointment/solutions to keep suture line clean; clots should certainly be cleaned. Dressings should not be left on for too long, and those with 'strike through' should ideally be replaced or 'reinforced'.

A skin wound is waterproof after 48 hours. Appropriate timing of stitch removal and avoiding tension is more important than the choice of suture. A delay will cause stitch marks that are caused by reepithelialisation along the suture tract that begins around day 7. Cross-hatching occurs when there is prolonged suture tension on the skin.

The general timings for suture removal are site-dependent.

- Face and neck: 5 days (3–4 days for eyelids)
- Scalp: 10 days (if necessary, sutures may be left longer, as the stitch marks will be hidden by hair)
- Arms: 10 days
- Legs and back: 10–14 days

When removing a suture, one end is cut flush with the skin to avoid pulling through a significant length of bacterial colonised stitch material. It should be pulled towards the incision line to minimise the chances of the wound reopening. Wound support with Steristrips or Micropore tape may be used as the wound only achieves 5% of its original strength at 1 week.

It is important to advise patients that the time for scar maturation may exceed 18 months no treatment is usually indicated in the absence of a functional problem.

Alternatives to sutures

- Staples allow rapid wound closure. In addition, there is a minimal inflammatory reaction and less skin ischaemia. Wounds

heal well but only if apposed properly (the trickiest part). Staples have gained bad press from being left in for too long, causing train track staple marks on the skin and may be uncomfortable when removed. However, if staples are removed before day 5, they do not form staple marks. They are especially useful in the scalp as they do not gather hair into the wound or tangle with it as sutures do
- Glue: Cyanoacrylates (Histoacryl and Dermabond) are adhesives that polymerise on contact, with a one-minute leeway for fine adjustment. It is cytotoxic and thus should be limited to the skin surface only. Glue is particularly useful for simple lacerations in children
- Steristrips are easy to apply, but weaker than sutures and vulnerable to the wet. Avoid placement under tension, especially in the thin-skinned elderly as traction dermatitis and blistering may result. They can also be used to approximate the skin edges prior to gluing

Further reading

Miller AG, Swank ML. Dermabond efficacy in total joint arthroplasty wounds. Am J Orthoped 2010; 39:476–78.

Related topics of interest

- Facial lacerations
- Local anaesthetics
- Vacuum wound closure

Tattoo removal

The rate of skin tattooing is on the rise, especially among the younger population. However, many suffer from buyer's remorse and a significant number will request removal when personal attitudes or professional circumstances change. Tattoos can be classified as:

- Professional tattoos: There is a uniform placement of pigment in the dermis. Modern tattoos can be bright or fluorescent, metallic or multi-coloured. Although the pigments are often iron-based, there is no standard formulation and may thus be modified with a variety of additives. This can cause unpredictable reactions to laser and thus test patching of the tattoo itself may be advisable
  - Ferric oxide (Fe_2O_3), which is reddish brown, may be instantaneously reduced to ferrous oxide (FeO), which is black
  - Titanium dioxide (TiO_2) is white, but turns black when reduced to titanium oxide (TiO) and is extremely difficult to remove
- Amateur tattoos: These are less consistent in depth, but are easier to remove. The favourable factors include the presence of less ink, use of blue-black ink that is susceptible chromophore and is relatively superficial (papillary dermis).
- Traumatic tattoos are extremely variable in their constituents and depth. There are often gravel and metallic components. Great care is required when dealing with firework injuries due to the potential embedment of flammable substances

Tattooing

During the tattooing process, the ink penetrates through basement membrane into the dermis and is found at several levels. Over the course of a month, the tattoo fades slightly due to clearing of the epidermal ink. Cells found within fibrous granulation tissue sequester the residual ink. When the basement membrane is re-established after approximately 3 months and epidermal ink has been lost through desquamation, ink is limited to dermal fibroblasts of the scar tissue in the perivascular regions.

Treatment options

Tattoo removal involves a combination of processes that clear pigment and obscure them by fibrosis. Even if the colour is cleared completely, there may still be residual textural changes and dyspigmentation of the skin.

Superficial destruction

These techniques remove the superficial layers of the skin to either remove the associated pigment with it or to prime the surface so that it is susceptible to other agents. Such agents include tannic acid, oxalic acid and urea paste, which function by leaching pigment with the exudate. They typically cause low-level inflammation that may promote phagocytic activity, but also carries a risk of significant scarring.

- Salabrasion with salt is one of the oldest methods of tattoo removal
- Dermabrasion and dermaplaning (shaving of partial-thickness skin layers)
- Thermal infrared coagulation produces a non-coherent, multi-spectral and ultimately non-specific thermal burn
- Liquid nitrogen
- Argon laser

Deep destruction

Scarring is inevitable if deep removal is required and a variety of one-stage procedures are available.

- Full-thickness excision and reconstruction with various techniques, most commonly skin grafting
- Ablative lasers such as CO_2 non-selectively vaporise the skin and its associated pigment

Q-switched lasers

Q-switched lasers are more selective for pigment destruction than the continuous wave CO_2 and Argon lasers. They are capable of delivering nanosecond laser pulses of high peak and short duration that raise the temperatures of the absorbant chromophore to >1000°C. This causes photomechanical fragmentation of the pigment that renders the particle size small enough for phagocytotic clearance. The ruby laser was the prototypical Q-switched laser.

- The effect of an individual laser is dependent on the absorbance of its target pigment (chromophore), which in turn depends on the laser wavelength. The wavelength of the laser must thus be optimally matched to the colour of the intended target pigment. Several different lasers are thus needed to deal with multi-coloured tattoos effectively **(Table 61).** Yellow/orange tattoos tend to respond poorly as a whole. Nd:YAG works well for black pigment as is ruby laser for green pigment
- Multiple treatments (6–8 weeks apart) are the norm. On average, 50% of patients have a 50% response rate after 10 treatments. As some tattoos may only be partially removed especially multi-coloured and fluorescent ones, it is important to counsel patients carefully. Laser treatment requires time (months to years) and is frequently incomplete

Aftercare

The treated area is covered with an ointment and an occlusive or light dressing that is changed twice daily. Patients must avoid the sun for a month and continue sunblock use for a further 2 months.

Complications of QS lasers

- Scarring is much less frequent and less severe than with other methods, but is still a possibility. There may be textural changes
- Incomplete response, particularly if the tattoo has a lot of yellow colour, which tends to reflect light
- Hypopigmentation (in around 50%) is usually temporary, but can be permanent in a minority, especially with ruby lasers. Hyperpigmentation is less common and is related to the native skin colour
- Allergies are rare but may be severe. Mercury is present in some red inks and cobalt or chromium in the inks may cause hypersensitivity when dispersed with laser
- The explosive splatter from Nd:YAG lasers can theoretically harbour infectious viral particles such as papillomavirus. Eye shields and facemasks are mandatory during treatment
- Darkening may occur, especially with red or flesh-toned tattoos. Tattoos that have an iron oxide (e.g. eyeliner tattoos) or titanium dioxide are prone to darkening (see above). Test patches are advisable

| Table 61 Suitable lasers for coloured tattoos ||
Target colour	Effective lasers
Green	QS ruby (694 nm red), QS Alexandrite (755 nm purple/ red)
Red	QS frequency-doubled Nd:YAG
Black, blue-black	Most tattoo lasers are effective to a degree, especially Nd:YAG (1064 nm)

Further reading

Choudhary S, Elsaie ML, Leiva A, et al. Lasers for tattoo removal: a review. Lasers Med Sci 2010; 25:619–27.

Related topics of interest

- Hair removal
- Lasers: principles

Tissue expansion

Tissue expansion is the process of increasing tissue surface area through plastic deformation.

It is classically achieved by gradual inflation of on implanted internal device, termed a tissue expander. It can also be done with an external device through the use of continuous suction, albeit less efficiently (BRAVA).

With gradual expansion, all the overlying layers are thinned with the exception of the epidermis, which is thickened. There is increased fibroplasia and elastin fragmentation of the dermis. A vascular capsule forms around the expander within a week and the resultant increased vascularity from it and the effective delay phenomenon makes tissue-expanded flaps more reliable. Two thirds of the increase in tissue is due to viscoelastic deformation from creep and stress-relaxation, and the remaining one-third from true tissue growth or biological creep.

Terminology

- Creep: Time-dependent increase in plastic deformation in response to a constant force
- Stress-relaxation: Time-dependent reduction in force required to maintain a given stretch
- Biological creep: Increase in tissue growth with stretch

Common indications for tissue expansion include:

- Breast reconstruction: Expanders can be used to expand the skin prior to replacement with a definitive implant
- Scalp reconstruction: Such as for alopecia and giant naevi. Expanders are placed in the subgaleal plane
- Pre-expanded flaps: Expanders can be placed under planned skin flaps to increase the amount of tissue that can be harvested

Advantages:

- It recruits local skin, which provides the best colour; contour and hair match (where important)
- The tissue can be functional with a robust blood supply and intact nerve supply

- It provides additional soft tissue, without the need for a remote donor
- Complications are not uncommon, but salvage is often possible, and the process can be repeated
- Does not burn bridges. Alternative reconstructive options are (usually) not sacrificed

Disadvantages:

The procedure may be a major undertaking for the patient.

- Multiple operations, usually two per reconstruction (one to insert, one to remove) along with multiple visits for expansion of prosthesis
- Carrying a disfiguring lump around for the duration
- With relatively high risk of complications

Contraindications: Patients who are unable to cope and tissues that will not stretch. Such tissue includes the previously infected, scarred, grafted or irradiated tissue, and areas that are inherently difficult to expand, such as the back. There have been no reports of increased complications in well-controlled diabetic patients.

There are a variety of expanders that come in various shapes and sizes, which can be tailored and chosen to suit requirements. Rectangular implants offer the largest increase in surface area per volume expanded (38% versus 32% and 25% for crescentic and round expanders respectively). There is a variety of predictive formulae available, but in practice, the largest rectangular expander (except in the breast) is at least as wide as the defect is inserted. Crescentic expanders tend to expand more in the centre than peripherally, and thus potentially allow a shorter donor scar. The volume marked on an expander is less relevant, since most will tolerate significant overinflation safely. However, there is a risk of leakage from the filling port if pressure is too high

- Suggestions for estimating the size of expander include:
  - Area of the base of expander should be 2.5 times the area of the defect for rectangular/crescentic expanders

- Diameter of the expander should be 2.5 times the width of the defect for round expanders
- Multiple smaller expanders are a useful technique and allow more expansion per operation, but where possible, avoid communicating pockets, which allow rapid spread of any infection
- Backing: Some expanders have a firm backing and can be used for areas, such as eyelid, to protect the underlying soft tissues from compression. On curved surfaces, the corners can 'point' due to increased localised skin pressure over these areas, which can potentially necrose
- Filling ports may be integral (have raised edges and magnetic, but with increased risk of accidental puncture of expander or skin necrosis) or distant. Smaller ports (micro/mini) are available in some implants but can be more difficult to feel and are able to withstand fewer injections (10 vs. 20 for standard sized ports). Distant ports can be internal or exteriorised. The latter is particularly useful for children, but the risk of infection is increased. Even low-level infection and inflammation can result in a poor scar (as compared to a second incision for placement of the port)

Incisions

- The expander is placed adjacent to the anticipated defect ideally through a separate incision, to avoid preferentially expanding the lesion to be excised. Tangential incisions are commonly used and can be made smaller, but will stretch significantly with expansion and have a higher rate of dehiscence. Remote radial incisions or incisions more than an inch away from the expander are less likely to rupture (less tension as they lie perpendicular to expansion forces), but require extra dissection, have longer scars and may theoretically compromise the vascularity
- Remember to inspect and test the expander. The soft tissue is usually dissected just above the muscle fascia (subgaleal plane of the scalp and subplatysmal plane of the neck). The

pocket needs to be at least 1 cm larger than the expander. Place the port, so that the tubing is straight and nearly taut
- Drains are optional. It is common to inject some fluid (with or without dye) to fill up the dead space. The expander should be evacuated of air prior to filling

Expansion regime

A fine needle is used because each injection pass cores out a piece of the port material. A 23G butterfly needle is better, as it reduces damage by the seesaw needle movement seen when a needle is directly attached to a syringe. The skin stretches to accommodate the increased volume over 6–12 hours, gradually reducing any initial discomfort or blanching.

- Individual regimes vary and can be tailored to the patient as much as practicable. Typically, expansion commences 1–2 weeks after insertion (allows wound healing, settling of oedema and for any problems with flap to become apparent, and before significant capsule formation) and the patient returns at approximately weekly intervals for repeated expansion (gauged by the response of the skin and patient comfort, avoiding blanching and pain) until the final desired volume is reached
- Smaller, more frequent inflation may be more efficient, but longer intervals are better tolerated. The effect of timing has not been consistently shown. Continuous expansion is theoretically best but is not practical. Rapid expansion refers to expansion every 2–3 days, based on theoretical creep and stress-relaxation times. Intraoperative expansion is of limited effectiveness

Utilisation of expanded skin

The point at which adequate expansion has occurred can be estimated. This can be done using a tape measure over the top: The gain is calculated by subtracting the base width from the length of the domal curvature. A degree of overexpansion is useful. A 4-week consolidation period may reduce stretch back (see below).

Whilst in most other instances, it is best to first define the defect; the converse delivers significant advantages with tissue expansion, if the condition permits. It is better to mobilise the expanded skin and then to resect the recipient site as much as allowed. When there is a shortfall, it is better to leave residual lesion and reinsert the expander for a further cycle of expansion.

A measure of success of tissue expansion is how efficiently the expanded skin is utilised in the form of local flaps. This translation of a 3D surface onto a two-dimensional one can be difficult to visualise.

- Rotation advancement flaps are common, particularly in the scalp. Place the expander in the region of back-cut of the proposed flap rather than adjacent to the defect. Although there is no increase in hair follicle numbers, the surface area can be doubled without significant evidence of hair thinning
- Transposition flaps are more efficient than advancement flaps. There is a compromise between flap mobility and efficiency of usage. With pure advancement (Pantographic principle), a narrower flap allows more movement, but some of the expanded skin on either side of the flap is unused and wasted
- Unfolded box model: This is a useful concept allowing more intuitive and effective use of most tissue expanders, particularly rectangular and round expanders. The expanded skin is viewed as five sides of a box that can be unfolded in a variety of ways, differing by the placement of the lateral wings, i.e. whether the sides of the box are incorporated into the proximal (least useful), middle or distal face (often the best option)

Overexpansion just prior to flap advancement/expander removal may result in a minor tissue gain, possibly from breaking up the capsule, but it is difficult to estimate and unlikely to be more than a few millimetres. The capsule is not removed, but may be scored for extra movement. Cutting at the base improves movement, but at the expense of blood supply. Progressive tension sutures (similar to quilting but for a different purpose) to progressively take up tension in the advanced flap and reduce retraction has been used, but cause temporary dimpling.

There can be a 'welling' effect with a build up of thickened capsule-like material around the base. Resorption may take up to a year, and thus usually removed intraoperatively. Expanded skin is less than expected/calculated/measured because:

- Only one third of the expanded skin is truly added to by growth. The remaining that is not plastically deformed will rebound back when the tension is released
  - Stretch back: Stretched skin will contract back quickly. Additional shrinkage will occur with time, which may lead to widening of scars or secondary deformations. This is one of the arguments against expanding forehead flaps for nasal reconstruction
- The inner diameter represents the amount of tissue available and is less than the measured outer diameter
- Not all expanded skin is available due to functional units/anatomic landmarks, such as eyebrows and hairlines

Complications

An overall rate of 5–15% is typically quoted, with a higher risk in:

- Children, especially the very young, those with burns or prior expansion or tissue loss
- Lower limb: 50% infection rate, attributed to the thinner skin and fewer perforators. Expansion is significantly less successful below the knee
- Limbs in general do not expand as well

Common complications

- Haematoma/seroma
- Expander rupture/migration/extrusion
- Wound dehiscence, which may be due to aggressive overexpansion or poor placement of the incision
- Infection despite the use of prophylactic antibiotics. However, due to good blood supply, infected expanders may still settle with intravenous antibiotics and allow completion of the procedure

- Skin necrosis may be due to overenthusiastic inflation or 'points' developing particularly over folds or corners, especially when using expanders with 'backing'

- Atrophy of neighbouring tissues, especially in young children, where the underlying bones can be deformed. The problem is usually reversible within months

Further reading

Ibrahim AE, Dibo SA, Hayek SN, et al. Reverse tissue expansion by liposuction deflation for revision of postsurgical thigh scars. Int Wound J 2011; 8:622–31.

Related topics of interest

- Breast augmentation
- Breast reconstruction
- Scalp reconstruction

Tissue fillers

Discussions of ageing have evolved somewhat from the simple concept of gravitational pull and sagging to a multifactorial problem. There are changes in the connective tissue, thinned dermis, loss of elasticity, shrinkage of soft tissue volume (including fat) and laxity of supporting ligaments. There remains disagreement regarding the degree of bony atrophy. Treatment is similarly multifaceted.

- Skin rejuvenation: Chemical, laser or other energies
- Botulinum toxin for dynamic wrinkles
- Volume restoration and static wrinkles with fillers
- Surgical lifts

Soft tissue ageing is a combination of soft tissue descent and volume depletion. Tissue fillers can improve the facial contour by volume restoration. Non-autologous fillers (such as HA) are only FDA-approved for facial wrinkles and folds. Their use in facial volume rejuvenation is off-label.

The ideal filler does not exist. Fillers are classified according to their composition and durability (temporary, semi-permanent or permanent), but the divisions are somewhat arbitrary. High quality data on the long-term effects and controlled comparisons between the different fillers are lacking.

Temporary fillers

Collagen can be derived from either humans or animals. Hyaluronic acid fillers have almost completely superseded them.

- Zyderm I and II, Zyplast: Bovine dermal collagen (98% type I, remainder type III) has been used around the world for several decades (FDA approval 1981) and lasts for 4 months on average. Test doses are advisable due to reports of allergy (1–3%)
- CosmoDerm I and II, CosmoPlast: This is purified human-derived collagen cultured from a single cell line of human dermal fibroblasts. These have had FDA approval since 2003. The lower immunogenicity (about 1%) alleviates the requirement for a test dose. There is a longer duration of action claimed (3–6 months), but definite evidence is lacking

Others

- **Cymetra (injectable Alloderm):** Decellularised human dermal matrix in the form of fairly large particles. It has limited aesthetic applications and is mainly used for laryngeal injections
- Fascian is made from micronised cadaveric fascia
- Autologen: Collagen prepared from the individual's own skin. It is expensive and takes 6–8 weeks to produce. Isolagen is cultured from autologous fibroblasts from a 3 mm punch biopsy

Collagen is the standard for comparative purposes (often being the control in trials of newer fillers). Its decreasing use is related to its short duration of action and potential complications, such as hypersensitivity.

Hyaluronic acid injection

Hyaluronic acid (*hyalos* from Greek for vitreous, where it was first isolated) is extremely hydrophilic and binds large amounts of water. It is responsible for skin hydration as well as its turgor. HA has an average half-life of 2 days (depends on the area of body) with one third of total body HA turned over daily. Modifications, such as particle size and cross linkage are used to increase their longevity (although Restylane has relatively low cross-linkage and its longevity is supposedly related to its high concentration). HA-based products are now the most commonly used tissue filler, reflecting their longer duration of action (6–12 months), ease of use, and good safety record with minimal risk of infection or allergy (all HAs are structurally identical across species). Complications are easily treatable as HAs can be dissolved with hyaluronidase. Non-cosmetic uses include nipple reconstruction, vesicoureteral reflux, female incontinence, vocal cords insufficiency and submucous clefts.

Semipermanent fillers

- Radiesse is made up of calcium hydroxyapatite microspheres in a gel carrier and lasts for 1 year in the face, as it is broken down to calcium and phosphate. It has been used in vocal cord insufficiency and urological indications, where it lasts up to 3 years. It is not osteoconductive and does not calcify or ossify. It is radio-opaque (it is sometimes used as a tissue marker) and does not interfere with diagnostic X-rays
- Sculptura (NewFill in Europe) is made of poly L-lactic acid microspheres in mannitol, and carbomethylcellulose in a freeze-dried preparation that is reconstituted with a lignocaine solution. There is a potential for granuloma or capsule formation
- Autologous fat (see below): Autologous fat is harvested from areas, such as the abdomen, thigh or buttocks by liposuction. Its main disadvantage is the unpredictable proportion of fat that survives in the longer term and difficulty in reversing overcorrected areas. Indications include breast augmentation and reconstruction, correction of contour deformities, and partial reversal of radiation damage (controversial)

Fat injection

Autologous fat is completely biocompatible with potential for full integration. However, early results were poor, and it was largely abandoned (particularly with advent of other fillers), until better results were demonstrated with changes in technique. Fat cells are very fragile and each step can potentially increase damage. Graft survival is extremely technique dependent (harvest, injection, site and level, etc.) and somewhat unpredictable, although quoted to be approximately 50–80% (stabilising after 4–5 months). Adipose derived stem cells (ADSCs) are 1000 times more plentiful than in bone marrow. ADSC-supplemented fat grafts may improve results (supposedly through improved angiogenesis and reduced inflammation).

Technical points

The optimal technique is unknown and there is no consensus. Most regard the Coleman technique (1997) as being the gold standard.
- Harvest: A blunt needle is used to infiltrate adrenaline (1:400,000 with or without lignocaine) into the sites from where fat is then harvested with low suction by hand
- Refine: According to Coleman, centrifugation at 3000 rpm for 3 minutes removes unwanted components from the fat that is then transferred into 1 ml syringes. Others leave the fat to stand and separate by gravity, whilst others use sieves/gauzes/Telfa rolling. There is no comparative evidence of showing superiority of one over another
  - 4 layers: Top 1–3 mm is transparent yellow with triglycerides, next is a thick whitish layer of several centimetres with lipocytes, followed by a pink/red liquid with tissue and blood components and at the bottom. The pellet is packed with red cells and large tissue fragments
- Placement: A 1 ml syringe is used for greater precision, while blunt cannulas allow movement in more natural tissue planes. The fat is injected on withdrawal in very small aliquots (< 0.1 ml) and in multiple planes. The aim is to maximize contact surface area for better graft survival and also to reduce irregularities

Permanent fillers

There are a variety of permanent fillers available, most of which are synthetic and thus are not easily degraded. Like semi-permanent fillers, these are often materials with proven use for other indications. One of the most commonly used permanent fillers is Artecoll, made from insoluble PMMA (polymethyl methylacrylate) fragments in a suspension of bovine collagen.

Complications of tissue filler injection

Results are operator technique and experience dependent. Temporary fillers have a low incidence of complications, and are easily treatable or reversible. Complications with semi-permanent and permanent fillers may be persistent, difficult to remove, and thus should be used very cautiously.

- Early: Infection, hypersensitivity (true hypersensitivity is rare), herpes reactivation, lumpiness, vascular occlusion and skin necrosis (compression of blood vessels due to excessive injection may also contribute), and light blue discolouration due to the Tyndall effect. The Tyndall effect arises due to light scattering by particles in a suspension.

Preferential scattering of the short-wavelengths (red) and transmission of the long-wavelengths (blue) occur when the particle cross-section (40–900 nm) approximate the wavelengths of visible light (400–750 nm)

- Late: Delayed hypersensitivity, infection, foreign body reaction/granulomas and migration. Nodules may represent a foreign body reaction (with other symptoms of inflammation, e.g. redness) or due to uneven or incorrect injection

Further reading

Serra-Renom JM, Muñoz-Olmo J, Serra-Mestre JM. Breast reconstruction with fat grafting alone. Ann Plast Surg 2011; 55:598–601.

Related topic of interest

- Skin rejuvenation

Ultraviolet light

Ultraviolet (UV) light causes skin photoageing that manifests as fine wrinkling, dyspigmentation and actinic keratoses. It is a major aetiological factor for non-melanoma skin cancer. Fair-skinned Caucasians living in regions of high and intense sun exposure are at the highest risk. The lifetime risk of a Caucasian Australian developing a non-melanoma skin cancer is 1 in 2. Public education is paramount. A tan is unhealthy and it represents skin damage.

The UV in sunlight can be classified by wavelength.

- More than 95% of the total UV radiation that reaches skin is ultraviolet A (UVA). More than 99% of UV reaching dermis is UVA as well, as its penetration is greater than UVB. It tends to cause tanning without burning. (UVA for tAn). PUVA (psoralen + UVA) treatment is shown to increase the BCC and SCC development risk by 7–11 fold but the data is conflicting with melanoma
  - UVA is subdivided into UVA1 and UVA2, the latter being similar to UVB and thus regarded as of greater carcinogenic potential. However, recent studies show that UVA1 (emitted by most sunbeds) has more carcinogenic potential than previously thought
- Ultraviolet B (UVB) (290–315 nm) is primarily responsible for sunburns and carcinogenesis, which may be related to it effects on immune function. It is most strongly associated with BCC but is also a proven risk factor for SCC and melanoma (UV**B** for **B**urn and **B**CC). Eye damage from UVB may lead to cataract formation
- Ultraviolet C (UVC) (200–290 nm) is completely absorbed by the Earth's ozone layer

The effect of UV varies with:

- Fitzpatrick skin type (1975), as shown in **Table 62**
- Gender: Different areas are more frequently exposed to UV due to different clothing and occupational exposure
- Genetics
  - Xeroderma pigmentosum is an autosomal recessive defect of DNA repair associated with an increased risk of skin cancer
  - Albinism is caused by a genetic defect in the tyrosinase enzyme that prevents the production of melanin. It affects both sexes and all races equally. Patients have an increased risk of BCCs and SCCs, but rarely melanomas

Sunblock

Conventional sunblock preferentially blocks UVB more than UVA. When properly used, sunblocks still provide useful protection. Sunblock use may engender a false sense of security and may encourage greater sun exposure, leading to an increased cancer risk. Patient education on being sun smart is of greatest importance. As 50% of lifetime UV exposure occurs before the age of 18, it

Fitzpatrick phototype	Colour of skin	Ultraviolet sensitivity	Reaction to sunlight
I	Extremely fair	Extreme	Always burns, never tans
II	Fair	Very sensitive	Always burns, sometimes tans
III	Medium	Sensitive	Sometimes burns, gradually tans
IV	Olive	Moderate	Occasionally burns, tans well
V	Brown	Minimal	Never burns, tans to dark brown
VI	Black	Insensitive	Never burns, tans deeply

Table 62 Characteristics of the Fitzpatrick skin types. This can also be used to predict the risk of hyperpigmentation after ablative treatments or skin resurfacing

is crucial that sun protection is applied to children.

- Minimise exposure at midday (10 am to 2 pm). UV intensity in the 3 hours on either side of this peak period is halved
- Wear tight-weave long sleeved tops and trousers, hats and sunglasses
- Note that water, snow and sand can reflect UV and increase exposure
- Avoid sunbed use

Sunblocks are classified by their properties:

- Chemical or absorptive sunblocks work by absorbing UV. PABA is the gold-standard and most commonly used but is a skin irritant and stains clothing, thus limiting its use
  - Benzophenones are newer agents that block both UVA and UVB (weaker). Avobenzone has stronger UVA absorbance
  - Broad-spectrum chemical sunscreens are formulated with a combination of agents to block both UVB and UVA
  - PABA esters, salicylates and cinnamates mainly block UVB
- Physical or reflective sunblocks work by scattering the UV radiation. Zinc oxide and titanium oxide are large particle agents that scatter high amounts of UV but are opaque and need to be rubbed in. Newer micronised preparations address the opacity problem by being less opaque, but confer less protection
  - Tinosorb S (Bemotrizinol) and Mexoryl absorb both UVA and UVB

Substantivity is the measure of resistance to sweat, water and exercise of a sunblock. Its effectiveness is quantifiably expressed as sun protection factor (SPF). SPF is the ratio of the minimum amount of UV required to produce minimal erythema with the sunblock applied to that required for reproducing it in its absence. Only sunblocks with a SPF of 15 or greater are recommended. Note that SPF only applies to UVB. The Japanese PA rating quantifies UVA protection.

- Apply generously 30 minutes before exposure in sufficient quantity. Reapply at least every 2 hours (more frequently if in water or if sweating)
- The protection conferred is time-based and is calculated by multiplying the SPF with your normal tanning or burning time. If a patient normally burns in 30 minutes, then an SPF15 sunblock will prolong this to 450 minutes (30 × 15). Note that reapplying more sunblock after this period will not allow prolong the onset of burning any further if the patient remains in the sun
- Daily sunscreen use (for 5 years) has been shown to reduce the rate of SCC and actinic keratosis formation but the evidence for BCCs is less compelling, This may be related to the longer lag time involved

Further reading

Tewari A, Sarkany RP, Young AR. UVA1 induces cyclobutane pyrimidine dimers but not 6-4 photoproducts in human skin in vivo. J Investigat Dermatol 2012; 132:394–400.

Related topics of interest

Vacuum wound closure

The terms vacuum wound closure, NPWT, TNP (topical negative pressure) and VAC (vacuum assisted closure, KCI) are synonymous but all misnomers. A vacuum is neither present, nor can pressure be a negative value as it is scalar quantity, not a vector. The inaccurate terminology is used here, as there is lack of a widely known accurate alternative.

The concept is that the application of subatmospheric suction pressure to selected wounds will speed up their healing but the exact mechanism of action is unclear. Theories include

- Negative pressure reduces stagnant oedema in the interstitial space. This chronic wound fluid contains debris, inflammatory mediators, matrix metalloproteinases and osmotically active substances that are deleterious to healing. Decreased oedema also decreases pressure on vessels and the diffusion distance
- Increases blood flow, which improves oxygen and nutrient delivery. Although there is enhancement of flow several centimetres away, there is actually hypoperfusion and ischaemia of the wound bed. This hypoxic stimulus may encourage angiogenesis and granulation tissue formation
- Reduction of bacterial count. Large clinical studies have suggested that any effect on bacterial counts is unlikely to contribute significantly to wound healing
- Deformational stress increases protein and matrix synthesis, the rate of angiogenesis and subsequent formation of granulation tissue (begins after a few days)
- Direct mechanical suction effect that encourages wound edge movement, similar to a tissue expander effect but in the opposite direction

Negative pressure wound therapy may not lead to complete healing for all wounds, but it can be a good intermediary step prior to definitive closure by improving the wound bed or acting as a manageable dressing.

Method

In principle, the technique is simple, as are the basic components. Proprietary systems using specific sponges, tubing and closed-loop programmable suction are reproducible and validated. Portable battery powered units are available for ambulatory patients with smaller wounds.

- The wound must be thoroughly debrided to remove gross necrotic tissue and to lay open any tracks or fistulae. NWPT is not a substitute for wound debridement and should only be used when the wound is relatively clean
- The wound is covered with a sponge/gauze dressing of the same size or slightly smaller. Suitable porosity and texture will allow the even transmission of suction pressure to the entire wound
- The sponge should not overlie intact skin to avoid maceration
  - Two types of sponges are offered for their different properties (VAC): A black polyurethane sponge (400–600 μm, more open and hydrophobic) claims to encourage granulation tissue formation. The white polyvinyl sponge (60–270 μm, hydrophilic and pre-moistened with sterile water) is more suitable for fragile tissues. A newer silver-impregnated polyurethane sponge has also been introduced
  - Applying a non-adherent dressing at the base of the wound may prevent ingrowth of granulation tissue into the sponge, which may make removal painful and bloody otherwise. The manufacturer does not recommend this as it negates the supposed advantages of the sponge pore size
- Non-collapsible suction tubing is inserted into the sponge and is connected up to suction
- The sponge is covered with an adhesive occlusive dressing with an overlap of at least 2.5–5 cm. The surrounding skin may be prepared with a hydrocolloid dressing as the base for adhesive sheet. This is

particularly useful for difficult, irregular or moist areas, such as perineum

- The dressing is changed every 48–72 hours. It is important to inspect the dressing regularly for air leaks that are damaging. Air leaks encourage wound dehydration and further necrosis

Pressure

Although something similar had been used/reported by Russian surgeons in the 1970s, the experiments by Morykwas in 1997 are often quoted as the first examples of this technique. The latter group showed (in animals) that the optimal negative pressure for improved blood flow was 125 mmHg (with a bell-shaped curve showing that pressures above 400 mmHg caused blood flow to be reduced below baseline), and suggested that intermittent suction (5 minutes on, 2 minutes off) was the most effective modality, particularly for encouraging granulation tissue formation. The reasons for this are unclear, but it may be that either the microcirculation or cellular response shuts off with continued stimulation. However, clinicians tend to favour continuous suction, as it is less painful and therefore better tolerated.

- Intermittent suction requires a dedicated machine to control the cycling. It is not suitable for heavily exudative wounds as the exudate collecting in the 'off' period may compromise the seal. It is also not the best modality in sternotomy wounds as the beneficial splinting effect will be lost during that time

Continuous pressure of 75–125 mmHg is used in the majority of cases (50–75 mmHg may be used for skin grafts or venous ulcers). More recent experiments in rabbits have suggested that 75–80 mmHg is optimal and the small vessels are damaged at 120–125 mmHg. Similarly, studies with laser Doppler in pigs demonstrate increased capillary flow with negative pressures several centimetres away from the dressing, but there is a zone of hypoperfusion at the wound edge. This varies between tissue types.

- Newer products available from Smith and Nephew (after buying Blue Sky Medical) use a lower level of vacuum with either gauze or sponge based on the Chariker-Jeter technique, 1989

Problems

- Suction can be painful, particularly with venous ulcers and may require analgesia; topical LA can be applied on the wound or injected through the tubing. Alternatively, suction is commenced at a lower pressure and increased slowly. If the pain is unbearable despite these measures, the treatment may have to be discontinued
- Excessive fluid loss may cause electrolyte or fluid disturbance in large exuding wounds
- Overgranulation into the sponge may lead to bleeding when the dressing is removed. Avoid leaving dressings on for too long
- Airleak (see above)

Contraindications

- The strongest contraindication is of tumour in the wound. The theoretical increase in blood flow may encourage tumour growth and suction may facilitate movement of malignant cells across tissue planes. Palliative wound control is the exception
- Excessive necrotic/infected tissue or untreated osteomyelitis
- Unexplored fistulae. Fistulae may cause large fluid losses, although vacuum therapy has been used to close fistulae in selected cases. This involves fitting a piece of foam into the fistula opening after exploration, then covering rest of the wound with more sponge, followed by occlusive dressing. A lower pressure (75 mmHg) is used and the dressing is changed every other day. An average of 4 weeks is required

Other relative contraindications include arterial disease, bleeding conditions and anticoagulation. There have been reports of significant bleeding into dressings in patients on anticoagulation despite normal parameters. In February 2011, the FDA issued a Safety Communication reporting deaths from bleeding as well as complications from use in infected wounds and retained dressings.

NPWT can be applied to a wide variety of wounds and its effectiveness is well established, but there is a lack of robust randomised data comparing it to standard methods. A common concern is the cost of proprietary systems, although some studies still find the overall cost in its favour, when compared to other methods.

Further reading

De Waele JJ, Leppäniemi AK. Temporary abdominal closure techniques. Am Surg 2011; 77:S46–50.

Related topic of interest

- Chest reconstruction

Vascular anomalies

The correct identification of vascular lesions is important as although they can appear very similar, they have very different clinical behaviours, particularly in their response to surgery. In addition, the usage of consistent and correct nomenclature is vital for meaningful discussion and comparison. Often, due to inadequate appreciation of the differences, the terms 'haemangioma', 'vascular malformation' and 'vascular anomalies' have been used interchangeably, leading to confusion. Many 'haemangiomas' described in the literature, particularly those in adults and those with bony overgrowth, were probably vascular malformations.

Mulliken and Glowacki (1982) studied the cellular components and flow characteristics of different lesions, providing the framework from which current standardised definitions are based.

Vascular anomalies comprise:

- Haemangiomas
- Vascular malformations

Diagnosis is primarily clinical. MRI is the gold standard investigation if required, but requires specialised radiological expertise for interpretation. Doppler ultrasound may demonstrate flow characteristics and is a useful first line investigation. A high vessel density ($>5/cm^2$) and high Doppler shift (>2 kHz) can be used as diagnostic criteria for haemangiomas, with 84% sensitivity and 98% specificity. Biopsy is not usually indicated.

Effective interaction with parents is important. The early rapid proliferation can be very distressing. While the patients themselves may be aware of the problem by 18 months of age, they do not usually perceive it negatively until after the age of 4.

Haemangiomas

These are the commonest tumours of infancy (1–3% of births with median appearance at 2 weeks of age) in Caucasians, with an increased incidence in the premature (up to 10–20% of babies under 1 kg birth weight). It is less common in Afro-Caribbeans. Most cases are sporadic and of unknown cause,

although it may display autosomal dominant type inheritance. The majority (60%) are found in the head and neck and 15–20% will have more than one lesion. Females are three times more likely to be affected.

The gross appearance is variable. With little overlying tissue, the lesion may appear bright red (strawberry naevus, 65%), but deeper lesions have a bluish colour (cavernous haemangioma, 15%). Histology shows hyperplastic endothelium with increased mast cell numbers and rapid endothelial cell turnover.

Infantile haemangioma

History is the most important differentiating factor. It is characteristically present weeks after birth, is disproportionately proliferative and has a fleshy feel on compression (more substance than venous malformations that tend to empty easily instead). Infantile haemangiomas have endothelial cells that are glucose transporter-1 protein positive.

- A herald patch (macule, telangiectasia or ecchymosis) may precede the haemangioma
- Proliferative phase: Typically occurs during the first 6 months to 1–2 years, followed by a stationary phase of variable length. Mast cell infiltration (numbers increase up to 40 times) is a feature of haemangiomas in the later phase of proliferation. They produce heparin that enhances cell migration
- Involutional phase: This begins with central pallor and increased laxity in the lesion
  - Rule of thumb: 50% of cases will involute by age 5, 70% by age 7 and 90% by age 9. Minimal involution is expected after the age of 12
  - 80% involute without serious sequelae, but one third will have a residual patch of grey fibrofatty tissue. The latter is more likely with late onset involution
  - Late onset involution is likely in deep lesions and lesions of the lip and oral cavity
  - There are no early indicators that are predictive of maximal size or final outcome

Congenital haemangioma

Congenital haemangiomas are rare lesions that are fully developed at birth and are glucose transporter-1 protein negative, distinguishing it from infantile haemangiomas. The two subtypes are characterised by their natural history:

- Rapidly involuting congenital haemangiomas (RICH) begin involution within weeks and are usually complete by 14 months
- Non-involuting congenital haemangiomas (NICH) never regress and grow proportionately with the child, mimicking a vascular malformation

Management

As most haemangiomas do involute, the usual treatment is active observation. On an average, < 20% require treatment but this may vary significantly.

- Bleeding less common than expected and is easily controlled. The Kasabach-Merritt phenomenon is a platelet consumption coagulopathy that arises from platelet and clotting factor trapping within the lesion. Patients are at risk of intracranial, pulmonary and gastrointestinal bleeding. It is extremely rare with simple haemangiomas but is a feature of haemangioendotheliomas and tufted angiomas, neither of which are true haemangiomas by current definition
- Ulceration (spontaneous) is the commonest complication (< 5%) and can be painful and lead to increased scarring. Pulse dye laser or steroids may be useful, but most can be treated with dressings
- Obstruction
  - Obstruction of the visual axis or direct compression of the cornea can cause permanent visual problems, such as amblyopia or anisometropia (failure to develop binocular vision) within one week of onset. It requires urgent treatment and referral to an ophthalmologist. The upper lid is affected three times more commonly than the lower lid
  - Airway obstruction: Neonates are obligate nose breathers in the first few

months. Acute airway obstruction is surgically treated urgently, although subacute obstructions can be managed with propranolol or steroid-induced involution
- Heart failure is rare except in multiple haemangiomatosis (mortality rate of 54%) or large visceral lesions

Early surgical debulking or excision may be contemplated for:

- Isolated lesions causing obstruction
- When the anticipated result of involution will be worse than the surgical scar
- Lesions located in prominent areas that cause psychological distress

The risk of intraoperative bleeding is not excessive and is neither a concern nor a contraindication to surgery. Staged surgery may be required for large involutional scars. Timing is one of the most controversial aspects of treatment as involution is unpredictable.

Medical treatment

The treatment regime can be multi-modality, individually tailored and modified by parental concerns and psychological issues. Aim to treat prior to school age.

- Propranolol: The serendipitous finding of its effectiveness was documented in patients who were treated with propranolol for hypertrophic cardiomyopathy. Response is rapid and involution is complete within days, but the mechanism of action remains unknown. It has now become the standard first line medical treatment. A stepwise dosage increase from 1 mg/kg/day to a maximum of 2–3 mg/kg/day is commonly used, but the optimal dose remains unknown. Significant side effects include hypotension, bradycardia, hypoglycaemia and bronchospasm, but are rarely severe enough to cease treatment. The safety of propranolol for cardiac conditions in the infant has been established for the last 40 years
- Systemic steroids: Steroids produce a response rate of 84% at doses of 2–3 mg/kg/day. Other studies claim only a 30% clear responder rate, with an equal rate of clear non-responders. Steroids only

work on actively proliferating lesions and their effectiveness is usually evident by 2 weeks. Use of steroids is declining with the popularity of propranolol

- – Intralesional steroid injections are not in common use and its effects are systemic, not local
- Subcutaneous interferon injections, such as IFN-2α (both a and b), are slower acting (20 months) than steroids. However, they work on steroid non-responders. The overall response rate is 50% and more effective if started early. It can cause haemodynamic compromise, fever, flu-like illnesses, neutropenia and neurological problems, such as dysphagia. Spastic diplegia may occur (10%) and can be permanent
- OK432 (denatured streptococcal protein) stimulates immunologic action and fibrosis. Other sclerosants include alcohol and sodium tetradecyl sulphate that are injected under ultrasound guidance. The results are better for vascular malformations than haemangiomas
- Embolisation of haemangiomas has very limited success due to the small diameter of vessels involved, but may be considered in large visceral lesions
- Laser treatment has a limited role due to its limited depth of penetration (PDL 1–1.8 mm, Nd:YAG up to 5–6 mm). They are useful for reducing pain in ulcerated lesions (at the risk of scarring and hypopigmentation) and for treating sequelae, such as post-involutional telangiectasia

Vascular malformations

These are errors of development and are therefore, present from birth. Lesions of small size or deep location may only be clinically evident at a later age. Vascular malformations show no gender preference and characteristically grow in proportion to rest of the body. Although the overall architecture is abnormal, the ultrastructure of the endothelium is normal (stable, mature and non-hyperplastic). These lesions do not regress or involute. Chemotherapy and anti-angiogenic treatments are ineffective. With the rare exception of spindle cell haemangiomas that demonstrate tumour-like growth, the majority of malformations expand (with blood pressure and flow) rather than grow.

Vascular malformations are classified according to the speed of the blood flow and composition of the vessels (Table 63), although many are mixed.

Low-flow lesions

Capillary malformations

Capillary malformations are found in 0.1–1% of newborns, more commonly affecting females and a positive family history is detected in 25%. The lesion is commonly referred to as a port-wine stain (PWS, naevus flammeus). PWS typically occurs in the trigeminal distribution (80% on face). It begins as a flat and red/pink patch, but with progressive vessel dilatation and ectasia, becomes nodular (cobble-stoned appearance) and darker, especially on the face.

There is a great heterogeneity in the vessel diameter and depth. Superficial capillary ectasia is a common feature, but deeper vessels in the dermis and subcutaneous tissue are also present. Tissue hypertrophy can occasionally occur and is postulated to be due to reduced sympathetic innervation.

The traditional treatment options of tattooing, scarification and primary camouflage have been superseded by pulse dye laser (PDL) treatment. There is evidence

Table 63 Comparison of low-flow and high-flow malformations	
Low-flow malformations – often combined	High-flow malformations
Capillary [port-wine stains (PWS)] malformation	Arterial malformation (AM)
Venous malformation (VM)	Arteriovenous [arteriovenous malformation (AVM),
Lymphatic malformation (LM)	arteriovenous fistula (AVF)]

that early treatment is more effective, as the vessels are smaller, less collagen scattering occurs and less melanin is present. PDL works by vessel heating to 60°C for 1 ms, causing endothelial cell contraction and vessel ablation. Even though PDL (585 ηm) has become the treatment of choice, only 10–20% will show near-complete response. The majority have an unpredictable and partial response, due to variations in geometry, vessel size and limited penetration. Poor response should be expected in darker lesions (more haemoglobin in total and a higher proportion of deoxyhaemoglobin) and extremity lesions.

- Purpura formation is the expected treatment end-point. It persists for 1–2 weeks and may produce hypopigmentation. Cooling may reduce this and also permit higher fluence usage
- Resistant lesions: Persistent vessels are larger in diameter and may respond to:
  - Larger spot sizes (from 5 mm to 7 mm or 10 mm) or 595 ηm PDL (Vbeam with long pulse) that may work in up to two-third of resistant cases
  - KTP 532 ηm penetrates deeper and may be useful for thicker malformations, without causing purpura
  - IPL has been used for resistant PWS, but may have more complications
  - Combination laser systems such as Cynosure (PDL and Nd:YAG) and Gemini (Nd:YAG and KTP)

Venous malformations

Venous malformations (VMs) are also historically referred to as cavernous haemangiomas (avoid this terminology). They may not be noticed until later in life, where they appear as a faint blue patch that gradually transforms into a soft, non-pulsatile, compressible blue mass. VMs are typically isolated lesions that show a predilection for the lips and tongue and may affect adjacent tissue growth (over or under growth). They occur sporadically, but may be occasionally autosomal dominant.

- Blue rubber bleb naevus syndrome with visceral as well as cutaneous lesions (vide infra)
- Turner syndrome: Patients may have lesions of the gut and feet

Vascular malformation versus haemangiomas

- VMs grow in proportion to rest of the child
- Their colours tend to be consistent, while haemangiomas change from bright red to deeper colours
- VMs are compressible and are easily emptied and will slowly refill or engorge in the dependent position. Haemangiomas are of a firm and doughy texture
- Skeletal deformities and tissue overgrowth are more common in malformations, especially lymphatic

Low flow versus high flow vascular malformations

- The CT appearance of VMs is heterogeneous, whereas haemangiomas are well circumscribed and homogeneous. Phleboliths are the pathognomonic sign of VMs, but may only appear later in life. The T2 MRI appearance of a phlebolith is a dark hole, enclosed by the hyperintense signal of the VM (Table 64)
- MRI signal voids indicate high flow. A no flow signal indicates a capillary

Table 64 Radiological features of vascular malformations (VMs)		
Low flow	VM	T2 hyperattenuation, no flow voids on MRI **Phleboliths on CT** Septated hypoechogenic on US
	Lymphatic malformation (LM)	MRI T2 hyperattenuation Hypoattenuated CT with no enhancement Septated hypo/echogenic on US
High flow	Arteriovenous malformation (AVM)	**Flow voids on MRI** Contrast enhancement on CT Hypoechogenic on US and continuous flow on Doppler

malformation. MRA can be useful and avoids the use of contrast
- VMs have no parenchyma, unlike haemangiomas

Treatment
- Compression garments may alleviate pain and oedema
- Sclerotherapy causes immediate coagulation, intense inflammation with late fibrosis. Assessment and repeat treatments should be delayed for several months to allow for this. Injections of 95% alcohol or sodium tetradecyl sulphate may be used. Although high recurrence rates are quoted, the procedure can be repeated easily and safely
- The outcome of surgical resection may be better in patients who have had prior sclerotherapy or embolisation
- Laser (Nd:YAG) is not curative but is a useful debulking modality, especially for intraoral lesions. The results from intralesional laser have been variable

Lymphatic malformations
Lymphatic malformations (LMs) classically transilluminate. They are subdivided by predominant size of the component cysts. However, many head and neck lesions are a combination of both micro and macrocystic disease. Furthermore, LMs commonly have a significant venous component, and such lymphovenous lesions can be difficult to manage.
- Microcystic: Commonly called lymphangiomas, and tend to be diffuse lesions that cross tissue planes
- Macrocystic: Commonly referred to as cystic hygromas. They commonly occur in the neck, especially the posterior triangle, and may extend into mediastinum. Macrocystic lesions tend to respect tissue planes and remain localised, making them more amenable to surgery. It is common to wait until child is older for this, when surgery is technically easier. Macrocytic lesions are often separate from the normal adjacent lymphatics, suggesting a process of abnormal sequestration

Lymphatic malformations do not involute and sudden increases in size may occur from infection. Bacterial clearance is slow and antibiotics should be continued for 3 weeks after clinical resolution of infection. Hygiene and avoidance of insect bites are important.

Treatment
Nonsurgical options include sclerotherapy followed by compression. They may cause a prolonged (sterile) inflammatory reaction. Injections can be repeated as necessary and tend to be less effective for microcystic disease.
- Pressure garments may be helpful.
- Radiotherapy is uncommon.

Surgery: Total resection is the only potentially curative treatment, but the recurrence rate is high if incomplete. The presence of skin vesicles indicates dermal involvement, with communication to underlying subcutaneous cisterns. These must be included in the resection. LMs can be associated with tissue enlargement, such as congenital macroglossia, macrocheilia and microtia. Excessive mandibular growth may require resection.
- Preoperative MRI is used to delineate extent. Subfascial lesions are usually intertwined with nerves, vessels and muscles, and tend to be unresectable. Suprafascial lesions may be injected as a primary treatment or prior to definitive surgery.
- Wound infection and delayed healing is common. Infections should be treated aggressively.

High-flow lesions
Arterial and arteriovenous malformations are often discussed together.
- Arterial malformations (AMs) include stenosis, hypoplasias, duplication or tortuosity. They are often asymptomatic
- Arteriovenous malformations (AVMs) most commonly occur in the head and neck. They often show collaterisation and pseudokaposiform features. The shunt is at the capillary level and is of low pressure. Angiography should be performed before surgery. The epicentre of the AVM is called a nidus

AVMs tend to present later in infancy as a pulsatile lump (sometimes bruits can be heard) and enlarge and darken around puberty to become symptomatic. They may become painful, ulcerate or bleed. In advanced cases, the high flow can cause high-output heart failure. They may cause hypertrophy and erosion of adjacent bones. The parasitic steal phenomenon (proximal diversion) may cause ischaemia to the distal structures.

The two general types are:

1. Macrofistula: Greater ischaemia
2. Microfistula: Usually multiple, found in the lower limb, and does not cause ischaemia

Schobinger staging (1990) for AVMs:

- Stage I: Quiescent—Blue skin patch
- Stage II: Expansion—Mass with thrill/bruit
- Stage III: Destruction—Mass with bleeding/ulceration/pain
- Stage IV: Decompensation—Stage III with heart failure

In general, the treatment is aimed at stage III/IV lesions. The value of early treatment is unclear, except for discrete lesions that can be excised easily. Watchful waiting with compression garments is a common strategy. They are often stable, but may exhibit unpredictable growth phases. Definitive treatment options are limited and curative treatment is unlikely.

- Ligation of proximal feeding vessels increases the collateral supply and often leads to rapid recurrence. It is not an option in modern practice
- The lesion recurs after selective angiography and superselective embolisation, but at a slower rate. Repeated embolisation is a useful way to delay surgery (on an average 2–8 years). It can also be used just prior to surgery (24–48 hours prior but not more than 72 hours) to reduce bleeding. However, there is no reduction in the resection size. Embolisation can also be used for symptomatic relief, such as pain, heart failure or bleeding
- Arterial lesions require complete excision

Syndromic lesions

- Klippel-Trenaunay-Weber syndrome: The diagnosis requires two of the three symptoms of the triad of vascular malformations, varicosities and hypertrophy (bony and soft tissue). It usually affects an extremity (95% lower limb)
  - Capillary-lymphatic-venous malformations (CLVMs) are often multiple and contiguous (patchy in Parkes–Weber syndrome). Abnormal lateral leg varicose veins (with abnormal valves of variable length; pathognomonic marginal vein of Servelle) may be present in up to two thirds, and can be thrombophlebitic. The literature traditionally recommends preservation of these veins, as they may be the only venous drainage for the limb. This is challenged by recent experience that demonstrates safe resection as the deep veins are present in most cases but may not be easily demonstrated with conventional techniques. Syndactyly and lymphoedema (50%, usually hyperplastic) may be present. The treatment is generally conservative with compression garments and limb length monitoring. Limb hypertrophy may treated functionally with limb shortening or epiphysiodesis. Eventual resection/amputation may be needed
  - Parkes–Weber syndrome appears similar, but has a significant AVF or cerebral arteriovenous malformation (CAVM) with uniform hypertrophy and haemodynamic compromise. The overall morbidity and mortality is greater. Surgery is contraindicated
- Osler-Weber-Rendu (hereditary haemorrhagic telangiectasia) syndrome is an autosomal dominant condition, in which small bright-red AVMs are found in the perioral skin, mucous membranes and occasionally in the central nervous system. Neurological symptoms may be present with latter involvement. Epistaxis is the commonest mode of presentation
- Sturge-Weber syndrome is classically a triad of facial PWS, intracranial vascular malformations (parieto-occipital leptomeningeal angiomatosis) and ocular choroidal malformations. There may be

epilepsy in the first year of life (80%), mental retardation (60%) and eye disease, such as congenital glaucoma. The risks of CNS involvement are:

- V1 and V2 involvement: 80% risk of eye or CNS involvement (overall rate is 9% in contrast), 45% risk of glaucoma
- V3 without V1 or V2: No ocular or CNS involvement

All patients with a V1 PWS should have ocular and neurologic evaluation.

- Blue rubber naevus syndrome (usually sporadic): Painful blue blebs that represent multiple venous malformations of the skin. It may also affect the gut. Blebs can be treated with excision, sclerotherapy or laser. Steroids are ineffective
- Maffucci syndrome is the occurrence of venous malformations with enchondromatosis. The bones are deformed and shortened with exostoses, particularly affecting the fingers and toes.

Visceral malformations are also present. The malignant transformation rate is up to 20%

- Proteus syndrome: Capillary, lymphatic, venous and capillary-venous malformations in association with macrocephaly, macrodactyly, lipomas and naevi

Pyogenic granuloma

The exact aetiology is unknown, but is often attributed to trauma. It may be associated with PWS and pregnancy. Treatment options include surgery, cryotherapy, silver nitrate ablation, diathermy or laser therapy with an overall recurrence rate of 5%. Surgery is reported to have a lower recurrence rate (3.6%), but poorer cosmesis as compared to laser. Sud (2009) demonstrated reasonable results with shave excision before PDL for larger lesions. PDL monotherapy requires >6 sessions for eradication.

Further reading

Sud AR, Tan ST. Pyogenic granuloma: treatment by shave-excision and/or pulsed-dye laser. J Plast Reconstr Aesth Surg 2010; 63:1364–68.

Related topic of interest

- Lasers

Zygomatic fractures

The typical patient is a young (age 20–30 years) male (80%) involved in an altercation or road traffic accident. The classical tripod fracture actually has four components:

- Zygomatic bone at the ZF suture. This is the strongest part of the 'tripod' and may be incompletely fractured. A fracture here should prompt the active exclusion of other fractures
- Temporal bone along the zygomatic arch 1.5 cm posterior to the zygomaticotemporal suture
- Zygomaticomaxillary buttress in the orbital margin/floor and anterior wall of the maxillary sinus
- Inferior and lateral orbit through greater wing of sphenoid. All zygomatic fractures involve the orbit, except for isolated arch fractures

Fractures can pivot about one point. Therefore, not all fracture fragments are necessarily displaced. It may be impacted due to direct blows, is often comminuted and the deep temporal fascia may act to prevent displacement of bones. A quarter of patients with zygomatic fractures will have other additional facial fractures, and almost always involves a component of the orbital floor. As the zygoma itself rarely breaks, fractures may be more appropriately viewed as 'malar fractures' or 'zygomatic separation'. Many fractures are minimally displaced and surgery not required.

Assessment

The assessment of a trauma patient should proceed in the standard fashion. Many of these patients will have polytrauma, and hence serious concomitant injuries must be excluded as a priority.

- Palpate the bony margins. There may be flattening of malar prominence with a bony step along the infraorbital margin (lateral portion is inferiorly displaced and orbital volume is usually increased). The zygoma has many articulations and the masseter is a major deforming force. This can pull the fragment in complex ways; typically medial, inferior and posterior,

leaving a depressed lateral canthus and palpebral fissure
- Soft tissue bruising and swelling
- Functional
  - An ophthalmic consultation is important as 5% have a significant eye injury, which increases to 20–40%, if there is an orbital floor fracture
    - Diplopia (30%) is commonly due to limitation of upward gaze from entrapment of the inferior rectus, contusion, muscular oedema or nerve paralysis. Entrapment can be confirmed by the forced duction test, which is best done under GA
    - Enophthalmos
    - Subconjunctival haematoma with no posterior limit, subcutaneous emphysema and decreased visual acuity may imply retinal detachment
  - Mouth opening: Trismus may be due to a depressed zygomatic arch fracture, impeding movement of the coronoid process or due to masseter spasm
  - There may be paraesthesia in the infraorbital nerve territory. Lack of numbness and/or periorbital/ subconjunctival haematoma makes diagnosis of fracture unlikely

Diagnosis

- History and examination is the mainstay of clinical fracture diagnosis
- Plain radiographs generally offer poor views of the zygoma due to temporal bone shadows. They are thus generally insufficient for decision-making and have largely been replaced by CT (facial views cost almost as much as CT)
  - Waters series (30° occipitomental, chin to plate) view for the zygomatic arches and maxillary sinus is the single most useful view. It rotates the temporal bone below the sinus and allows visualisation of the maxilla/sinus, orbits and zygomatic arch, i.e. upper facial (**Figure 17**)
  - Submentovertex or Titterington views can show zygomatic arches, and also condyles

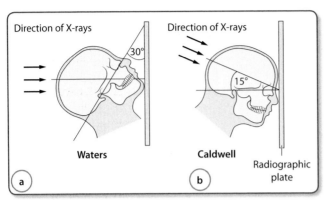

Figure 17 Common 'trauma' views. The Waters view (a) demonstrates the zygomatic arches and maxillary sinus well whilst the Caldwell view (b) is a postero-anterior view that demonstrates the ZF suture.

- PA and lateral
- Townes
- Caldwell view (forehead to plate, 15°) shows the ZF suture well and is useful for the frontal sinus, orbital/floor and mandibular ramus
- Fine-cut CT (coronal and axial) is useful for preoperative assessment of the injury, particularly of the orbital wall. 3D reconstruction may be useful for more complex injuries, whilst some surgeons have reported experience with intraoperative CT for more accurate fragment reduction.

Management

One needs to consider:

- Functional problems, e.g. jaw opening, visual disturbance
- Cosmetic issues, e.g. asymmetry

Conservative treatment (analgesia, nursing head-up, soft diet, protection and no nose blowing for 6 weeks) is a suitable option for stable and undisplaced fractures with no functional problems. ORIF is the mainstay of modern treatment and is required in 80–95% cases. However the exact indications for surgery are not rigid. Those with less severe deformities may not require treatment. Recent studies have shown that low impact fractures involving the infraorbital rim that were not treated, did not have any significant long-term problems. Some advocate that at least two fractures be plated. Davidson found that fixation is stable with plating of ZF suture

fracture and one other fracture site. Single-site fixation is acceptable in certain situations, but increases the risk of leaving rotational deformity. The use of multiple fixation points reduces the chances of fragment rotation and retrusion, which may be difficult to judge with overlying swelling. Formal/complete three-point fixation is actually indicated only in rare circumstances.

The surgical principles (as with all fractures) are:

- Adequate exposure
- Precise reduction
- Accurate stabilisation

The fractures may be accessed by:

- ZF suture via lateral brow incision (or upper lid crease, upper blepharoplasty incision) with a Dingman retractor placed posterior to the body of zygoma. The lateral orbital rim/wall is a good guide to ensure good reduction
- Infraorbital rim via subciliary or transconjunctival lower eyelid incision. Placing the plate above the rim rather than in front of it, as it makes it less palpable. Resuspension reduces tissue drooping
- Zygomaticomaxillary via upper buccal sulcus incisions. The actual need for fixation here is controversial except in complex and comminuted fractures. The fracture line can be explored.
  - Bone grafts may be needed if gaps of more than 0.5 cm are present in the buttress areas
- A coronal incision/approach may be needed for severe zygomatic fractures or open fixation of zygomatic arch fractures

Gillies lift for a depressed zygomatic arch fracture (generally a 'W-shaped' fracture): A 3 cm incision is made in the hairy temple 4 cm superior to the zygomatic arch and posterior to the temporal hairline. Dissect through the silvery white deep temporalis fascia to see the muscle, slip the Rowe's elevator above the muscle and below the arch. Care needs to be taken to avoid causing a secondary fracture of the temporal bone, when using the bone as a pivot. The lift only works, if the arch is not comminuted and has an intact periosteum. An alternative is a direct percutaneous lift with a clip or hook.

- Fixation is usually unnecessary in isolated arch fractures as the periosteum and muscle splints the fracture. Unstable fractures (such as long standing fractures with soft tissue contraction) may need ORIF (wiring)
- Some have suggested inflating a Foley catheter under the arch and left *in situ* for 5 days after radiological confirmation of reduction

Timing of surgery

A zygomatic fracture without eye signs and symptoms is not an emergency. If surgery cannot be performed before oedema sets in, it can be safely postponed until practical to do so, within 2–3 weeks. Late surgery (weeks) will be hindered by the healed fracture/callus and soft tissue fibrosis.

Complications of surgery

- Bradycardia may occur due to the oculocardiac reflex (V1 to reticular formation to vagus, leading to bradycardia, nausea and syncope)
- Nerve injury to infraorbital occurs in up to 20% of patients and is usually transient
- Eye injury
  - Persistent diplopia: 10% have diplopia at presentation with up to half of these becoming persistent (usually affecting upward gaze only). This should be followed closely and a CT may be required
  - Blindness (0.3%) is very rare. It may be due to bone fragments, haematoma or oedema impinging on the optic nerve or retinal detachment. Orbital exploration in the presence of globe rupture or hyphaema can exacerbate injury. Traumatic optic neuropathy is rare (1–2%) and is often undetected, as the mildest form may cause only slight colour blindness. Steroids are often used
  - Enophthalmos is rare (3%), but can be severe, if it involves the posterior part of orbital cavity (relative to the coronal axis of globe)
- Late complications
  - Mechanical plate failure
  - Deformities, such as scleral show/ectropion may be due to tissue drooping (malar fat pad) and bony migration. It is particularly common with comminuted fractures. They may be reduced by periosteal suspension and fixation respectively. Those with only a two-point (wire) fixation around the orbit may have an axis, about which the zygoma can rotate under the powerful contractions of masseter

Further reading

Zhang QB, Dong YJ, Li ZB, et al. Minimal incisions for treating zygomatic complex fractures. J Craniofac Surg 2011; 22:1460–62.

Related topic of interest

- Mandibular fractures

Index

Note: Page numbers in **bold** or *italic* refer to tables or figures, respectively.